FRAMES OF REFERENCE IN PSYCHOSOCIAL OCCUPATIONAL THERAPY

FRAMES OF REFERENCE IN PSYCHOSOCIAL OCCUPATIONAL THERAPY

Mary Ann Bruce MS, OTR
Barbara Borg MA, OTR

SLACK Incorporated, 6900 Grove Road, Thorofare, New Jersey 08086

Printed in the United States of America

Library of Congress Catalog Card Number: 86-42868

ISBN: 0-943432-97-9

Published by: SLACK Incorporated
               6900 Grove Rd.
               Thorofare, NJ 08086

Last digit is print number: 10   9   8   7   6   5   4   3   2   1

CONTENTS

Introduction   xx

1. HISTORICAL OVERVIEW OF PSYCHOSOCIAL OCCUPATIONAL THERAPY   **1**

Occupational Therapy in Psychiatry and the Mental Health System   1
Defining Terms in Occupational Therapy   5
     Paradigm and Frame of Reference   5
     Patient or Client?   5
Other Social Influences   7
Marker Events in the Occupational Therapy Profession   7
Specialization as It Affects Psychosocial Occupational Therapy   10
Chapter Summary   11

2. THE FRAMEWORK OF THERAPY IN OCCUPATIONAL THERAPY   **15**

The Therapeutic Relationship   15
     Defining the Therapeutic Relationship   16
     What Is Therapy?   16
     The Occupational Therapist's Role in the Therapeutic Relationship   17
     Summary   22
Groups in Occupational Therapy   22
     Occupational Therapy Groups   23
     What Is a Group?   25
     The Role of the Occupational Therapist in the Group   26
     Styles of Leadership   26
     The General Group Format   28
     Documentation of Occupational Therapy Groups   30
     Summary   31
"Purposeful" Activity   31

Contents

"Purposeful Activity" in the Framework of Therapy 33
The Role of the Occupational Therapist with "Purposeful" Activity 33
Chapter Summary 35

3. THE OBJECT RELATIONS FRAME OF REFERENCE **39**
Definition 39
Theoretical Development 39
The Influence of Freud 40
The Influence of Jung 47
Input from Existential Humanism 49
Freudian Psychotherapy and Ideology Today 52
Altered View of the Role of Past History 53
New Conceptualization of the Development of Gender
Identity: Altered
View of Femininity 53
Challenging the Supremacy of Biological Determination 54
Prephallic Experiencing 54
Geriatric Psychiatry 55
Shortened Length of Treatment 55
Current Practice in Occupational Therapy 56
The Person and Behavior 56
The Role of the Occupational Therapist 57
The Function of Activities 57
Theoretical Assumptions 60
Evaluation 61
Treatment Goals 68
Treatment Process 69
Chapter Summary 74
Disenchantment with Freud 75
Occupational Therapy — Not Psychoanalysis 76
Contribution of the Object Relations Frame of Reference 76
Limitations of the Object Relations Frame of Reference 78

4. THE BEHAVIORAL FRAME OF REFERENCE **85**
Theoretical Development 85
How Learning Occurs 86

Classical Conditioning   87
Operant Conditioning   88
Kinds of Reinforcement   89
Schedules of Reinforcement   90
Punishment   91
Shaping   92
Building Chains of Behavior   92
Modeling   93
Token Economies   94
Desensitization   96
Biofeedback   96
Difference Between Feeling-Oriented and Behavioral Approaches   97
Current Practice in Occupational Therapy   98
    The Person and Behavior   98
    The Role of the Occupational Therapist   99
    Function of Activities   102
    Theoretical Assumptions   103
    Evaluation   104
    Treatment Goals   111
    Treatment Process   113
Chapter Summary   119
    Contributions   120
    Limitations   120

5. OVERVIEW OF THE COGNITIVE PROCESS   **127**
Theoretical Conception of Cognition   128
    Information Processing View of Cognition   128
    The Structural-Organismic Perspective   129
Infancy (Birth to Two Years)   132
    Physical Knowledge   132
    Symbolic Representational Knowledge   133
    Social Cognition   133
    Summary   134
Early Childhood (Two to Six or Seven Years)   134
    Physical Knowledge   134
    Establishing Simple Relationships   135
    Symbolic Representational Knowledge   136
    Social Cognition   136

Contents

Summary	138
Later Childhood (Seven to Eleven Years)	138
Physical Knowledge	138
Symbolic-Representational Knowledge	139
Social Cognition	140
Summary	140
Adolescence and Adulthood (Twelve Years and Older)	141
Physical Knowledge	141
The Scientific Period	141
Symbolic-Representational Knowledge	142
Social Cognition	142
Summary	143
Perception, Metacognition, and Memory as Cognitive Processes	143
Perception	143
Selective Attention	144
Attention Span	144
Metacognition	144
Memory	145
Problem Solving	146
Cognition in the Context of Therapy	147
The Psychiatrist's Assessment of Cognition	147
The Psychologist's Assessment of Cognition	148
Psychological Testing for Brain Damage	148
The Occupational Therapist and the Concept of Cognition	149
6. THE COGNITIVE-BEHAVIORAL FRAME OF REFERENCE	**155**
Definition	156
Theoretical Development	156
Occupational Therapy Literature	156
Cognitive-Behavioral Literature	156
Current Practice in Occupational Therapy	168
The Person and Behavior	168
The Role of the Occupational Therapist	169
The Function of Activities	171
Theoretical Assumptions	172
Evaluation	173
Assessment Instruments	176
Treatment	177

Treatment Goals   177
Occupational Therapy and Cognitive-Behavioral Strategies   178
  Listening for Musts   178
  Homework   179
  Building Knowledge Through Reading   179
  Patients Learn Their Rights   179
  Films and Visual Media   180
  Modeling and Role Playing   180
  Modeling and Physical Guidance   180
  Identifying Cognitive Distortions   180
  Testing Cognitions   181
  Educational Experiences   181
  Sample Psychoeducational Group in Occupational Therapy   182
Treatment for Peripheral or Deep Change   183
Chapter Summary   184
  Limitations   184
  Contributions   185

7. DEVELOPMENTAL FRAME OF REFERENCE   **193**
Definition   193
Theoretical Development   194
Theories of Life Span Development   196
  Life Stages   196
  Mediating Factors in Understanding Development   207
  Enabling Developmental Skills   208
  Mosey's Seven Adaptive Skills   208
  Theoretical Basis for Cognitive Development   209
  Theoretical Base for Moral Reasoning and Development
    of Social Perspective   212
  Issues of Moral and Social Reasoning as They Impact
    Occupational Therapy   215
  Theoretical Basis for Building Sensory-Integrative Skills   216
Current Practice in Occupational Therapy   218
  The Person and Behavior   218
  Function of Activities   219
  Theoretical Assumptions   221
  The Role of the Occupational Therapist   222
  Evaluation   223

Contents

Treatment Goals 227
Treatment Process 229
Cognitive Developmental Treatment 230
Building Cognitive Skills Related to Moral Reasoning
    and Social Perspective 234
Summary 235
Sensory-Motor-Integration Treatment 236
Building Other Adaptive Skills 237
Life Development Intervention 238
Chapter Summary 241
    Contributions 241
    Limitations 242

8. OCCUPATIONAL BEHAVIOR FRAME OF REFERENCE ... **251**
Definition 251
Theoretical Development 252
Current Practice in Occupational Therapy 254
    The Person and Behavior 257
    The Role of the Occupational Therapist 262
    The Function of Activities 264
    Evaluation 265
    The Treatment Process 268
Chapter Summary 271
    Contributions 273
    Limitations 273

9. ORGANIC MENTAL DISORDER **281**
Holism 283
Holistic Relationship of Functional Systems in the Brain ... 284
    Plasticity 285
    Bilaterality 285
    Central Nervous System Re-organization 286
Holistic Relationship of Physiology to Personality .. 287
    The Reticular Activating and Limbic Systems 287
    Depression 287
    Emotional Lability 288
    Apathy 289

Suspiciousness 289
The Individual in His Environment 291
Emotional Environment 291
Summary 292
Evaluation 292
Orienting to the Evaluation Process 292
Sensory Perception and Sensory Synthesis 293
Body Awareness Synthesis 295
Vestibular Kinesthetic Synthesis 295
Motor Synthesis 296
Speech Synthesis 297
Cognition 299
Attention 300
Concentration 300
Orientation 301
Knowledge 301
Memory 302
Judgment and Insight 304
Abstraction 305
Problem Solving 306
Affective States 307
Social Parameters 307
Assessment Process 308
Assessment Tools 309
Assessment of the Environment 312
Final Assessment Comments 312
Treatment Process 313
Establishing Treatment Goals 313
Making Treatment Meaningful 314
Simplification 314
Simple Retraining Through Repetition 315
Feedback 315
Amplification 316
Substitution 316
Modeling and Physical Guidance 316
Brainstorming and Guided Search 317
Generalization 317
Reality Orientation 318
Memory Strategies 319

Contents

Sensory-Integration   320
Responding to Affective Changes   320
Chapter Summary   322

10. THE SUICIDAL PATIENT   **327**
Current Understanding of Suicide   328
Demograpy of Suicide   329
Characteristic Emotion and Cognition of Suicide   331
Crisis Model Within a Broader Treatment Scope   333
Intervention   334
    Ambivalence   335
    Psychoeducational Model of Treatment   335
Maintaining the Therapeutic Relationship   337
Other Therapeutic Guidelines   339
Termination of Treatment   342

11. CONCLUSION   **347**
Multiframeworks for Education and Practice   347
Psychosocial Occupational Therapy   351
    Activity as Therapy   351
    Roles of the Occupational Therapist   352
    The Patient in Occupational Therapy   352
    Dynamic Interaction in Occupational Therapy   353
    Theoretical Principles   353
    The Promise: The Reality   354

APPENDICES   **357**
A. Principles of Occupational Therapy Ethics   359
B. Standards in Practice for Occupational Therapy Services
    in a Mental Health Program   366
C. Developmental Groups   369
D. Activity Groups   371
E. Defense Mechanisms   373

F. Person Drawings   375
G. Sample Psychoeducational Course Model   386
H. Seven Adaptive Skills   388
I. Commonly Assessed Sensory, Motor, and Cognitive Tasks and
    Analysis of Activity Complexity   391
J. The Apraxias, Agnosias, and Aphasias   397
K. Task Checklist   399

Index   **401**

Mary Ann Bruce MS, OTR
Adjunct Associate Professor
Program in Occupational Therapy
School of Allied Health Sciences
University of Texas Health Science Center
San Antonio, TX

Barbara Borg MA, OTR
Private Practice
Psychiatric Occupational Therapist and Counselor
Longmont, CO

ACKNOWLEDGEMENTS

The authors wish to express their appreciation to family and friends who have offered encouragement during the writing of this text; to patients, students, and colleagues who have shared life, treatment, and educational experiences with us; to Dr. Carl Keener for his advice and friendship; and to administrators of Quinnipiac College who supported the sabbatical leave during which much of the research for this text was done.

INTRODUCTION

Patient interactions, faculty, clinician, and student discussions as well as multiple career and life experiences have influenced the authors' conceptualization of psychosocial occupational therapy. This conceptualization is based upon beliefs about the patient and his capabilities, psychosocial disability, rehabilitation and the treatment process, and the roles and responsibilities of the occupational therapist in the mental health setting.

The authors are confirmed in their belief that occupational therapy has a useful body of knowledge based upon a history of theory and practice with multiple frameworks. We believe that each of the frames of reference in occupational therapy has value, contributes to the profession's history, and influences current practice. We believe that through the study of the history, the multiple frames of reference in occupational therapy, and the theoretical constructs that provide the basis for each framework, the reader will gain a breadth and depth of knowledge which can be applied in and strengthen practice.

We are aware of the current emphasis in the profession being given to the study of occupation and the priorities some place on avoiding in occupational therapy a repetition of concepts that are seen as in the "territory" of psychology or counseling. It seems to us, however, that we create false divisions if we attempt to understand human occupation apart from the "human." The individual does not simply collide with activities. He is constantly changing them and being changed by them. His engagement in activity is the means by which he gives life to his needs, wishes, fears, choices — it is the means by which he experiences himself. No meaningful understanding can be developed, we believe, without looking at the constant interrelationship of man, purpose, and occupation. For this reason, we have sought to explore in each framework the way in which man and activity are seen to define each other.

We believe that the occupational therapist needs a broad knowledge base in psychosocial occupational therapy in order to continue to meet the challenges of the multiple mental health settings in which she works, to individualize intervention strategies which are sensitive to the humanistic-holistic foundation of the profession and to design treatment programs with a theoretical base which could be validated through research. We are by no means convinced that any one frame of reference is best for all individuals.

Breadth and depth of knowledge of psychosocial occupational therapy come from the study of occupational therapy history and practice as well as from the study of the related fields of knowledge which have had an impact on the theoretical frameworks of the profession. Therefore, the authors have summarized the psychology and counseling literature from which psychosocial occupational therapy has gleaned major theoretical principles and which have affected occupational therapy practice. The literature summaries are then discussed within the context of occupational therapy and are exemplified by experiences that the authors have encountered during their professional career or in personal life, and the experiences of others as recounted in the occupational therapy literature.

Contrary to what is proposed in some recent occupational therapy literature, the authors believe that each frame of reference is relevant and therefore have not discarded any one frame of reference or seen any as irrelevant. Rather than hastily negate a framework, we have chosen to discuss contributions and limitations of each frame of reference, and through these discussions we seek to develop the critical thinking skills of the reader.

The authors feel that the humanistic attitude of the occupational therapist ultimately permeates each frame of reference as it is applied in practice. The humanistic attitude, which emphasizes the respect and dignity patients deserve, is referenced or discussed throughout the text. Examples of this attitude will reflect an "eclectic" approach and the sharing and mutual participation of the occupational therapist and patient that occurs in contemporary occupational therapy.

The authors hope that you, the reader, will begin the reading of the text with an "open mind" that will allow you to discover the wealth of knowledge and possibilities within occupational therapy theory and practice. Reflect upon your expanded knowledge, identify the possibilities and alternatives that each frame of reference presents for your setting or patient, and then formulate interventions based upon clinical judgment. We strive to help the reader acquire a clinical judgment which has multiple resources and which is flexible and adaptive to the individual needs of the patient.

The discussions of the frames of reference and the examples of evaluation and treatment are not all inclusive nor are they intended to be prescriptive. They are in the text to demonstrate possible ways of applying theory in clinical practice. The sample therapeutic approaches, activities, and techniques are presented as a source of information to be referred to by the reader in developing occupational therapy programs.

Frames of reference are seen by the authors as maps which give boundaries to and provide an overview of the territory to be covered by the patient and therapist. During the occupational therapy process, they provide direction and guidance for the patient and therapist as they journey together in search of the routes that lead to expedient re-entry into the community and a productive satisfying life.

For the experienced therapist, reading the text may be a review of those frames of reference which are maps with familiar routes that she has frequently traveled with her patients. However, even during familiar journeys we may see something new that has previously gone unnoticed, or we may satisfy our need to explore and try an alternate route. The traveler who explores may be refreshed by the alternative view or may affirm that the frequented route is the preferable choice.

The text is written for the experienced traveler as well as the novice explorer. The novice can get an overview of each of the theoretical maps that are in the realm of psychosocial occupational therapy. She can explore the possible routes in practice and begin to identify the criteria that will determine which routes she will frequent with patients.

In the overview, the reader will be able to identify the knowledge and skills needed to fulfill the professional roles and responsibilities of the occupational therapist which she uses as she travels with the patient to help him find himself and use his abilities as he finds his way to become an active participant in life.

For those readers who wish more than an overview of occupational therapy theory and practice, the authors suggest that the student or clinician conscientiously read the recommended or referenced texts.

For clarity in the text, the therapist is referred to as "she" and the patient is referred to as "he." This choice does not indicate prejudicial judgment nor does it reflect a "sexist" attitude.

Chapter 1

Historical Overview of Psychosocial Occupational Therapy

This historical overview of psychosocial occupational therapy is presented in order to highlight marker events within the occupational therapy profession as well as those in the mental health field which have influenced the boundaries of psychosocial occupational therapy, which have impacted theory and practice in occupational therapy and in mental health, and which have influenced the guidelines for education and research. Understanding the history of our profession, as in reflecting on each of our personal "histories," gives us insight into where we have come from and why we value what we do, and it helps us appreciate our paths in relationship to the larger society. The following events and trends should not be approached as facts to be memorized. Rather, the reader is given a flavor of the events and trends that have become a part of occupational therapy as a profession. The reader will be reminded of this history when she proceeds through the chapters in this book, for this text is organized in a way that is consistent with the chronological movement from the earliest (Freudian based) practice to the most recent frameworks of cognition and occupational behavior.

Occupational Therapy in Psychiatry and the Mental Health System

Throughout occupational therapy's history, whether it is viewed from within psychiatry or mental health systems, there is the philosophical influence of "humanism." From the early

1

writings to the present professional publications either the humanistic philosophy is "directly" acknowledged or its influence is evident in the manner in which the patient is described, in the importance given to the therapeutic relationship and the patient's contributions to the therapy outcome, and in the types of intervention strategies described to increase the patient's quality of life. In this text humanism is presented as a philosophy that is evident in or influences each frame of reference practiced in occupational therapy. Therefore it is not treated as an individual frame of reference, as has been done in some other occupational therapy literature.

Occupational therapy arose out of a "moral" concern for the mentally ill in the late 1800's and early 1900's. During this time two hospitals in the East (McClean Hospital and Frankfort Asylum) were noted for having treatment programs that were based upon a "holistic" philosophy in which patients were treated kindly and patients were involved in activities which were believed capable of helping them adapt to their culture. From these initial roots come the approaches of Meyer (concerned with the complex biological and psychological interactions of man which influence his social performance in daily life); Slagle (concerned with using purposeful activity to develop habits); Dunton (concerned with forming habits to help the patient work and socialize in his community); Haas (concerned with achieving competence and a sense of pride from activities completed in the workshop); and Bryan and Marsh (concerned with the use of industrial therapy to help patients continue to be productive members of society); (Kielhofner and Burke, 1977). These philosophies continued to be used and refined throughout the 1920's and 1930's.

After World War I, occupational therapy was developed to provide occupations for the "mentally" ill and to help them resolve "problems of living" (Tiffany, 1983). The occupational therapy used in this period was that developed by Meyer and others who were humanistic and sought to help the patient identify his capablities and use them productively. This form of therapy, as developed by Meyer, was practiced in the medical setting and was seen as augmenting medical treatment.

During the 1930's and 1940's the occupational therapist provided services through the use of activities selected to aid in diagnosis, to facilitate adjustment to the hospital, to supplement other therapies that the patient received, and to develop constructive habits (Tiffany, 1983).

Following World War II, during the late 1940's, and throughout the 1950's there was minimal legislation for mental health. The occupational therapy profession invested energy primarily in developing more scientific approaches to treatment and in expanding the services offered the physically disabled (Tiffany, 1983). Some viewed this "scientific movement" as a denegation of humanism and a movement away from the original philosophical base of the profession. However, an alternate view of this change in theoretical focus would be to see it as an expansion of theory and practice to include principles of both science and humanism in a "holistic" or biopsychosocial approach.

In psychiatric occupational therapy during the 1950's the understanding of psychodynamics and principles of interpersonal psychology influenced occupational therapy practice. The incorporation of information from psychiatry and psychology has broadened occupational therapy's understanding of the therapeutic relationship, strengthened our understanding of the meaning of activities for patients, pointed out the need for sensitivity to nonverbal communication and its potential for increasing understanding, and enabled social and interpersonal communication to be increasingly influential in and beneficial to the treatment process.

One major negative outcome of the scientific movement was in the categorization of patients and activities in such a way that attempts were made to "match" a particular activity to the treatment of a particular diagnosis or to relieve specific symptoms. Thus, activities were used in a restricted manner, and there was often an unrealistic attempt made to "cure" a patient who had an illness rather than help him to use his capabilities to solve problems in living and adapt to his life situation. The "symptom-activity match" process tends to eliminate the personalization of treatment and the appreciation of the interpersonal context in which activities occur. However, this negation of the interpersonal context of activity is minimized in contemporary practice. While certain activities may be seen as more appropriate given the limitations related to symptomatology, activities are not like pills given to "cure" symptoms.

This scientific influence was also felt in psychiatry as psychopharmacology evolved and psychiatrists sought to control patient symptoms through the use of medication. From the 1940's until the present, medications have been used in moderation or extensively depending upon the psychiatrist's philosophy. The type and dosage of medications are controversial and, though noted, these issues are not elaborated on in this text. The occupational therapist is sensitive to the effects of medication on patient performance and reports her findings to the psychiatrist and other treatment team members. In some situations the use of medications minimizes patient symptoms and makes patients more amenable to treatment. An important exception to this seems to be with overly or heavily medicated patients and when long term usage brings about detrimental side effects.

From 1943 to 1954 there was increased support from the community at large and from within occupational therapy to develop vocational rehabilitation programs for psychiatric patients. This support promoted prevocational evaluation and programing and led to patient employment within treatment settings (Dunton in Willard and Spackman, 1963). The employment of patients in treatment settings was furthered by the development of sheltered workshops and through contractual agreements made between mental health settings and community businesses during the 1960's. However, patient work programs were called into question during the 1970's as patient advocacy grew and as work unions classified jobs and limited the boundaries of employment to the confines of the institutional setting.

During the 1960's the community mental health movement was a strong force that contributed to the growth and development of mental health practice, occupational therapy practice, and applied psychology in general. The community mental health movement introduced new terminology, expanded treatment settings and treatment strategies, suggested new responsibilities for mental health professionals (with some "role blurring"), heightened public awareness of mental health issues, and requested an empathetic response from the general public to the "mental" patient. These changes helped bring about legislation from the federal, state, and local levels which called attention to "patient's rights," legal responsibilities of institutions, and standards criteria for patient care and quality assurance.

The impact of the community mental health movement is evident in the professional journals published since the 1960's. One of the first observations made from a review of the occupational therapy literature is a change in the terminology used for defining the realm of practice. Early writing refers to "psychiatric occupational therapy," a term which is tied to psychiatry, a medical specialty. Writings of the last 20 years have continued to reflect psychiatric-medical ties but have also suggested an expanded concept of theory in the use of the terms "psychosocial occupational therapy" and "occupational therapy in mental health." The change in terminology reflects the expansion of practice beyond the traditional hospital or medical setting to the community mental health, school, and home settings. In mental health practice occupational therapists were asked to develop occupational therapy services for day treatment programs and for residential community living or transition centers, and to design prevention programs. The occupational therapist's role evolved to include that of educator and consultant, and the responsibilities and expertise that she offered in these new roles allowed her to be viewed as a "peer" with other professionals on the treatment team rather than as an aide to the psychiatrist (see end note 1).

The broadening of the occupational therapist's role to include patient education and prevention influenced the philosophical base of practice. Some old concepts were renewed while new ideas were incorporated to form "health" concepts and treatment approaches that would strive to utilize the patient's "healthy side" (the patient's strengths), remediate psychosocial problems, treat symptoms, promote adaptation, provide patient education, and increase the patient's quality of life.

One outcome of this expansion was the evolution of "activities therapy." In an "activities therapy" program, occupational therapists, recreational therapists, dance therapists, art therapists, music therapists, and sometimes horticultural therapists were employed. Each therapist came with her own professional training and offered a particular speciality, as suggested by her title, which contributed to treatment within the therapeutic milieu. The therapists used creative-expressive media, work oriented experiences, recreational activities, activities of daily living, and interpersonal communications experiences to improve psychosocial functioning. The activities therapy movement has had great impact on the growth and development of psychosocial occupational therapy. It is also one which continues to influence and perhaps limit occupational therapy's future. While each of the therapies listed may be viewed as one kind of "activities therapy," there is no professional training specific to an individual calling herself an "activities therapist." Economic constraints and the limited resource pool of qualified occupational therapists have in some instances promoted the hiring of "activities therapists" rather than occupational therapists.

The expansion of practice not only gave rise to a proliferation of therapeutic approaches and called into focus multiple frames of reference, but led to a diverse use of terminology, controversial issues regarding the role of the occupational therapist, and questions regarding what is unique to occupational therapy and how the profession can be unified.

Defining Terms in Occupational Therapy

Paradigm and Frame of Reference

In occupational therapy, there are multiple definitions and/or interpretations for the terms frame of reference, model, and paradigm. Rather than repeat these definitions, the authors will summarize the terms as they have been used in the recent professional literature.

The work of Kuhn (1970) is often cited in the discussion of the term *paradigm*. As applied to occupational therapy, a paradigm would contain the guiding premises and theories behind the profession as a whole. As such, a paradigm identifies the theories that have been or need to be tested and which will lead to the creation and organization of knowledge.

A frame of reference refers to principles behind practice with specified patient or client populations. It includes a statement of the population to be served, guidelines for determining adequate function or dysfunction, and principles for remediation.

In psychosocial occupational therapy there are multiple frames of reference which have been organized in numerous ways. Recently, Llorens presented a chronological discussion of occupational therapy frames of reference and common theories upon which they are based. She identified the following frames of reference applied in occupational therapy practice: "humanistic, psychoanalytic, behavioral, developmental, acquisitional, neurodevelopmental, neurobehavioral, spatiotemporal adaptational, occupational behavior, occupational performance, and neurorehabilitation" (Llorens, 1984, p. 8).

In this text the frames of reference presented were chosen by the authors because collectively, the frameworks represent a diverse reflection of the body of knowledge in psychosocial occupational therapy over the past 85 years. When reflecting upon the evolution of practice, recent theoretical developments that broaden or change the emphasis of current practice can be seen. Given the multiple arenas of practice, we have chosen frameworks which are applicable in multiple psychosocial settings in occupational therapy with a broad range of patients and patient problems. The frameworks are presented in this text in a manner which allows the reader to see the evolution of psychosocial thinking in occupational therapy, and thereby shows how each successive framework incorporates some of the ideas that in the preceding frameworks emerged as important.

Patient or Client?

An outcome of the community mental health movement was to call into question the use of the term "patient." Mental health professionals felt that the term "patient" reinforced the "sick role" of the individual and supported his pathology or illness, and his need to be taken care of by health professionals. Mental health professionals, wishing to minimize the "sick role," focus on problems of living, not illness, and encourage the individual to assume responsibility for his own health and care and thus choose the term "client." A *client* is someone who "seeks a service but not a medical service" (Gillette, 1971, p. 100). The reader should note that the use of the term "client" is not supported by most psychiatrists who continue to treat "patients."

In occupational therapy both terms, "client" and "patient," are used depending upon the treatment setting or perhaps the preference of the occupational therapist and/or the treatment team with which she works. However, recently in the occupational therapy literature there has been a controversy over the use of the two terms.

Until recently, the choice of the term "patient" rather than "client" was probably made with little consideration given to the legal, ethical, and moral issues involved in the choice. However, these issues as well as the far reaching implications for the profession were brought to the occupational therapist's attention by Reilly (1984) and have recently been studied and summarized by Sharrott and Yerxa (1985).

Sharrott and Yerxa justify the continued use of the term "patient," citing the following reasons: (1) the term is based upon a "moral-ethical tradition" rather than an "economic-legalistic foundation" and the occupational therapy profession has a moral-ethical base; (2) the term is compatible with the Meyerian philosophy of the profession; (3) the term connotes the ethical stance of moral treatment of the nineteenth century; and (4) the term supports opportunity for health care regardless of the patient's ability to provide financial renumeration (Sharrott and Yerxa, 1985).

For those therapists who support the use of "client" to equalize the responsibilities in treatment, Sharrott and Yerxa use Veatch's conceptualization of medical ethics to identify how responsibilities can be equalized in the patient-therapist relationship. Briefly, Veatch proposes that medical ethics be based on a covenant code. "A covenant is a contract that emphasizes moral bonds and fidelity and requires right action by both health professionals and the lay public." Medical ethics are designed to apply to "patient-health professional relationships." The fundamental principles of the covenant are: "(1) Keeping promises and commitments to one another, (2) treating one another as autonomous members of the moral community free to make choices that do not violate other basic ethical requirements, (3) dealing honestly with one another, (4) avoiding actively and knowingly the taking of morally protected life, (5) striving for equality in individual welfare and equality in the right of access to health care, and (6) producing good for one another and treating one another with respect, dignity, and compassion" (Veatch, 1981, pp.327-328, in Yerxa and Sharrott, 1985, p. 403).

In this text the authors have chosen to use the term "patient." The term is congruent with occupational therapy's philosophy and history. It supports a moral-ethical base for practice; it is compatible with mutuality of respect and responsibility vital to the patient-therapist relationship; and it supports occupational therapy's advocacy role for quality care for those we treat regardless of the disability or the treatment setting. However, the authors recognize the necessity to function within one's environment and are aware that use of the words "client," "student," or "resident" may be dictated by the setting in which the occupational therapist works. Regardless of the term applied, the material presented in the text is viable in practice.

Other Social Influences

In addition to the community mental health movement of the 1960's, there are other socioeconomic events which have influenced mental health practice. These include the civil rights movement, the women's movement, changes in criminal law and increased use of "insanity pleas," and society's changing views about disease, mental health and illness, and deviance. These trends have led to legislation and legal decisions in support of patient rights and patient advocacy and the 1963 Community Mental Health Act, which established community mental health centers and mandated that the following services be made available: inpatient, outpatient, day treatment, emergency service, and community consultation and education.

These changes have contributed to the heightened "social conscience" of occupational therapists. For example, occupational therapists have reconsidered the classification of activities as male or female oriented and are more aware of the legal implictions that affect treatment and the need for professional liability insurance as well as the need to consider the greater interests of society.

Marker Events in the Occupational
Therapy Profession

We have briefly considered some of the changes within society, medicine, and the mental health community and their influence in the history and development of psychosocial occupational therapy. Next we review briefly the administrative decisions made by the governing body of the occupational therapy profession which have influenced theory, practice, education, and research in psychosocial occupational therapy. In general the administrators and governing body of the American Occupational Therapy Association have supported, individually or jointly with other organizations, educational and research activities which promote the growth and development of psychosocial occupational therapy.

In the 1950's the Mental Health Study Act (1955) and a grant to the American Occupational Therapy Association from the National Institute of Mental Health provided funds that led to the Boiling Springs Pennsylvania Conference (1956). Leaders in the field of psychiatric occupational therapy met to discuss the influence of recent developments in psychiatry and psychology on occupational therapy practice. In the published proceedings West (1959) notes the outcome of the conference as heightening the awareness of the benefits of a holistic approach to treatment, of occupational therapy as a component of the therapeutic milieu, of the collaborative efforts of the occupational therapist and other members of the treatment team, and of the increasing use of groups in occupational therapy treatment (Tiffany, 1983).

One of the events that occurred within the profession and simultaneously with the community mental health movement was the Social Rehabilitation Services Grant (1964), which led to the establishment of 14 regional institutes and 21 national institutes for the purpose of providing continuing education experiences in group process, object relations theory, and principles of administration and supervision (Tiffany, 1983).

In 1966 the National Institute of Mental Health funded research to study and design occupational therapy programs in comprehensive community mental health. The study indicated that there had been a shift from in-hospital to community settings for treatment, a decrease in the average number of treatment days utilized per patient, an expanded role for the occupational therapist which required her to assume more leadership responsibility and use administrative-supervisory and consultation skills, and a change in the activities used — i.e., activities which were shorter term and which required fewer heavy tools and equipment and instead more portable tools because of the multiple settings in which occupational therapy occurs (Howe, 1966).

In 1967 in Albion, Michigan, a symposium was held in which seven leaders in the field of psychosocial occupational therapy met to consider the theories in psychiatric occupational therapy and to try to integrate them into a "mind-body" theory which would be "meaningful" and "applicable" to occupational therapy. At the conclusion of the symposium it was felt that (1) the seminar had unrealistic expectations; (2) educators and clinicians needed to study the body of knowledge that exists and to identify the relationships that exist in this knowledge; (3) the relationships identified needed to be researched; (4) a frame of reference was needed which would utilize a holistic approach; and (5) occupational therapy had two major paths of theoretical development — one for physical disabilities and one for psychiatry (Mazer, 1968).

The next marker event began with an invitation in 1968 extended by the American Occupational Therapy Association's Consult in Psychiatric Rehabilitation to clinicians to submit papers describing frames of reference used in psychiatric occupational therapy. There were numerous responses, and several papers were selected for publication in the *American Journal of Occupational Therapy.* The three theories presented were: (1) a theory based upon psychoanalytic ego psychology and learning theory (Diasio, 1968), (2) a theory based upon learning theory (Smith and Tempone, 1968), and (3) a theory based upon developmental theory (Mosey, 1968; Mazer and Mosey 1968). The 1970's were characterized by workshops and task forces to study occupational therapy in mental health, and administrative decisions which further governed practice. The events of the 1970's sought to identify the status of practice and the underlying theories in practice, to refine the standards and ethics of practice, to identify the boundaries of practice, and to identify the assessment and intervention strategies used — all with the intent of unifying the profession. Among the events identified were a symposium held in Boston in 1970, entitled "The Skill Continuum from Play Through Work." The major goal of the symposium was to "develop a philosophy . . . for viewing human activity as a continuum and the productive behavior of later life as a development from the foundations established during childhood" (Johnson, 1971, p. 308).

The papers presented at the Boston meeting were published in the September 1971 issue of the *American Journal of Occupational Therapy*. The articles sought to heighten the clinician's awareness of the following: (1) the patient's desire for competence as a motivating force for behavior (White, 1971); (2) the relationship between intrinsic motivation and the growth and development of the child through play (Florey, 1971); (3) the necessary elements in a milieu that promote play (Takata, 1971); (4) the value of play in treatment to promote "learning," "coping," and "adapting" to change (Michelman, 1971); (5) the relationship between the play of a child and the creativity of the adolescent and the adult (Michelman, 1971); (6) the role of work and play in the development of occupational behavior (Matsutsuyu 1971); (7) the childhood and adolescent developmental experiences which influence work behavior (Maurer, 1971; Bailey, 1971); and (8) the redefining of work to the broad concept of "activity" and the role of activity in the rehabilitation process (Johnson, 1971).

During the 1970's the Representative Assembly became a policy making body for the profession. This Assembly approved such documents as the Ethical Statement of the profession in 1976 (see Appendix A), Standards of Practice in Mental Health in 1978 (see Appendix B), and Uniform Terminology in 1979.

Since early in the profession there has been concern expressed for the lack of valid and reliable assessment tools in mental health practice. Again this concern was brought to the forefront in 1977 by the mental health specialty section of the American Occupational Therapy Association. This concern led, in part, to the meeting of an "assessment institute" held in 1979 prior to the annual conference in Detroit. Before convening the institute, occupational therapists were invited to present assessments that they used in practice. Assessments were reviewed and recommendations were made regarding further development and research potential. One of the outcomes of this institute was the presentation of the Bay Area Functional Performance Evaluation (BaFPE) and recommendation for its further development and research design. Today this assessment battery is used in many mental health settings and continues to be studied to determine validity and reliability standards. (See the description of the BaFPE in this text.)

In addition to approving documents, the Representative Assembly sent members to participate in meetings or symposia with educators and clinicians to discuss education, practice, and research issues. One such meeting occurred in 1978 at Scottsdale, Arizona. Ten leaders in the field presented papers on the current status of practice, the history and philosophy of the field, and the future of occupational therapy. Participants at the meeting reaffirmed the philosophical base of the profession, recommended support for research, and suggested that the association reassess the entry level requirements for the profession (Tiffany, 1983).

In San Diego, California, at a special meeting of the Representative Assembly in 1978, leaders in the profession were invited to discuss the philosophical base, the status of practice and education, and credentialing issues. From the discussions that occurred a philosophical base of the profession was identified, and "occupation" was identified as the common core of occupational therapy (Hopkins, 1983).

The events, concerns, and ideas that characterized the 1970's continue to be of concern in the 1980's and shape current discussion, legislation, theory development, practice, education, and research. Some of the key events of the 1980's were as follows: (1) In 1980 an Ethical Statement for the profession was adopted (see Appendix A). (2) In 1980 the Educational Essentials for Occupational Therapy Professional Education were revised, changing the mandate for a three month field work II experience in a psychosocial (mental health) setting (six months of field work with various disabilities and ages is now required). (3) In 1980 the American Occupational Therapy Association was invited by the Commission on Psychiatric Therapies of the American Psychiatric Association to identify the therapies that exist in practice. A committee chaired by Gail Fidler studied the issue and responded with a report in 1981 (Tiffany, 1983, p. 282). (4) In 1981 two other major documents were supported and accepted: the Uniform Occupational Therapy Evaluation and the Entry Level Role Delineation Study. (5) In June 1984 a Research Symposium was held in Boston, sponsored by the American Occupational Therapy Association and the American Occupational Therapy Federation. The meeting was held to call together educators and clinicians to discuss possible collaborative research, to establish the need for a data base for occupational therapy in mental health, and to support research proposals in psychosocial occupational therapy.

Other events in the eighties which have affected practice are the use of Diagnostic Related Groups System (DRGS), the Strategic Integrated Management System (SIMS) of the American Occupational Therapy Association, the Conference in New York which concerned the Future of Occupational Therapy in Mental Health (1984), and the forthcoming mental health-occupational therapy continuing education program, SCOPE (Strategies and Concepts: Opportunities for Program Development and Evaluation), which was developed by the American Occupational Therapy Association (1985-1986).

Specialization as it Affects Psychosocial Occupational Therapy

The education, research, and practice in the field are also reflected in and influenced by the literary contributions in the field. The multiple publications which have contributed to occupational therapy's body of knowledge include many textbooks, the *American Journal of Occupational Therapy,* as well as two juried publications which have originated during the past decade, the *Occupational Therapy Journal of Research* and *Occupational Therapy in Mental Health.* When one reviews the list of publications in psychosocial occupational therapy, one is struck by the jump from a new book every 15 to 20 years to multiple texts within the last 10 years. The increase in publications reflects the growth of the profession and its knowledge base and parallels the trend toward specialization in the occupational therapy profession and the movement in professional education to masters and doctoral level preparation for therapists.

Also the development of *Occupational Therapy in Mental Health* and the *Journal of Research*, which occurred in 1980 and 1981, respectively, broadened the arena available for professional exchange beyond that made available by the *American Journal of Occupational Therapy*, which was the primary juried publication in the field until these juried publications appeared. These additional professional journals are another indication of the expanded role of psychosocial occupational therapy within the profession, and they serve as one means by which the growing body of knowledge pertinent to psychosocial practice is being disseminated.

The profession has also facilitated communication among psychosocial occupational therapists through the *Occupational Therapy Newspaper* and the *Mental Health Specialty Section Newsletter.*

Chapter Summary

From the cursory review of occupational therapy history and from the professional literature, major theoretical and practice issues have emerged. Posed as questions, these include the following:

(1) What are the legitimate boundaries of occupational therapy mental health practice?

(2) What are the legitimate tools for evaluation and treatment?

(3) Do we treat "patients" or "clients" or "residents" or "students"?

(4) How can we best organize occupational therapy's body of knowledge? As a model? As a frame of reference? As a paradigm?

(5) How should we categorize the models of practice in the field?

(6) Should there be only one frame of reference for practice?

(7) Is there a unifying theory of occupational therapy?

(8) What is unique to occupational therapy?

(9) How can we best standardize assessment?

(10) Can and should we unify the treatment strategies utilized in the field?

(11) Where are the greatest needs for research in psychosocial occupational therapy?

(12) What will further enhance needed research in education and in practice?

(13) How can the profession meet the demands of psychosocial practice with the limited number of occupational therapists in the professional pool?

(14) How do we prepare for the future needs of the mental health profession and assure the continued endorsement of psychosocial occupational therapy practice?

There is no simple solution to any of these problems and perhaps some of these questions do not or should not have a definitive answer. The authors' intent in this text is to summarize the body of knowledge that exists in psychosocial occupational therapy and encourage the reader to give careful consideration to the wealth of theory and practice that exists. Question it; discuss it with colleagues; propose research; or just think about what you read. Most important, avoid making a hasty decision or giving a quick answer to one of the above questions when such an answer would limit patient care under the guise of professional unity.

End Note

1. Being an "aide" to the psychiatrist was the predominant role for the occupational therapist as well as for other health professionals who worked in psychiatric hospitals during the 1950's.

References

Bailey D: Vocational theories and work habits related to childhood development. AJOT 25(6):298-302, 1971.

Diasio K: Psychiatric occupational therapy: Search for a conceptual framework in the light of psychoanalytic ego psychology and learning theory. AJOT 22:400-414, 1968.

Dunton D: Psychiatric occupational therapy. In Willard H, Spackman C (Eds): Occupational Therapy. Ed 3. Philadelphia, Lippincott, 1963, pp 57-74.

Florey L: An approach to play and play development. AJOT 25(6):275-280, 1971.

Gillette N: Occupational therapy and mental health. In Willard H, Spackman C (Eds): Occupational Therapy. Ed 4. Philadelphia, Lippincott, 1971, pp 51-132.

Hopkins H: An historical perspective on occupational therapy. In Hopkins H, Smith H: Willard and Spackman's Occupational Therapy. Ed 6. Philadelphia, Lippincott, 1983.

Howe M: The role of occupational therapy in community mental health. AJOT 22(6):521-524, 1968.

Johnson J: Considerations of work as therapy in the rehabilitation process. AJOT 25(6):303-308, 1971.

Kielhofner G, Burke J: Occupational therapy after 60 years: An account of changing identity and knowledge. AJOT 31(10):675-689, 1977.

Kuhn TS: The Structure of Scientific Revolutions. Ed 2. Chicago, University of Chicago Press, 1970.

Llorens L: Theoretical conceptualizations of occupational therapy: 1960-1982. Occup Ther Ment Health 4(2):1-14, 1984.

Matsutsuyu J: Occupational behavior: A perspective on work and play. AJOT 25(6):291-294, 1971.

Maurer P: Antecedents of work behavior. AJOT 25(6):295-297, 1971.

Mazer J (Ed): Toward an integrated theory of occupational therapy. seminar, Aug. 26-31, 1967, Albion, Michigan. AJOT 22(5):451-456, 1968.

Mazer J, Mosey A (Eds): Special section — Theories of psychiatric occupational therapy. AJOT 22(5):398-450, 1968.

Michelman S: The importance of creative play. AJOT 25(6):285-295, 1971.

Mosey A: Recapitulation of ontogenesis. AJOT 22(5):426-438, 1968.

Mosey A: Occupational Therapy — Configuration of a Profession. New York, Raven Press, 1981.

Reilly M: The importance of the client versus patient issue for occupational therapy. AJOT 38(6):404-406, 1984.

Sharrott G, Yerxa E: Promises to keep: Implications of the referent "patient" versus "client" for those served by occupational therapy. AJOT 39(6):401-405, 1985.

Smith A, Tempone V: Psychiatric occupational therapy within a learning theory context. AJOT 22(5), 415, 1968.

Takata N, The play milieu: A preliminary appraisal. AJOT 25(6):281-281, 1971.

Tiffany E: Psychiatry and mental health. In Hopkins H, Smith H: Willard and Spackman's Occupational Therapy. Ed 6. Philadelphia, Lippincott, 1983, pp 267-334.

Veatch R: A Theory of Medical Ethics. New York, Basic Books, 1981.

White R: The urge towards competence. AJOT 25(6):271-274, 1971.

Chapter 2

The Framework of Therapy in Occupational Therapy

If we continue with the metaphor proposed in the introduction, we can imagine that in the journey through this text, we will travel the major routes of occupational therapy practice. As we use a particular frame of reference or map for our journey, we will encounter common structures in our environment that serve as the framework of the occupational therapy process. This framework provides the structure within which practice occurs. In actual practice life comes into this sterile framework or structure via the everyday personal encounters between (1) the patient and therapist, (2) the patient and the activity, and, often, (3) among several patients and treatment staff within a group milieu. In this chapter we briefly review the nature of the therapeutic relationship, the group milieu, and the purposeful activity in order to help the reader better understand the contribution that each makes to the occupational therapy process and to set the stage for discussing the frames of reference that encompass the major portion of this text.

The Therapeutic Relationship

As educators, we have stood before eager students early in the semester, seeking to convey not only "fact" but also our feelings about the significance and special nature of the therapeutic relationship. Enthusiastic ourselves, we nevertheless were in something of the same dilemma as a person trying to talk about a melody. We spoke about rhythms, characters, and intonations that admittedly fell far short of the actual experiencing of the "melody" in the relationship.

Here, again, we wish to discuss what for us have emerged as essential aspects of the therapeutic relationship, recognizing that we have been selective in the values or attributes we discuss. We know, too, that just as the notes in a song must be heard in relationship to each other, so must be the elements in a personal relationship.

As you read, we hope that you will recognize in the values and behaviors described some reminiscences of relationships you have known in your own life. From your own experience you bring both intuitive and well-formed ideas about the kinds of interpersonal conditions you find helpful and those you do not. Pausing to reflect upon your own experiences may help bring to life the discussion that follows.

Defining the Therapeutic Relationship

The therapeutic relationship is a unique coming together of two people whose expressed purpose is for one to assist the other in dealing with internal or external stress, maturing, and meeting personal needs in a more satisfying way. The therapeutic relationship is between those two persons whom we refer to here as patient and therapist; other terms may be used in a context that is not medically oriented. In the therapeutic relationship, the patient is at the center. It is the mutual understanding of his thoughts, values, fears, needs, and aspirations that is the focus, and it must be his goals for himself that ultimately define treatment.

After familiarizing oneself with the major frameworks in which therapy is conceptualized, it becomes clear that there are some differences of opinion about what is "therapeutic," and the role of the therapist can be coined in quite different terms, depending on the treatment frame. What is particularly evident, however, is that professionals from a variety of helping disciplines and treatment models recognize that for treatment to "work," there must exist a sound relationship between patient and therapist. Further, whether the primary therapeutic agent is seen as physical exercise, leisure activity, verbalization, or medication, there are many commonly held beliefs regarding the therapeutic relationship that cut across the so-called boundaries of differing treatment philosophies and modalities. We have selected for elaboration here therapeutic conditions that, in some instances, were given initial emphasis within the humanistic-existential movement (see discussion in Chapter 3, Object Relations Frame of Reference). However, we have chosen for discussion conditions that are consistent across the frameworks discussed in this text. To look further at what constitutes a therapeutic relationship we need to pause and reflect, "What is therapy?"

What Is Therapy?

Therapy is a process by which a patient in distress can come to experience himself in new ways, ways that are more personally satisfying and that help him to relate more positively in his world. At its heart, therapy facilitates change — be it a change from dis-ease to increased "ease" or physical well-being; expanded ideas, attitudes, or skills; or changed ways of approaching events and tasks. A person seeks therapy when he is ineffective in making desired changes by himself.

In occupational therapy, activities are seen as an essential therapeutic agent. It is through his involvement with activity that a patient will learn new skills, or mobilize the physical body, or learn more about himself and others. He does not only talk about what he wishes to change (although reflecting upon his experiences may enhance his ability to learn from them); he tries out and practices new behaviors.

It must be recognized that many of the activities in occupational therapy are not unusual or new — they are often the "stuff" life is made of. Yet in both mental health and physical medicine we see time and again the patient who can not imagine himself trying, much less succeeding at, the activities which are so familiar and available to him. For him, therapeutic activity remains inaccessible until such time as he is able to picture himself in a role different from a previous one, or until he is willing to risk changing — or a combination of both. The therapeutic relationship serves to open windows and widen pathways when, within its support, encouragement, caring, and guidance, risks are taken.

The Occupational Therapist's Role in the Therapeutic Relationship

When we risk change, we risk failure as well as success. We risk upheaval and uncertainty; we move to unfamiliar ground. In order for someone to let go of the old and familiar, he must first feel safe, and it is an essential role of the therapist to ensure safety.

Safety. Think for a moment about the situations in which you were willing to test a new idea, or experiment with an activity that was quite foreign to you. We suspect that you needed to feel emotionally safe. Few of us have such self-assurance that we will easily risk ridicule, or tempt criticism. Perhaps someone assured you that if you faltered, he would be there to offer support. A patient, as with all of us, needs to know that he will not be shamed or shame himself. Beyond that, he needs to know that he will not be forced into going further than he wishes, that the boundaries he sets will be respected. Sometimes that means allowing the patient to go very slowly even when we might be wanting to "get the ball rolling" quickly. The patient must also feel physically safe. If he fears loss of control or physical harm, he needs to know that he will not be allowed to harm himself or others.

Coming from and providing a firm knowledge base enables the therapist to establish an environment of safety. Being knowledgeable about the patient's physical and emotional needs, and about the demands and limitations within a broad range of human endeavor, is a requisite if a patient is to feel safe within our care.

Providing the patient with information helps him gain power and control in relation to his own "safety" or well-being, and is an important part of the continuing effort we make to enhance the patient's ability to be effective and appropriately self-reliant.

While we cannot predict the outcome of therapy, when we as therapists behave in a manner that is consistent and predictable, others tend to feel more safe with us, for they know what they can expect from us and what is expected of them.

We all hear about professionalism and may mistake it for starched shirt stuffiness or distancing maneuvers. In fact, in our being "professional" we strive to be consistent, ethical, dependable, and knowledgeable, and we make a statement of our commitment to the best in care. Such a commitment helps in establishing the sense of safety necessary if another is to entrust us with his efforts at change.

Trust. An essential part of the therapeutic relationship lies with the ability of the therapist to foster trust, a trust which is integral to the sense of safety we have just addressed.

There are different aspects of trust between two persons, three of which we emphasize here. One aspect relates to one person knowing that another will be honest — that his conduct is based on moral integrity. We have probably all been in situations in which we were not certain whether our confidences would be kept; or perhaps we have been unsure whether someone has been truthful. In such situations we tend to close up rather than open up, feeling a need to protect ourselves and our thoughts and feelings.

There is also trust based on finding the other person to be authentic or "real." That is, there are certain values and characteristics that emerge consistently in his interactions. We do not find him to be a chameleon. Our patient is more likely to experience us as "real" when we are, as described by Rogers, "congruent" (Rogers, 1972, p. 13). Congruent in this usage means that our words, affect, and actions go together to give a clear and consistent message.

Being "real" and congruent requires that as therapists we be aware of our beliefs and values. As stated by Rogers, ". . . if I can form a helping relationship to myself — if I can be sensitively aware and acceptant toward my own feelings — then the likelihood is great that I can form a helping relationship toward another" (Rogers, 1972, p. 14). Knowing what we ourselves believe helps us to keep our needs separate from those of our patient, helps us to be clear about our own boundaries and limitations, and allows us to behave in a manner that is consistent and begets trust.

Trust is nurtured also when we as therapists behave openly, as if we trust ourselves and believe in the worth of our therapy and in our own worth. This includes acknowledging when we do not have all the answers and showing that we are willing to risk our own failures. When a patient can see that we are willing to be vulnerable and open to learning, he finds that one does not have to be "perfect" to be trustworthy and he finds that he has a powerful example or model from which he can learn.

Another important facet of trust exists when a patient trusts that we give his well-being the highest priority. He trusts that we care about him.

Caring. Devereaux describes caring as the heart of the therapeutic relationship and notes that "its presence enriches all other aspects of the relationship" (Devereaux, 1984, p. 796). As she notes, being cared about is the opposite of anonymity within and disconnectedness from the rest of the world. If you ask prospective or practicing therapists about their desire to be therapists, they will very often cite their wish to "help" or "care about" others. Brammer refers to the need to care as a valuing of altruism (Brammer, 1979, pp. 30-32). He reminds us that in our reaching out to others, we fulfill our own need to feel valuable and connected to others. In recognizing that as therapists each of us gains something important for ourselves, we are better able to keep our motives and beliefs separate from the aims of our patients.

We each have our personal ideas about how caring can best be expressed, and, indeed, each human relationship will bring special circumstances and unique opportunities for caring. Basically caring means that we believe that our patient is valuable, that we desire to know him in a real way, and that his needs, feelings, and aspirations direct our service. Caring is not to be confused with "mothering" or infantilizing our patient. Rather, in caring for our patient we seek to help him be independent and better able to care for himself.

It is ironic that many patients who seek treatment (or are directed with reluctance into treatment) state that they have no need to change because, as they say, "No one cares about what I do." When we let our caring show, we do not act as a substitute for friends, parents, spouses, et al., but we do provide a person-to-person relationship in which someone *does* care. This, at times, acts as an evocative challenge to long held suppositions as the patient may confront the possibility, "Perhaps someone does care. Perhaps I am worthy of being cared about."

Open Communication. Safety, trust, and the confirmation of caring all depend for their vitality on open communication within the therapeutic relationship. When there is open communication, both the patient and the therapist can express themselves, make their concerns known, clarify areas of doubt or ambiguity, and move toward the common goals of therapy.

There has been much written about specific skills and therapist attitudes believed to enhance communication (see note 1). When, for example, we as therapists maintain good eye contact, indicate verbally and nonverbally our interest, and avoid a judgmental stance, we increase the likelihood that our patient will trust us with his thoughts. But open communication implies something deeper than encouragement to talk. It depends on there being an attitude of true permission for our patient to be himself with us. Can you recall any instances when a parent, teacher, or friend said, "Tell me what you *really* feel" or "Be yourself"? Yet when your response was received as challenging, the permission to be honest was rescinded. An essential part of open communication is allowing our patient to experience negative as well as positive feelings and to share those that he chooses to share with us. That is not always as easy as it sounds.

Patients may be angry with us when we feel they have no cause; they may express "romantic" feelings; they may behave unpredictably and threaten our personal need for order and control. While not making ourselves targets of abuse, when we "hear out" those feelings that may make us uncomfortable, we let the patient know that our caring about him does not come and go with his ability to please us, and we increase the likelihood that the patient can better understand his own concerns and feelings. In the process, we may learn more about who we are. It is not that we have to agree with or feel the same way that our patient does. In fact, communication is a reciprocal process — and often includes our stating when and how things look different from our vantage point. Open communication requires that both the patient and the therapist have a respect for the right of the other to feel as he does, and it provides an opportunity for each to gain insight into the perceptions of the other.

Understanding. Open communication is necessary if the patient is to believe that he is understood, that the therapist really *knows* him. Depending on the conceptual model, we as therapists may seek specific kinds of information from the patient, but it is important not only that we gain information that we believe is necessary from our viewpoint, but also that the patient know that we understand what is important in his eyes.

Often a patient who is going through a particularly difficult time will feel isolated by his experience. For example, a woman newly divorced might say, "No one can know how I feel." Or an amputee, being encouraged to put pressure on a painful stump, might say, "It's easy for you to tell me to bear down; you don't feel the pain I do." In a way, both patients are correct; we cannot know exactly how each feels. But if we can draw upon our own experiences and attempt to look and listen in order to understand, we can go a long way towards appreciating the frustration and pain each experiences. In so doing, we increase our ability to communicate caring and to serve the best interests of our patients. Further, our encouragement to the patient to take risks does not become an insensitive demand.

Valuing Change. In the therapeutic relationship, the patient sees the therapist as someone who values change and who believes in his ability and potential for positive change. While each individual is ultimately responsible for taking his own risks, each of us is encouraged when someone we trust says, in essence, "I really believe you can do this."

There is much in the recent literature about the devastating effects of parenting in which a child is told over and over again, "You are inept. You'll never amount to anything." And as therapists we are unlikely to imagine ourselves making such statements. Yet in our efforts to "care" or "help," we may give our own detrimental messages. When, for example, we overprotect a patient in order to prevent him from failing, or because his reliance on us serves to make us feel important, we communicate, "I don't believe in your ability to take care of yourself, or to be successful."

At times we must use careful clinical judgment to determine whether an actual risk of physical harm exists, and to assess how it can best be managed. Much of the changing and risk-taking in the psychosocial realm relates, however, to emotional risk-taking. We may find ourselves wishing to protect our patient from disappointment, failure, or rebuffs. The clinical judgments we make in these instances are some of the most difficult. If, however, we have established a sound therapeutic relationship, we enhance the ability of our patient to handle disappointments or to experience them as more manageable. When we let him know that we will value him regardless of what he has accomplished, we facilitate risk-taking.

Accepting Tentativeness. In order for the relationship to be therapeutic, both the patient and the therapist must accept some tentativeness in therapy. A patient may, understandably, seek to limit ambiguity and perhaps ask for assurances that "everything will go according to plan." If we generalize this, it is not unlike the wish that most of us have had at some time that "life would go according to plan." Learning to cope with the everyday vicissitudes depends on the confidence that each of us, patient and therapist, has in ourselves, our knowledge and skills, and the degree to which we are aware of the uncompromising values that give us our bearings.

As therapists we need to realize that while treatment plans give us direction, some of the most memorable learning occurs when we and our patient can respond spontaneously to unscheduled events or unexpected feelings. If we remember our initial premise that therapy facilitates change, we can better realize the essential need to accept tentativeness as part of the therapeutic process.

Dealing with Limitations. Finally, the therapeutic relationship is one in which the therapist recognizes and abides by its limitations. Some of the limitations in therapy relate directly to the nature of the patient's problems and the extent of resources. What we wish to address here are the more general limitations integral to the nature of the relationship itself.

Therapy is a temporally bounded process: it cannot and will not go on endlessly. Helping a patient be cognizant of the probable duration of treatment enables the patient and the therapist to establish reasonable expectations of what can be accomplished. If therapy is a process that facilitates change, we might speak metaphorically of therapy as serving as a bridge into unfamiliar terrain. The therapist serves as the guide, but once the bridge is crossed, there exists a point at which the guide departs, and the patient continues without her. With this in mind, it behooves the patient and the therapist always to be considering ways in which, as Devereaux states, we can "create opportunities for reconnecting the patient with other human beings and the environment" (Devereaux, 1984, p. 794).

There are other limitations related to the structure of therapy. These include mutually agreed upon boundaries regarding the length of each treatment session, the therapist's availability at times other than those scheduled, and the responsibilities specific to patient and to therapist as they work together in therapy. Whether the structure of therapy is handled informally or formally (i.e., through a verbal or written "contract"), it is important that we as therapists recognize what purpose such structure serves. In part the creation of this structure works to enhance predictability in therapy and increase the level of safety, as discussed earlier. It also provides expectations by which we can judge whether the goals of therapy are being met. Just as important, such a structure provides a mechanism that helps keep us from slipping into patterns of relating that could keep our patient perpetually and increasingly dependent on us. There may be special instances in which dependency will appropriately be fostered, especially, for example, when a patient has had extreme difficulty in allowing himself to ask for or accept any help from anyone. What we caution against here are those times in a therapeutic relationship when a therapist becomes so involved in "helping" that she loses sight of the others in the patient's world who could effectively (and better) relate to the patient in regard to given needs.

Beyond the obvious ethical boundaries prohibiting the therapist from compromising the emotional or physical well-being of her patient, the therapist must make it clear also that she is not a "friend." While our patients may understandably feel friendly towards us and us towards them, a friendship is not created for the purposes of therapy, nor therapy for the purpose of friendship. We will like many of our patients very much, but when therapy ends, so does the therapeutic relationship. If a patient can be helped to recognize the qualities that have made it possible for him to feel good about himself with us, then he can begin to see in himself the potential he has to build friendship. He does not need to feel "cheated" when therapy ends; rather, he is better able to relate meaningfully in his world.

Summary

In his description of self-actualization, Arthur Combs asked, "How can a person feel liked unless someone likes him? How can a person feel acceptable unless somewhere he is accepted? How can a person feel he has dignity unless somewhere someone treats him so? How can a person feel able unless somewhere he has some success?" (Combs, 1972, p. 121). The answers to these questions, said Combs, contain the guidelines to the "encouragement of growth and development everywhere" (Combs, 1972, p. 122) and the basis for the conditions of therapy.

In this brief review we have sought to illustrate that each therapeutic condition is related to the integrity and substance of the whole relationship. When one therapeutic element is lacking, the entire relationship is jeopardized. As you read further in the text, try to identify the way in which the therapist operating within each of the different frames of reference will affirm the therapeutic conditions described and incorporate these into her own practice.

Groups in Occupational Therapy

The discussion of group treatment and group dynamics in this chapter will briefly review the more general theoretical principles that are applicable in occupational therapy practice. This general overview will identify the characteristics that make a group therapeutic, highlight the process for forming a group, identify the role of the occupational therapist in the group, and discuss the function of group dynamics in occupational therapy groups. The coverage of group treatment and dynamics in this chapter does not provide expertise in skills necessary for leading or for processing a group, but it will give direction for further study in this area. The reader is encouraged to study the psychology, sociology, and occupational therapy literature pertaining to group development and process, leadership styles and their impact, roles within a group, group strategies and responses, and the use of treatment groups in the multiple arenas of occupational therapy practice. The material available which pertains to group theory and application merits a text in itself. Although not covered in depth, group principles are exemplified throughout this text. Sample activities, skills, and techniques used by the occupational therapist during treatment groups are described within the context of each of the major frames of reference presented.

Since the early 1900's social scientists have been interested in groups and how people function in group situations. In the late 1930's, the study of groups became an identified field of inquiry, and Kurt Lewin popularized the term "group dynamics." Later, in 1945, an organization was established for the research and study of group dynamics. Since this time, the application of group theory and dynamics in treatment and education has evolved to the formation of the multiple group treatment formats and educational strategies that are available today. In addition to the academic interest in group theory and its clinical application, the development of group treatment has been fostered by the community mental health movement, the increased patient load and scarcity of mental health professionals (the lack of occupational therapist is included), and the expansion of psychological and sociological theories that support the use of group intervention.

Occupational Therapy Groups

In occupational therapy, patients have been treated in groups since the profession's origin. However, the systematic application of group dynamics in activity groups for the purpose of heightening therapeutic progress came to the forefront during the 1960's. The two figures who have made major contributions to the application of group theory in occupational therapy are Gail Fidler and Ann Mosey. In addition to publications by these therapists, there are numerous other articles that exemplify occupational therapy group treatment in mental health as well as in other specialty areas of the profession.

Task Groups. In 1963, Fidler called attention to the group "phenomena" in occupational therapy treatment and in the working relationships that occupational therapists maintained with other professionals. In her book she acknowledged the relationship between patient groups, staff groups, and the family group. She gave an overview of the roles and functions of the occupational therapist within the treatment group and suggested responses that the occupational therapist can make which help to establish rapport between the therapist and patients. Fidler acknowledged the influence of group development, leadership styles, group characteristics, and therapist and patient responses upon the activity process and the outcome of the treatment experience. Six years later Fidler expounded further her initial discussion of group treatment and identified the "task-oriented group" and its purpose in occupational therapy. The theory that supported task groups was a "meld" of sociologic, psychoanalytic, and learning theories (Fidler, 1969, p. 43).

The theory can be summarized as follows: Interpersonal, intrapsychic, and environmental forces influence affect, learning, and behavior. Therefore, these forces are explored in a "here and now" atmosphere to identify patient stresses, to explore conflict and problems, to elicit interaction among patients, and to facilitate learning and change. Exploration and learning in the "here and now" occur in occupational therapy task groups. During group activities the psychosocial forces and their influence are evident. Thus activities can be used to explore stresses and conflicts, to remediate problems, and to increase learning through "doing." The activity itself as well as the processing of activities during groups promotes function in the treatment environment and prepares the patient for performing in daily life. Occupational therapy is described as a "learning lab" in which the patient develops skills for life and the "work world" through task experiences (Fidler, 1969).

Task-oriented treatment groups as described by Fidler were developed at the New York Psychiatric Institute. The original group was composed of eight patients, selected because they were unable to be productive in life, they had limited independent function, and the

23

therapist determined that they were ready for the group experience (readiness criteria were not identified). The group met for 1½ hours four times per week and worked on a common task that was achieved through group effort and consensus decision making (Fidler, 1969). Fidler states that the task can be "any activity or process directed toward creating or producing an end product or demonstrable service for the group as a whole and/or for persons outside of the group." Some examples given are "publishing a newspaper, cooking, gardening, a patient council, ward decorating" (Fidler, 1969, p. 45).

The purpose of the task-oriented group is to "provide a shared working experience wherein the relationship between feeling, thinking and behavior and their i   :t on others and on task accomplishment and productivity can be viewed and explored. Alternate patterns of functioning can be considered and tested within the context of the here and now, to the end that such learning may induce ego growth and improve function. Task accomplishment is not the purpose of the group but hopefully the means by which purpose is realized" (Fidler, 1969, p. 45). Stated another way, the task group as described by Fidler has a strong emphasis on group process, a term which we will encounter again in the discussion of an object-relations treatment framework.

The task is used to identify group cohesiveness, group problem solving strategies, the group and individual patients' views of reality, cause and effect relationships, the communication patterns in the group, and the relationship between the roles and functions in a group and the patient's community responsibilities (Fidler, 1969)

Since the publication of the task-oriented group theory, occupational therapists have used group treatment in mental health as well as physical medicine, pediatric, and geriatric settings. Today the task-oriented group continues to be a viable form of treatment that is frequently used in occupational therapy. It also continues to influence other group treatment approaches that have emerged.

Developmental Groups. Mosey's contributions to group treatment in occupational therapy were published in 1970, 1973, and 1981. She discusses developmental groups, roles within a group, group skills, group process, activity groups, and a tentative taxonomy for activity groups.

The concept of developmental groups originated with Wilbauger and was further developed and presented by Mosey in the book, *Three Frames of Reference for Mental Health* (1970). The developmental groups identified were: (1) parallel group, (2) project group, (3) egoecentric-cooperative group, (4) cooperative group, and (5) mature group. The groups were correlated with developmental age spans and necessitated identifiable interaction subskills. Each group is briefly defined in Appendix C.

Activity Groups. In 1973 Mosey further contributed to the occupational therapy body of knowledge regarding groups through her discussion of group dynamics and group processes in *Activities Therapy*. In this publication she defined a group and discussed group membership roles (task and social-emotional roles); decision making in groups; the communication process; and group goals, cohesiveness, and group norms. She provided this information in order to increase the activities therapist's understanding of small groups and how they can

24

be used to provide learning situations for patients in treatment groups which will prepare the patient to live more independently in the community.

In an activity group, individuals relate around a specified task or activity. This may be for the purpose of assessing patient function, as well as a way to implement treatment goals. If one is to understand the interaction within the group as well as its outcome, one must look at the characteristics of the activity (medium and process) as well as be acquainted with principles of small group interaction.

Mosey stresses that what an individual can do within an activity group is representative of what he can accomplish within other (nontreatment) groups in which he participates. As such, the activity group acts as a microcosm of the larger environment, as we shall examine further in our discussion of the object-relations framework for practice.

Mosey notes that activity groups tend to be classified according to the goal of the group and she feels that this "leads to confusion" (Mosey, 1981, p. 110). Thus she proposes a "tentative" taxonomy of activity groups. The groups identified in the taxonomy are: evaluation groups, task-oriented groups, developmental groups, thematic groups, topical groups, and instrumental groups (Mosey, 1981, pp. 110-112). The reader is referred to the original source for the discussion of these groups. The groups are briefly defined in Appendix D.

What Is a Group?

Groups have been defined generally as a coming together of two or more people for a specific purpose. This definition has been further expanded by the psychologist and the sociologist, and the following elaborated definition is presented by Cartwright and Zander (1968, p. 48). A set of people constitutes a group when "one or more of the following statements will characterize them: (a) they engage in frequent interaction; (b) they define themselves as members; (c) they are defined by others as belonging to the group; (d) they share norms concerning matters of common interest; (e) they participate in a system of interlocking roles; (f) they identify with one another as a result of having set up the same model-object or ideals in their superego; (g) they find the group to be rewarding; (h) they pursue promotively interdependent goals; (i) they have a collective perception of their unity; (j) they tend to act in a unitary manner toward the environment."

Knowles depicts the difference between a collection of people and a group in Figure 2-1. The schematic representation of a collection of people graphically shows the lack of boundaries, lack of a shared goal, lack of group consciousness, undefined membership, and multiple directions of its members. No lines of interaction and interdependent communication exist.

In our lives we each belong to a number of groups. We are members of a family and may be members in religious, social, political, or community groups. Although we benefit from these interactions, the previously mentioned groups differ from therapeutic groups. Treatment groups usually have a more specific objective(s), usually within the framework of learning, remediation, or change, and have an identified time period for existence. In therapy, a group consists of a specific number of persons who come together because of common concerns and

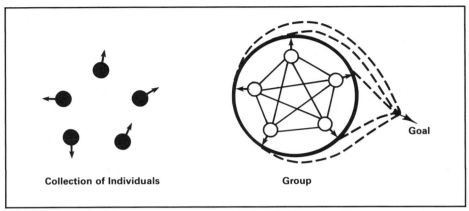

Figure 2-1. Reproduced with permission, Knowles, M and Knowles, H: *Introduction to Group Dynamics.* Cambridge Adult Education Co., New York.

stresses, or problems in living. The goals for remediation, learning, coping, or change may be formulated by the group members, or they may be established by the treatment staff.

In occupational therapy, patients come together daily or several times a week for the specific purpose of changing the way they think, feel, or behave in their daily lives. Patients may work on individual projects within a group, may work collectively on a particular task, may participate in role playing experiences, or may learn from academic tasks that are presented and processed in small groups. Since particular activity groups are exemplified throughout the book, we will speak generally of the role of the therapist and the manner in which a group experience can be used to enhance the goals of therapy.

The Role of the Occupational Therapist in the Group

The responsibilities previously identified in the discussion of the therapeutic relationship apply to the therapist's participation in group treatment but are expanded beyond the patient-therapist dyad by the complexity of interaction that occurs among patients during the group experience. The therapist continues to assure physical safety for all patients in the group and reflects her attitude of acceptance, caring, understanding, and valuing change. She also promotes and facilitates these attitudes among patients within the group and tries to elicit expression of caring, acceptance, and support for change by patients for each other. How this is accomplished is influenced by the therapist's leadership.

Styles of Leadership

Like any leader of a group, the occupational therapist has a choice of leadership style. She can choose to be an authority in the group, plan and present the activity, and set and enforce the boundaries for interaction. In general, as an authority she assumes the responsibility for determining the activity, delegating the task procedures, identifying the patient roles, controlling the group process, and limiting interactions in order to achieve an outcome that she has determined to be desirable.

In contrast, she may assume a democratic role in which she facilitates group member interaction and a sharing of leadership. Consistent with the democratic style of leadership, she delegates to the patients shared responsibility for selecting the activity and/or implementing the task and processing the experience. She encourages the patients to participate in the decision making process and to identify the roles they wish to assume, and she encourages the free exchange of ideas among patients.

A third possible leadership style is one called laissez-faire. This leadership approach allows the patients to assume full responsibility for identifying and assuming a goal and for planning and implementing the strategies for accomplishing the goal and allows the occupational therapist to be in the background, still making minimal contributions to the group experience (see note 2).

The leadership style that an occupational therapist assumes is determined by the task to be accomplished, the characteristics of the patient group, the desired outcome and the purpose of the group experience, and the day to day happenings that affect patients' feelings and behavior.

It is the authors' view that regardless of the leadership style, the occupational therapist has a role of "gate keeper." As a gate keeper she is available to provide safety and facilitate trust, caring, communication, understanding, acceptance, and change (key elements in the therapeutic relationship which can be enhanced by group interactions). Needless to say, this is not an easy task and one which is not taken lightly. As a gate keeper the therapist utilizes her knowledge of group dynamics and process and her understanding of individual patients in accordance with her chosen treatment frame of reference.

Safety and Trust. When the occupational therapist initiates a group, she helps to establish a sense of safety by stating the purpose and boundaries of the group, ethical principles of group interaction, and rules of confidentialty. Further, she identifies the group structure and any formal "rules" for group interaction. Some of the "rules" for group interaction can be conceived as less formal, because patients learn from observing each other and the therapist and learn acceptable ways to provide positive or negative feedback, constructive means to gain attention, and the like.

In addition to the development of trust between patients and herself, the therapist seeks to establish trust among patients. The group process as well as the outcome depends on patient interactions based upon trust among patients as well as trust between the individual patient and the therapist. The occupational therapist continually seeks to encourage patients to respond to each other in a constructive manner rather than allowing them to use her as the authority and primary respondent or channel of communication. When, for example, a patient indicates to her that he has felt slighted by another in the group, the therapist might ask him to redirect his communication to the appropriate other. Or, when a patient states that he felt clumsy or inept doing the group task, she might ask the group to respond, asking, "Who in the group has felt this way?" or "What have others done in similar situations?"

Universality. As patients interact during treatment groups, they learn that others have had similar experiences, problems, needs, and feelings. They realize that they are not alone. When patients share and learn from each other, there comes a sense of mutual caring and concern, a lessened feeling of isolation, an increased confidence in one's own ability to cope with life, to accept oneself and accept stress. Many social scientists believe that it is the ability of a group experience to make the individual more aware that his concerns and "problems" are universal that makes a group activity particularly helpful (Yalom, 1975).

Communication. Trust, caring, safety, and understanding depend upon the verbal and nonverbal communication among group members during the group and activity experience. The occupational therapist (at times acting as a model) facilitates interactions which promote acceptance among patients and open communication that results in a constructive outcome. This does not mean that patients are always "happy" and comfortable during the occupational therapy groups. It does mean that the therapist and patients will provide the support necessary for patients to take risks and make change, and to cope with the discomfort that is experienced during learning and the group activity.

The theory and strategies related to the effective use of interpersonal communication and group dynamics for the purpose of building trust, promoting care and empathy, and enhancing safety and change are not discussed in depth here, and the reader is encouraged to gain a more thorough understanding of these areas to heighten her effectiveness as a gate keeper, group leader, or group facilitator.

When looking at the interpersonal communication that occurs during occupational therapy groups, the therapist is aware of the content and process of a group. The *content* refers to the statements that patients make and to the specific behaviors that occur as the outcome of the identified task. One might think of the content as the "what" of the group activity. The *process* of the occupational therapy group is the "how" of the activity or the dynamics that occur as the group ensues: i.e., the interactions between patients; the nonverbal behaviors that occur in response to the activity, other patients, the occupational therapist or the setting; and the unspoken elements that occur that seem to influence individual patient behavior, the activity, and the group outcome.

The General Group Format

The manner and the extent to which the occupational therapist chooses to discuss the group and activity process depends upon the needs, skills, and limitations of the patients; the goals of the group; and the skill and expertise of the therapist. However, regardless of the depth of or manner of processing, the authors suggest the following general format as a guide for the therapist leading a group. This format is organized around three stages in the group process: (1) opening a group, (2) developing the group experience, and (3) closing a group.

Opening the Group. The occupational therapist states the name of the group (when appropriate) and perhaps defines it, identifies the time frame of the group, explains the purpose and goals of the group, and explains what the patient may expect from the experience. She may discuss how the patients were chosen for the group. To illustrate:

OTR: "Welcome! Today in occupational therapy we will be together for the next hour and a half to learn about how we use time and how we manage time. First we will draw a 'pie of life'" (an experience described by James and Jongeward, in *Born to Win,* 1971). The therapist then asks a patient to give to group members the materials needed to complete the task.

Group Development. After the "pie" is drawn, the therapist facilitates discussion of how patients use their time. A round robin format may be used; i.e., each patient is given a turn to tell how he uses his time. Or the therapist may ask for patients to volunteer to talk about their drawing. As individual patients describe the way they use their time and the feelings they have about the way their time is spent, the therapist may highlight the similarities that exist among group members. She may say, for example, "I notice several of you have indicated that you spend 80 percent of your time with nothing to do. Perhaps learning to use our unstructured time would be a useful goal in future group activities."

During the group activity and during the discussion that follows, the therapist will note patterns of participation. There is no one best pattern; in general the broader the interaction pattern, the better. In other words, it is generally desirable to have many patients actively participate. While it is true that individuals can learn by "listening" or watching when many or all members actively participate in the group, there is a greater "pool" of ideas from which all can draw, patient interest tends to be greater, and participants tend to feel a stronger investment in the group. The therapist will help patients communicate both their ideas and feelings in a effort to increase their understanding.

The therapist takes note of nonverbal communication such as that reflected by the patient's posture, facial expression, gestures, and where he sits in (or perhaps outside of) the group. She will observe how the patients work together, and she may, at times, reflect her observations back to the group in an effort to make the group more aware of its own process. As the activity ensues, the therapist will typically promote cooperation and participation. This often results in a cohesive or "team" feeling. She tries to minimize subgroup formation or cliques such as adults versus teenagers or old members versus new members. Cliques can interfere with the activity process and group outcome, decrease cohesiveness, and lessen the likelihood that patients will feel that they can learn from the experiences of others. The therapist is exhorted to promote an atmosphere of warmth, helpfulness, responsibility, friendliness, and cooperation. Toward this end, she will often need to help patients set standards for courtesy, productivity, tolerance, and support. Periodically, the therapist may need also to help the group identify procedures which will enhance the activity process and facilitate goal accomplishment. Goals must be clear and understood by each member in the group throughout the activity experience and in relation to the time left to complete the group task. The "content" of the group in the above example includes the ideas and feelings shared by patients regarding the way they spend their time. The "process" in the group includes the participation pattern — who participates and who responds to whom, the nonverbal behaviors of the group members, the style of leadership that was needed by the group, and the general reaction of the group to the experience.

Group Closure. In order to bring closure, the occupational therapist summarizes the group experience. When summarizing, the therapist restates the purpose of the group, identifies or clarifies the learning outcome of the experience, and/or reinforces the therapeutic benefit of the experience. She allows the patients to share with each other their perceptions of the experience and to give each other feedback, as well as to give suggestions regarding future group activities.

In addition to summarizing and reflecting upon the group experience, the occupational therapist tries to connect the experience to the environment outside the treatment setting. She may refer to past experience, analogous experiences in the patient's natural environment, and/or expected similar situations which could be encountered in the future.

A sample summary of group closure may be something similar to the following "pie of life" group summary:

OTR: "Today in occupational therapy, we have drawn a 'pie' to help us look at how we use our time (goal restatement). During the discussion of our drawings we learned that most of us don't know what to do with our free time (a statement of the learning outcome). Learning to use our free time can be one of the benefits of your hospital stay and can help you when you return home (a statement that identifies the link between hospital and community). In future occupational therapy groups we will do activities that can help you develop new interests, and learn about your community and resources you can use to fill your free time when you return home (a statement which sets the stage for future treatment activities)."

Documentation of Occupational Therapy Groups

Once the group is completed, the occupational therapist documents the experience in each patient's chart and/or in a more central location such as a staff or department communications notebook or log. The purpose of group documentation is to communicate patient progress as well as to keep other treatment team members informed of the significant patient interactions and learning that occur in occupational therapy. The sample group note here gives the reader a possible format for documenting groups. However, the documentation format may vary in order to meet the needs of the health setting and the documentation protocol established.

Sample Occupational Therapy Group Note.

Date: November 28, 1985

Group Title: Activities of Daily Living/Time Management

Group Goals:

1. Each patient will draw a "pie of life."

2. Each patient will identify how he uses time — the proportion of time used in self-care, work and leisure activities.

3. Each patient will communicate with group members regarding his use of time as depicted in the group drawing experience.

4. Each patient will identify one change he wishes to make in regards to how he uses time.

Occupational Therapy Activity: The "pie of life" is a paper and pencil task. Activity Experience: The patients met for 90 minutes. They were instructed to draw a circle and divide it into pieces that represent the portion of time during the week that is devoted to being alone, with friends, with family, at work, doing recreation activities, and doing self-care activities.

Patients in Attendance: (Here the therapist lists the names of those patients who attended the occupational therapy group.)

Summary of the Group Experience: (Content and process observations are noted) Ten patients participated in the Daily Living Group. All in attendance completed the "pie of life" drawing. J.S. and P.V. (patient initials) refused to share how they use time but listened to the comments by others. During the discussion of time use and management, "How to use free time" (while in the hospital or when at home) emerged as the primary concern among the majority of participants. Among the issues related to use of free time the patients identified the following: (1) patients have few interests, (2) patients are unfamiliar with resources in the community, (3) patients lack sufficient funds for transportation to community recreation facilities, and (4) patients would like more in-hospital activities on weekends. K.N. and L.V. (patient initials) volunteered to plan weekend activities with staff assistance.

The occupational therapist suggested that future daily living groups could be used to plan weekend events and will also provide activities to help patients develop interests, contact community resources, and incorporate activities to assist patients in learning to use "free time."

In general there was a spirit of cooperation and sharing in the group. The two new group members, L.G. and C.T., were introduced by K.N. who throughout the group experience showed initiative and promoted group interaction.

Summary

Not all occupational therapy is carried out within a group context. When therapy does occur in a group setting, there can be greater opportunity for patients to function in every day kinds of social experiences. Within these group experiences, the patient has increased resources from which he can learn, gain feedback, and gain support. In order for the group to be a helpful learning experience, the therapist must maintain the therapeutic relationship she has established with each of her patients, while assisting patients to relate to each other in a way that is honest yet accepting of individual differences and in a manner that supports risk-taking and change.

"Purposeful" Activity

The third component of the framework for therapy is the activity in which the patient and therapist participate in order to bring about change. In the occupational therapy literature there are multiple terms to describe activities that bring about change and among them multiple definitions of "purposeful" activity. Some of the terms used in the literature to describe activity include "purposeful activity" (Fidler, 1969; King, 1978; Mosey, 1981), "therapeutic activity" or "treatment activity" (Willard and Spackman, 1971), "goal directed activity" and "purposeful task" (Willard and Spackman 1963), and "occupation" (Fairman, 1968; Hopkins, 1983).

In each of the preceding definitions (with the exception of "occupation") the existence of a *goal* is implied. That is, the activity used in treatment has a specific objective. The term "occupation" also has many definitions, but in general it has been defined as how an individual occupies time. Until recently neither goal directed behavior nor purpose has necessarily been implied by the term occupation. However, in 1983 Fine in a paper approved by the Executive Board of the American Occupational Therapy Association in regards to practice, quotes a 1972 *American Journal of Occupational Therapy* article, "occupation in the title [Occupational Therapy] is in the context of goal-directed use of time, energy, interest, and attention to foster adaptation and productivity, to minimize pathology and to promote the maintenance of health" (American Occupational Therapy Task Force, 1972). However, in this text we use the term "purposeful activity" with its goal directed focus, rather than the term "occupation," which is most popularly identified with the occupational behavior frame of reference.

In addition to the Fine paper, the American Occupational Therapy Association submitted a position paper to clarify the use of the term "purposeful activity." The paper stated that an activity becomes "purposeful" when it has "unique" meaning for the patient; when it utilizes the patient's abilities; when it helps the patient fulfill his life roles; when it helps the patient achieve his personal goals; and when it increases the patient's feeling of competence and mastery in self-care, work, and leisure. Purposeful activities are tasks or experiences used in occupational therapy evaluation and treatment to assess, facilitate, restore, and maintain physical, emotional, and cognitive function (Hinojosa, Sabari, and Rosenfeld, 1983).

As used in this text, "purposeful activity" is conceived in accordance with its definition as presented by Fidler and Fidler (1978), supported by the American Occupational Therapy Association (1979), and reiterated by Mosey (1981). "An activity is purposeful only if it is congruent with 'the individual's sensory, motor, cognitive, psychological and social maturation . . . developmental needs and skill readiness...and recognized by [the individual's] social and cultural groups as relevant to their values and needs' (Fidler and Fidler, 1978, in Mosey, 1981, p. 99). Purposeful activities are doing processes that involve 'investigating, trying out and gaining evidence of one's capacities for experiencing, responding, managing, creating and controlling'" (American Occupational Therapy Association, 1979 in Mosey, 1981, p. 99).

It is not the author's intent to argue how to best define "purposeful activity," or to determine what are the commonalities in the definitions, or to identify one definition as more accurate and applicable to practice. Rather, the reader should note that multiple definitions exist which have and will continue to influence the theory and practice of occupational therapy.

The intent of the following discussion of "purposeful activity" is to highlight the contribution of activity to the framework of therapy and to present "purposeful activity" as an agent of change and to emphasize that activity becomes "purposeful" when it is utilized within the context of the person and his environment. Examples of the person-environmental use of activities are provided throughout this text. Purposeful activities which have been used by occupational therapists with individual patients or in activity groups are used to exemplify frames of reference in occupational therapy practice.

"Purposeful Activity" in the Framework of Therapy

In the therapy experience the patient is the center within the group and/or activity experience. The dynamic interaction of the patient with other patients, with the occupational therapist, and with the activity produces change. It is through this dynamic process that the activity becomes a change agent. To facilitate change, activities allow a patient to gain knowledge, acquire new skills, relearn to use his capabilities, identify his abilities and limitations, change and/or develop his interests, learn to use his time effectively, broaden his opportunities for recreation and work, and increase the network of people with whom he interacts.

The Role of the Occupational Therapist with "Purposeful" Activity

The role and responsibilities of the occupational therapist identified for the therapeutic relationship and in group treatment also apply when the occupational therapist uses purposeful activity to facilitate change. The therapist communicates the ideas that activities have value; that activities provide a safe vehicle for learning and change; that participating in activities can increase self-knowledge and knowledge of others; that activities can facilitate understanding, communication, and problem solving with others; and that activities in treatment can provide the bridge to the community.

Safety and Purposeful Activities. When the occupational therapist provides a safe environment for activity, she is concerned with the physical and emotional safety of the patient. The therapist is alert to the precautions necessary for fire prevention and general safety as she ensures a safe physical environment. She provides a clean and organized environment. She informs the patient of how to safely use materials and equipment and provides the necessary supervision mandated by the patient's abilities.

The therapist supports the patient's emotional safety by guiding the patient's choice of activity. She tries to help him choose an activity which is sufficiently challenging to allow him to learn and change and which will not be beyond his ability and capability. She generally seeks to avoid a failure experience and promote success. The degree to which the therapist actively intervenes to promote success will vary according to the patient's needs and the practice frame of reference.

To facilitate emotional and physical safety, the occupational therapist uses her knowledge of people and activities and her knowledge of health, growth and development, psychosocial disability, psychological theory, and activity analysis. She must apply this knowledge and her therapeutic skills within the context of a particular frame of reference. The therapist's personality, beliefs, knowledge, and skills give a unique quality to the use of "purposeful" activity and the manner in which factors related to emotional safety are interpreted and applied.

Valuing Purposeful Activity. Regardless of the knowledge and expertise of the occupational therapist, the use and effectiveness of "purposeful activity" will be constrained if the therapist does not believe in activities.

As discussed previously, many individuals who seek treatment find it difficult to see themselves trying new activities or succeeding at familiar activities. This may be especially evident when a patient lacks confidence, has limited information and/or skills, or has diminished "energy" because of a history of stress, conflict, failure, and/or depression. Different therapists prefer different kinds of activities (crafts, ADL, activities that stimulate sensory integrative function, etc.), owing in part to personal preference and in part to biases related to their chosen frame of reference. Whatever activities she utilizes, it is imperative that the therapist value the activities that she makes available to her patients. Sensing that the therapist believes in the ability of given activities to help him achieve his goals encourages the patient to expend the energy and take the risks involved in active participation.

The Boundaries Created by Purposeful Activity. Activities provide boundaries that can serve to increase a patient's sense of safety, as well as make more evident the successes he has achieved. This occurs because inherent in many of the activities used by occupational therapists are concrete or specific guides for behavior and interaction. These boundaries may be more readily apparent to a patient when a given activity is familiar to him, when the activity is around a tangible object or stair-stepped task, and/or when an activity has definable rules. When a patient can conceptualize the skills required in a given task, there is less ambiguity and uncertainty, and he can more easily anticipate what he can expect to gain from his participation. Many activities provide their own instantaneous and consistent "feedback" to patients — as, for example, with sewing, making a clay pot, and potting a plant — in which the patient can see the results of his efforts. Activities also provide a vehicle around which he can receive immediate feedback from patients, staff, and friends regarding his performance.

The structure inherent in most activity groups can also ease the discomfort the patient feels as he tries to learn social skills. For example, it may be more comfortable to practice social skills and work with others around planning a patient party or organizing a game of softball than to attempt socializing in a patient day room. In the dayroom, he might feel unsure regarding what are "safe" topics of conversation, or wonder if others even want to interact with him.

Purposeful Activity and the Treatment Outcome. In addition to the specific goal of the activity for the individual patient, how the therapist uses "purposeful activity" influences the treatment outcome. She may choose to emphasize the use of activity to produce a specific end product, an end product such as a woven wall hanging, a homemade cake, a painting, a wood project, a successful party, or a well written resume. Or she may choose to focus on the learning and the process that occur during the activity. The activity process is analogous to the process that occurs during a group experience. The *"process"* of the activity relates to the personal meaning the activity has for the patient; what the patient learns about himself and others as he works during the activity; the problem solving and work habits he acquires as he participates in the activity; the interactions which occur between the patient and therapist or the patient and other patients as the activity ensues; and the relationships he forms between the treatment experience and the knowledge and skills needed to interact in daily life. The activity process may not be readily evident to the patient. The occupational therapist shares with the patient her observations regarding the activity process in order to highlight the benefits of the activity experience, to facilitate change, and to provide the bridge between treatment and his daily environment. The sharing of these observations is given in a manner which is sensitive to the patient's cognitive, social, and emotional abilities and needs.

Purposeful Activities as a Bridge to the Community. When activities are purposeful, they serve as the bridge to the community. That is, the activities have meaning to the patient because they relate to a goal he has for the future, and/or the activity relates to the roles he assumes in the community and the tasks that he seeks to accomplish. In the context of activity, the patient gains knowledge, learns skills, and increases his self-confidence. The interaction between patient, therapist, and activity gives the treatment experience meaning and builds the bridge to the community. The learning and successful experiences in occupational therapy which come from purposeful activity help give the patient a sense of power and control in relation to the demands he will encounter in his everyday world.

Chapter Summary

The therapeutic relationship, group experience, and purposeful activity have been identified as providing the encounters through which therapy occurs. While in discussion each has been treated as a separate relationship, the reader will recognize that these relationships occur simultaneously during the therapeutic process. These relationships interact and constantly shape each other in a way that is unique with each therapeutic experience, and no two therapeutic experiences will be identical. In the remainder of this text, we see how the interaction of these three therapeutic elements takes on a special character in accordance with the values and beliefs imposed by each of the frames of reference.

End Notes

1. Some of the more frequently cited books that describe helping behaviors include:
Avila D, Combs A, Purkey W: Helping Relationships: Basic Concepts for the Helping Professions. Boston, Allyn and Bacon, Inc., 1971.
Bandura A: Principles of Behavior Modification. New York, Holt, Rinehart and Winston, 1969.
Benjamin A: The Helping Interview. Boston, Houghton Mifflin, 1969.
Brammer L, Shostrom, E: Therapeutic Psychology: Fundamental of Actualization Counseling and Psychotherapy. Ed 3. Englewood Cliffs, NJ, Prentice-Hall, 1977.

Brammer L: The Helping Relationship: Process and Skills. Englewood Cliffs, NJ, Prentice-Hall, 1979.

Carkhuff R, Berenson B: Beyond Counseling and Psychotherapy. New York, Holt, Rinehart and Winston, 1967.

Carkhuff R: Helping and Human Relations. Vol 1 and 2. New York, Holt, Rinehart and Winston, 1969.

Egan G: The Skilled Helper. Monterey, CA, Brooks/Cole, 1975.

Huss J: Touch with Care or a Caring Touch. AJOT 31(1):11-18, 1977.

Ivey A: Microcounseling: Interviewing Skills Manual. Springfield, IL, C.C. Thomas, 1977.

Krumboltz J, Thorenson C: Counseling. New York, Holt, Rinehart and Winston, 1969.

Mayeroff M: On Caring. New York, Perennial Library, 1971.

Perls F: Gestalt Therapy Verbatum. Lafayette, CA, Real People Press, 1969.

Rogers C: Client Centered Counseling. Boston, Houghton Mifflin, 1951.

Truax C, Carkhuff R: Toward Effective Counseling and Psychotherapy. Chicago, Aldine, 1967.

2. In some groups (outside the occupational therapy setting), the laizzez-faire leadership style may be a virtual abdication of leadership. However, given the nature of occupational therapy activity groups and their purpose, the authors feel that the occupational therapist continues to serve as a "gatekeeper" and does not allow the "chips to fall where they may" — short of chaos.

References

American Occupational Therapy Association: The philosophical base of occupational therapy. AJOT 33(11):785, 1979.

American Occupational Therapy Task Force: Occupational therapy: Its definition and functions. AJOT 26(4):204-205, 1972.

Avila D, Combs A, Purkey W (Eds): The Helping Relationship Sourcebook. Boston, Allyn and Bacon, Inc., 1972.

Brammer L: The Helping Relationship: Process and Skills. Englewood Cliffs, NJ, Prentice-Hall, 1979.

Cartwright D, Zander A: Group Dynamics — Research and Theory Ed 3. New York, Harper & Row, Publishers, 1968.

Combs A: Some basic concepts in perceptual psychology. In Avila D, Combs A, Purkey W (Eds): The Helping Relationship Handbook. Boston, Allyn and Bacon, Inc., 1972.

Devereaux E: Occupational therapy's challenge: The caring relationship. AJOT 38(12):791-798, 1984.

Fairman C: Response to Smith and Tempone, Psychiatric occupational therapy within a learning context. AJOT 22(5):422, 1968.

Fidler G, Fidler J: Occupational Therapy — A Communication Process in Psychiatry. New York, Macmillan Co., 1963.

Fidler G: The task-oriented group as a context of treatment. AJOT 23(1):43-48, 1969.

Fidler G, Fidler J: Doing and becoming: Purposeful action and self-actualization. AJOT 32:305-310, 1978.

Fine S: Occupational Therapy: The Role of Rehabilitation and Purposeful Activity in Mental Health Practice. White Paper. Rockville, MD, American Occupational Therapy Association, Inc., 1983.

Hinojosa J, Sabari J, Rosenfeld M: Purposeful activities. AJOT 37(12):805-806, 1983.

Hopkins H: A historical perspective on occupational therapy. In Smith H, Hopkins H (Eds): Willard and Spackman's Occupational Therapy. Ed 6. Philadelphia, Lippincott, 1983.

Hopkins H, Smith H (Eds): Willard and Spackman's Occupational Therapy. Ed 6. Philadelphia: Lippincott, 1983.

James M, Jongeward D: Born to Win: Transactional Analysis with Gestalt Experiments. Reading, MA, Addison-Wesley Publishing Co., 1971.

King L: Toward a science of adaptive responses. AJOT 32(7):429-444, 1978.

Knowles M, Knowles H: Introduction to Group Dynamics. New York, Association Press, 1972.

Lewin K: Field Theory in Social Science. New York, Harper & Row, 1951.

Mosey A: Three Frames of Reference in Mental Health. Thorofare, NJ: Charles B. Slack Inc., 1970.

Mosey A: Activities Therapy. New York, Raven Press Publishers, 1973.

Mosey A: Occupational Therapy — Configuration of a Profession. New York, Raven Press, 1981.

Rogers C: The characteristics of a helping relationship. In Avila D, Combs A, Purkey W (Eds): The Helping Relationship Sourcebook. Boston, Allyn and Bacon, Inc., 1972.

Willard H, Spackman C (Eds): Occupational Therapy. Ed 3. Philadelphia, Lippincott, 1963.

Willard H, Spackman C (Eds): Occupational Therapy. Ed 4. Philadelphia, Lippincott, 1971.

Yalom I: The Theory and Practice of Group Psychotherapy. Ed 2. New York, Basic Books Inc., 1975.

Chapter 3

The Object Relations Frame of Reference

Some of the most commonly accepted as well as soundly criticized beliefs about the nature of personality, the function of activity, and the therapeutic relationship have their basis in the tenets of those theorists whose ideas lay the foundation for the object-relations framework. Key figures in the evolution of this framework include Freud, Jung, Alexander, Carl Rogers, Maslow, May, and Perls in psychology and Yerxa, Azima, Fidler and Fidler, and Mosey in occupational therapy. Since no theorist can be covered in detail in this text, the reader will perceive, rather, a selection and synthesis of related postulates that have spanned the entire twentieth century to the present. At its heart, the object relations framework is one that legitimizes personal, subjective experience and challenges the premise that any experience can be understood apart from the bias of its beholder.

Definition

The object relations frame of reference, an eclectic frame of reference, is the theoretical approach which views persons, media, and activities as objects invested with psychic energy. Interaction with these objects is necessary to satisfy personal needs and promote psychosocial growth and ultimately leads to self-actualization. The activities are explored through a communication process in occupational therapy evaluation and treatment designed to lead to an understanding of behavior and problems and to increase self-awareness and self-understanding.

Theoretical Development

The object relations frame of reference is an outgrowth of the early psychoanalytic and communication process approaches in occupational therapy which were developed and described by Azima (1959) and Fidler and Fidler (1963). Ann Mosey expanded upon these early approaches to include neo-Freudian and humanistic influences and in *Three Frames of Reference for Mental Health* describes the object relations frame of reference as having an "eclectic" theoretical base (p. 37). An *eclectic* approach is one in which there is the integration of several theories to formulate a new and disciplined approach. It provides a rationale for evaluation and treatment which is based upon identified theoretical concepts and clinical techniques. It is not a license of total freedom for the clinician to do as she pleases, nor is it a simple common sense approach. The object relations frame of reference as an eclectic approach represents the integration of principles from Freudian, neo-Freudian, existential-humanistic, social, and ego psychologies.

The Influence of Freud

Since the mental health field as a whole and the object relations theory in particular continue to owe so much of their practice to the ideas professed by Sigmund Freud, a brief summary of these principles is provided in order that we might comment on some key concepts that influenced traditional psychoanalytically oriented occupational therapy and that continue to bear on current object relations practice. For those students who feel that they need a further review, the *Primer of Freudian Psychology* (Hall, 1954) is recommended. We must, however, stress that Freud lived and wrote many years ago, and his ideas have been subject to change, as new information is gathered by contemporary theorists. Object relations theory is not a mere recitation of Freud's thinking.

Society and mental health treatment have come a long way since Freud first elaborated his beliefs in *Interpretation of Dreams* (1900). If his peers and eventually the citizenry were outraged then by his emphasis on the role of sexual feeling in unconscious thought and conscious behavior, they nonetheless were given a way to conceptualize human thought, feeling, and behavior that had not existed in quite this way before. Today we talk about our "feelings" as if they have a value and substance of their own; we describe thoughts as being "conscious" or "unconscious" or "subconscious" and expect others to understand what we mean by these terms. We may substitute our term "hang-up" for Freud's "complex," but we discuss our "hang-ups," "neuroses," and "paranoias" and those of our friends as if they have influence, purpose, and some basis in our personal history. While Freud might be accused of opening a Pandora's box of self-examination, we must emphasize that he and those who followed gave us the concepts, the vocabulary, and the license to talk about and understand ourselves in a way that we now take for granted. Further, within the field of mental health treatment, Freud expanded the realm of the medical profession from a strictly physiologic approach in which aberrant behavior had to be treated with medication or typically not at all, to include a psychological approach in which a patient's thoughts and feelings could be dealt with in and of themselves.

Libido. Freud saw man as a closed energy system, the energy he labeled *libido*. He saw this energy or libido as limited, as directed inward (to self) or outward (as to other person's or objects). (In everyday terms, we may hear someone say, "This project is important to me; I've put all my energy into it" or "I'm so worried about my children's problems, I have no energy left for anything else.") Man's libido was seen as instinctual in origin and pleasure-seeking. To extend an analogy suggested by Hall (1954), we might think of a newborn infant, exemplifying ourselves, as having 16 ounces of libido. (Please note: one can not actually see, touch, or "weigh" libido!) The newborn infant experiences hunger, thirst, and pain, and he will cry vigorously when he is uncomfortable. Our rather typical infant will have caring parents who act to meet his needs, and the infant literally gets the picture of the kind of people and nonhuman objects that make him cozy and content. Soon he is able to imaginatively long for mother, bottle, soft toys, and any other objects experienced as enjoyable. Unfortunately, his 16 ounces of libido can only be used for *reflexive* physical activity and for wishing or picturing . While libido is pleasure seeking, it is not, of itself, able to distinguish between a real object (baby bottle) and fantasy (thoughts about the bottle). Thoughts about a bottle will not stop hunger pangs, and our infant is confronted with the need to develop greater powers of differentiation and control. In order to describe how this occurs, Freud conceptualized as follows:

That portion of the mind or psyche that was unable to differentiate between reality and fantasy was said to reside in a portion of the self he called the *id*. *Id-energy* or *id-libido* knows what it wants but not how to get it. Out of necessity, some id energy leaves the id and develops into another intrapsychic area Freud termed the *ego*. Ego-libidinal energy also seeks to satisfy, or bring pleasure, but it has the advantage of being able to realistically assess the outside world. As Freud said, the ego functions help the individual perform a task by "becoming aware of stimuli, by storing up experiences about them (in memory), by avoiding excessively strong stimuli (through flight), and . . . by learning to bring about expedient changes in the external world to its own advantage (through activity)" (Freud in Stafford-Clark, 1966, p. 134). The reader should be aware that there are no actual boundaries in the brain or elsewhere between the id, ego, and superego, to be discussed. Rather these terms are a "shorthand way" of conceptualizing and identifying different processes within the personality (Hall, 1954, p. 35).

The ego is considered to be the "organizer" of the personality. It is that part of the person able to state and feel that "I am myself, I am real, I am not part of anyone else. It is the logician and the mathematician; it can focus attention on one part of experience (the foreground), while putting the rest into the background. The ego is aware of time and sequence and is given the job of postponing gratification. The ego can also use libido to plan actions capable of removing obstacles to satisfaction in a function Freud called aggression. When the ego collects data, prioritizes it, and puts a plan of action into effect to see whether the plan works, the ego is said to be doing *reality testing* (Hall, 1954, p. 29).

Thus, the ego uses its share of libido to decide which needs will be satisfied, when, and how. Our developing child, now two years old, has some sense of self as separate, calls that self by a name, knows what it wants, and, possessing a functioning ego, does not need to cry in the hope that a bottle will magically appear. With determined ego direction, he can use a one-fourth ounce of libido to crawl up to mother with an empty bottle, pull the family cat out of mother's lap (aggression), and ask for his bottle to be filled (using a primitive form of sign language or insistent whines so typical of the young child). Since libido is limited and our child has only 16 ounces to invest, should he direct too much of his efforts daily to his bottle, there might be too little left to meet new challenges.

Applying her understanding of id and ego influence, the occupational therapist working within this frame of reference was very concerned regarding what we might term flexibility and broadness when looking at a patient's object relationships. Did the patient have energy invested in a wide enough variety of objects so that a full range of needs was being met? When an object (thing, event, person) was no longer need-satisfying, could this patient pull back energy from it and reinvest the energy in a productive, socially acceptable way? When the patient was involved in tasks, was the ego in control or was the id need for immediate gratification leading to impulsive, chaotic behavior? The occupational therapist was concerned about her patient's ego function, for it was that part of the psyche that allowed him to identify his needs, weigh alternatives, circumvent or remove obstacles, and act on decisions in his daily life.

If man were not a social being, the id and the ego might be effective in carrying our child into adulthood. However, libidinal energy had to be extended to one other intrapsychic area, the area that Freud called the *superego*. Because our child depends on his very survival for the love and approval of his parents initially, and ultimately other social contemporaries, some energy is used in assessing which objects and courses of action will bring parental approval and which actions his parents will think are "bad." He develops what is commonly called a "conscience," and with it an inner voice that influences his actions by telling him that he needs to feel "guilty" if he has displeased others, and proud if he has done what is "right."

Now the id, ego, and superego must share that "16 ounces" of original libido. All three portions of the psyche want pleasure for the person and must find a way to work together in relative balance and harmony in order that each part can do its necessary work. For what we might call "efficiency" of operation, some knowledge that our infant has gained — knowledge that might be interesting but of no practical value — may be pushed out of current awareness or consciousness into the area Freud termed the *unconscious*. Likewise, knowledge or thoughts that our child's evolving superego deems as "shameful" may be pushed from consciousness into the unconscious, or may never have been allowed into conscious awareness at all. Much material that is held in the area of the unconscious is composed of thoughts that we would be ashamed of were we conscious of them. Though they are in an area of nonawareness, they continue to exert a powerful influence over behavior. Freud believed that only a small part of thought or mind lies in the realm of the conscious. Identifying an in-between area of awareness, Freud suggested that some thoughts reside in the *preconscious* where they are not in current awareness but are able to be recalled (Freud, 1950, p. 465; see note 1).

Development of the Personality. Complementary to his theories about id-ego-superego and conscious-unconscious, Freud conceptualized that, while a person is pleasure seeking in essence, the objects and events that would be experienced as especially pleasurable would change as the individual matured. Freud began with the newborn and delineated stages of psychosexual and psychosocial development that would carry him into adulthood. He attributed special importance to the first three developmental stages, which span the first five years of life, citing prototype object choices and key patterns of psychosexual interaction which he believed influenced the individual's interactions for the rest of his life. It is in large part this belief that leads Freudian therapists to focus as extensively as they do on a patient's very early history.

In *Three Essays on Sexuality* (1901-1905) and in subsequent works, Freud noted that as the child develops, specific areas or zones of the body become especially sensitive to touch or stimulation, and that touch to that zone is very pleasurable. Freud termed all bodily pleasure as sexual pleasure and did not limit his use of the term sexuality to genital sexuality as we tend to do today. The first area to be significantly pleasure-related is the mouth and surrounding area, or the *oral zone*; this is followed by the *anal* zone and then the *genital or phallic* zone. Thus, activities which stimulate these various zones, which come to be associated with these zones and/or the way they function, will be experienced as need-satisfying. As the person matures and new body zones take on special importance, the old pleasure zones are still pleasure related but are seen as having less relative importance.

Stage Theory. As each of the body zones are experienced as a focus of pleasure and sensitivity, there exist significant persons and social interactions that become associated with the way in which pleasure is achieved. For the infant newly born to about the age of two, the oral zone is the focus of pleasure and it is said that he is in the oral stage. For him, activities that stimulate the mouth, such as those involved in sucking at mother's breast or biting, are favored. Mother is the most important person-object, and the abilities to receive nurturance and to learn to trust that needs will be satisfied are important social developmental tasks. For the child at about age one to three years, now experiencing the anal zone as especially sensitive, activities associated with excreting, particularly in terms of mastering control over excrement, will be satisfying. At this anal stage, mother and father are important as nurturers, but the childs relationship with them is changing. He has learned to say "No!" and seeks to gain a sense of autonomy and control over his environment, while not alienating parents. When the child is three to five years of age, he is in the third stage of development, the early genital or phallic stage.

Freud viewed the early genital stage as the key period for appropriate gender identification (Eichenbach and Orbach, 1983). He considered the male or female child as essentially bisexual (demonstrating traits of both sexes) until this stage, when young children become physiologically and cognitively more aware of their own genitals. Freud saw the boy child as becoming desirous of mother, and therefore in conflict with father — now a "rival" for mother's affection. The boy resolves this potentially disastrous rivalry by identifying with (seeing himself like) father, repressing his wish for mother, thus moving further away from mother in increased independence, and laying the foundations for his own eventual heterosexual relationship with a woman of his own.

The girl-child, Freud postulated, sees herself as like mother, and disappointed in the discovery that she lacks the male genital apparatus. Thus, she moves further from mother, and substitutes the wish for a penis with a wish to bear children, at first for father and then for a man of her own. It should be noted that the early genital phase was especially important for Freud in three areas: (1) the movement away from mother, called *separation-individuation*; (2) the child's translation of his longing for the parent of the opposite gender into an eventual wish for a heterosexual adult partner; and (3) the identification of the child with the same-gender parent and the suitable incorporation of "masculine" or "feminine" behavior (see note 2).

It is also during the early genital phase that the child continues to incorporate parental ideas about "good" and "bad" and firms up his evolving superego. Parents continue to be a primary object choice, but this is also the period in which a superparent or "hero" is sought.

From about ages five to 12 the child is in the *latency stage*; there are no new physical zones that take on significance, and the energy associated with seeking physical pleasure is rechanneled into learning new skills and forming peer friendships.

During adolescence, the last or late genital stage, the genital area is again experienced as especially pleasure-related, and there is movement toward adult heterosexuality. The heterosexual love object takes on special significance. It should be noted that the age boundaries given for each developmental stage are not really boundaries but flexible conceptual divisions which allow for the overlapping of stage-related behaviors. However, frequently the individual will get "stuck" or *fixated* at a certain level of psychosexual development. His behavior, object choices, and symbol production will reflect this fixation. In this case, an excess of libido will be directed toward trying to meet needs at a specific level, and the individual will not successfully move on to the next stage. The result will be an immature or restricted manner of dealing with self, others, and things. For example, an adult fixated at the oral stage will select objects and activities (perhaps symbolic) that reflect an over-reliance on oral pleasure, e.g., eating. In relationships he may seek to be mothered rather than engaging in a mature adult-adult relationship. Or the person might be overly "anal" in his object relationships. He might deal with objects or media in an overly messy or in an overly controlled manner. He might be unable to give and take comfortably in a love relationship, seeing the relationship, rather, as a continual struggle for control. A failure to be clear about one's sexual identity and sexual roles might be a reflection of an inability to deal effectively with the tasks of the early genital stage.

Being fixated at any given psychosexual stage of development tends to limit the range of need satisfying objects and ways of dealing with the environment. Being cognizant of norms of psychosexual development, the occupational therapist could look at a patient's object choices, ways of handling media, and manner of relating and begin to determine whether too much energy was being "spent" to accomodate immature psychosexual development. Table

Table 3-1

CONTRASTING RATIONAL EMOTIVE THERAPY (RET) and COGNITIVE THERAPY (CT) NORMAL PSYCHOSEXUAL DEVELOPMENT

Age	Zone of Special Sensitivity	Pleasurable Activities	Object Choice	Therapy Implications
Birth - 2	Oral Stage (a) early oral (b) late oral	(a) sucking, encorporating, swallowing; (b) biting, destroying	Self; oral object Maternal Figure	Characteristics of adult fixated at this stage: May be clingy; overdepenendent or unrealistically independent; enjoys talking, finds comfort in food, smoking, etc.; unable to form close relationships.
1-3	Anal Stage (a) early anal (b) late anal	(a) Excreting, touching excrement, being messy (b) Controlling, retaining, holding on to excrement; being very neat	Parent Figure; Anal object	Early: Might be overly messy; enjoys paints, clay etc. Late: Finds being messy repugnant; enjoys being the organizer, the collector. Generates conflicts over who is in charge.
3-5	Early Genital Stage (phallic)	Touching or exploring genitals; learning about own and genitals of opposite sex	Parent; superparent (hero)	May have difficulty accepting appropriate roles, manner of dressing, etc., or may have exaggerated sex role behavior. May be most comfortable with same sex relations or fear them due to homosexual concerns. May appear to be without conscience or remorse for antisocial behavior.
5-12	Latency (no new zone)	Sublimation of energy into learning new skills	Companion of same sex	
12-18	Late Genital Stage (adolescence)	Touching, investigating, fantasizing about own genitals and genitals of opposite sex	Self; Emergence of love for companion of opposite sex	Struggles with issues of independence versus dependence. May appear especially concerned regarding own physical appearance; may be preoccupied with matters of genital sexuality. May experiment with homosexual and heterosexual activity.

3-1 outlines briefly Freud's stages of psychosexual development and suggests some implication for working with adults in occupational therapy.

Exploring the Unconscious. Believing that the unconscious portion of the psyche exerted a powerful influence over behavior, Freud attempted to determine thoughts that were held in the unconscious. One way he did this was to look in depth at the individual's symbol production via free word association, his "slips of the tongue," and exploring with him his dreams. In reading *The Interpretation of Dreams*, one can discover that Freud interpreted symbols on a case by case basis, and a great many dream symbols were not interpreted sexually. However, when Freud did summarize his beliefs regarding symbols (see especially pages 242-258, *The Interpretation of Dreams,* 1950), there was a strong focus on the sexual aspect of dream symbols. For example, he suggests,"elongated objects, sticks, tree-trunks, umbrellas . . . all sharp and elongated weapons, knives, daggers, pikes represent the male member. . . . Small boxes, chests, cupboards, and ovens correspond to the female organ; also cavities, ships, and all kinds of vessels. . ."(p. 242, Freud-Brill, 1950). "Steep inclines, ladders, and stairs and going up or down them, are symbolic representations of the sexual act" (p. 243, Freud-Brill, 1950).

A further listing will not be given here; rather, the interested reader is encouraged to read Freud's work. What seems too often to occur upon the "listing" of Freudian symbols is a communication of the notion that a therapist need only compare her patient's symbol production to such a list and come to some valid conclusions. A symbol cannot be taken from the personal context in that manner, but must be related in a meaningful way to the individual's personal experiencing.

Anxiety. Freud stated that the healthiest person would be that individual who was aware of and willing to invest in a broad number of need-satisfying objects in a variety of socially acceptable ways. He felt that frustration and anxiety resulted when these needs could not be met or when the individual feared that he would commit an act that would be harmful or guilt-inducing. This would be especially likely to occur when ego strength was diminished and/or when demands on the ego were increased. The ego might try to deal with anxiety by trying to "deny, falsify or distort reality" (Hall, 1954 p.85) via special constellations Freud termed *defense mechanisms;* these are summarized in Appendix E on defense mechanisms. While we all employ some defenses, over-reliance on them, Freud said, limits our perceptions of realistic object choices. Given the influence of psychosexual development, a person was believed to develop characteristic ways of trying to meet personal needs, overcome obstacles, and deal with anxiety. Together these are reflected as *personality.*

The Therapy Process. While Freud felt that some thoughts about the self and the environment could be kept *repressed* (out of current awareness), use of any defense mechanism took libidinal energy. The process of therapy would seek to free up libidinal energy, allowing it to be voluntarily invested in a variety of need-satisfying object relationships. The process by which Freud himself attempted to do this he called *psychoanalysis.* He saw his role as one in which he could be neutral and allow the patient to play out on the "therapist screen" the unresolved conflicts and unconscious dramas that needed to be remediated. The major activity of psychoanalysis was interpretation, especially interpretation of the patient's behavior and affect during his sessions with the analyst, plus interpretation of dreams recounted by the patient. This interpretation was designed to increase insight and understanding. While the past was inevitably recounted in the psychoanalytic process it was the patient's memory of the past ["the world of reconstructed subjective experiences" (Michels, 1983 p.66)] that was considered important — the accuracy of such memory was not a primary concern. It is interesting to note that Freud viewed personality as tending to stabilize as one reaches maturity (in the early twenties) and as more and more libido is "tied up." Thus, the older adult (age 50 or older) was not seen as a good candidate for change or for psychoanalytic treatment (Sadler, 1978, p.5).

Traditional psychoanalysis was typically carried out by medical doctors who then gained specialized training in psychiatry and/or psychoanalysis. The traditional or Freudian occupational therapist, under the close direction and supervision of the physician, used activities as a means to assess personality structure, learn more about unconscious content, provide opportunity for the ego to learn more about the self, and provide opportunity for the ego to improve in its problem solving ability. Much emphasis was placed on understanding the patient's history, especially those significant events that were being held by the unconscious and tying up an undo amount of libido.

The occupational therapist used activities in which the patient could *project* aspects of his unconscious into the visible therapeutic milieu. Patients were encouraged to use such unstructured media as paints, clay, and collage, since these tended to facilitate symbol production — especially personal, unconscious symbols, which could be then seen and integrated into consciousness. Activities were also selected to help determine the ability of the ego to organize and problem solve and, eventually, to provide an opportunity for the ego to incorporate new, more successful means of problem solving. Seeing the therapist-patient relationship as implicitly reminiscent of the parent-child relationship, the occupational therapist followed the physician's cue in allowing the patient to *transfer*, or put onto the therapist his feelings (often unconscious) about his own parents. The therapist then helped the patient to understand and potentially re-experience aspects of this parent-child relationship. The occupational therapist believed that man was influenced by the past, but that he had a will and the ability to choose.

The Influence of Jung

Since the early literature pertaining to practice in occupational therapy makes so little mention of Carl Jung, it is difficult to assess how this man, who was a contemporary of Freud's and a ground-breaker in the field of psychology, influenced beginning object relations practice. It is not within the scope of this text to discuss Jungs's constructs in depth, and the reader is referred again to the bibliography. However, several concepts in current practice owe their inception to Jung, and it is on these that we will comment.

Polarities in the Self. Jung was himself well versed in and influenced by Eastern philosophy. The image of man as struggling to balance many opposing forces, as is conceptualized in the eastern image of the yin-yang, is key in Jungian thinking. Agreeing with Freud that much memory and thought is unconscious, Jung felt that the predominant tension in the unconscious was created by the pull of opposite forces that exist in the self. Some opposing forces identified by him included: the tendency of the self to be *introverted* (focused on the self) versus *extroverted* (focused on others); the tendency of the individual to gain information through tangible "seeing" versus the tendency to favor gaining information through intuition; a striving in the self for material comfort versus a striving for spirituality; and the existence in a man of *latent* or unexpressed feminine qualities and in a female, latent masculine qualities (see note 3).

Jung felt that all these polarities in the psyche needed to be developed and given expression in a person's life. This process he called *individuation*. Further, he conceived of a governing structure that would strive to bring all these polarities into balance and work toward the goal of wholeness. This force he called the *transcendent function* and the process, the ultimate goal of personhood, he called *transcendence*. It is interesting to credit Jung at this time for introducing concepts that have found a great deal of contemporary acceptance among a generation that is concerned about achieving a personal "balance" and inner harmony, and that is now turning to the field of psychology not just for advice about illness but also for assistance with personal growth.

Changes in the Second Half of Life. Whereas Freud's concept of psychosocial development tends to stop with the advent of a person's adulthood and sexual maturity, Jung spoke at length regarding the changes that occurred in self-perception, values, and social roles throughout the life process, to death. In conjunction with his belief that both men and women carry within themselves latent qualities of the opposite sex, Jung felt that in middle age, after relative success in meeting societal role expectations, each sex could allow himself or herself to give expression to some of these qualities. For example, a rather passive 40 year old mother might become more assertive in her relationships, and might seek a significant role in the business community. In contrast, the fortyish man, up till now a bit ruthless in his business pursuits, might start to feel that perhaps business is not so important and seek to spend more time in nurturing his children. Both sexes at middle age would, said Jung, tend to turn from materialistic concerns to spiritual concerns. As indicated by Hall and Nordby, Jung is one of the few psychologists until recently who has tried to understand the psychology of the middle years (Hall and Nordby, 1973, p. 93). In an evocative passage Jung states, "A human being would certainly not grow to be seventy or eighty years old if this longevity had no meaning for the species. The afternoon of human life must also have significance of its own and cannot be merely a pitiful appendage to life's morning" (Jung, 1971, p. 17).

Jung felt that "middle age" extended well into the fifties, sixties, and even seventies — old age to him really implying senility or a return to the unconscious. It was predicted by him that it would be the older person who would have achieved real wisdom and wholeness. Implicit is the premise that Jung valued the roles and accomplishments of the older person, in contrast to Freud's inference that older age brings rigidity and little growth. With so much of our population now in middle or older years, it is not surprising that a very widely read, lay psychology book popular in the late 1970's, *Passages,* by Gail Sheehy, was a restatement and popularization of Jungian philosophy. The occupational therapist working in the traditional or in today's object relations setting, if cognizant of Jungian theory, has had the opportunity to help patients understand their values, roles, and unconscious content in a much broader light than the strictly Freudian therapist. The occupational therapy literature documents the use of values clarification and women's awareness groups as meaningful activities used in contemporary occupational therapy.

The Collective Unconscious. In a final comment about Jung, we will raise a controversial aspect of Jungian thought. Jung conceived of the psyche as being conscious and unconscious in content, as did Freud. However, he went further in suggesting that the unconscious held not only thoughts and reflections of personal experience, but images and ideas and a predisposition to seek certain experiences in a way that our ancestors had. These universal images and predispositions, thought to be racially inherited, were called *collective* and said to be stored in the collective unconscious. Pointing to similar themes and content in mythology, religion and cross-cultural art, and finding the same themes in the symbolic expression of his patients, he looked at symbols in a much broader way than Freud. *Man and His Symbols* (we suggest the hardcover edition) is an excellent introduction for understanding symbols. The occupational therapist who is well acquainted with cross-cultural themes in art, mythology, and religion has the opportunity to help a patient to understand his own unconscious process in terms of broad themes, and in so doing may provide support in pointing out the patient's common threads with all mankind.

Input from Existential Humanism

With its roots in the writing of such articulate philosophers as Sartre, Camus, Tillich, Kafka, and Heidegger and in the neo-Freudian therapies of Horney, Sullivan, Klein, Adler, Rank, Fromm, and Erikson, existential humanism has evolved over the past 40 years to exert a significant influence in philosophy, psychology, and education. Generally included as part of the existential humanistic movement are those theories or therapies referred to as Gestalt or field theory, organismic theory, phenomenology, Rogers' "client centered" therapy, Frankl's logotherapy, as well as a broad range of psychologies referred to as "existential" or "humanistic." We will focus here on the elements common to existential humanism as they have contributed to the object relations framework for occupational therapy.

While it was primarily in the 1960's and early 1970's that the existential humanistic approach to psychology was elaborated in the literature [see especially Rogers (1951, 1961), May (1950, 1953, 1969), Maslow (1968, 1971), Jourard (1971), Perls (1969), and Moustakas (1956, 1961)], with the perspective of the 1980's, one can discern the continued influence of existential humanism across a broad range of theoretical frameworks and across many disciplines.

Existential humanism has brought considerable thought to bear on the issues of what is the essence of the human condition — and how one individual might best help another. Believing, as Freud, that the therapist must understand and appreciate the subjective experiencing of the individual, the existential humanistic professes a much different concept of what constitutes an optimum therapeutic relationship. It has been in this unique conceptualization of the therapeutic relationship that existential humanism has been especially evident in the field of occupational therapy. Existential humanism conceived of a very different "human nature" from that conceived by Freud, a view also quite consistent with the generally positive posture taken by occupational therapists. Existential humanism has also been a part of the movement across our society encouraging the individual to be "true to himself" and to act with integrity rather than with blind conformity. One result, evident in the practice of many contemporary occupational therapists, has been the re-evaluation of age and sex stereotypes, especially as regards role behavior and object choice.

The Nature of the Therapist-Patient Relationship. Most originally schooled in Freudian ideology, existential humanists challenged Freud's premise that a therapist needs to be passive and impersonal, and that she needs to facilitate a re-enactment of the parent-child relationship or the doctor-patient relationship. As Rogers stated, "I was asking the question, 'How can I treat, or cure, or change this person?' Now I would phrase the question in this way:'How can I provide a relationship that this person may use for his own personal growth?'" (Rogers, 1961, p. 32). The humanists suggested that the therapist and individual were each responsible for their own behavior and the ultimate outcome of therapy.

Existential humanists stressed that the individual has the ability for self-awareness and, with it, freedom to choose his own actions and determine his own destiny (Corey, 1982, p. 34). With this freedom of choice comes the responsibility for one's own behavior, a responsibility that includes a need to acknowledge one's effect on and relatedness to others. The aim of existential humanistically oriented therapy is to assist the individual to become more aware of his own needs, feelings, options, and goals — and to realistically understand the needs and feelings of others and facilitate his acceptance of personal responsibility for his own life.

Existential humanists believed that to assist the individual in meeting his own goals, the therapist needed to understand the subjective-experiencing or *phenomenal world* of the individual. They suggested that the individual was most able to be honest with the therapist and honest with himself in the context of a relationship in which the therapist herself was *authentic* (expressing honestly her own attitudes and feelings) and openly concerned for the individual, and in which the individual did not fear that the therapist would reject him upon "really knowing" him (Rogers, 1951, 1961). Rogers coined the term *unconditional positive regard* to describe the therapist stance (Rogers, 1951, 1961). Unconditional positive regard did not mean that the therapist necessarily agreed with or "liked" everything the individual did, but that she continued to value the individual and respected his right to feel different from her.

Existential humanists focused on the "wholeness" of the individual, in contrast to what they perceived as a psychoanalytic tendency to compartmentalize the person. In addition to seeing the individual as functioning as a holistic unit, they conceived of the individual as needing always to perceive "wholeness" (or to discern meaning from fragments, ambiguity, or "nonmeaning"). This operates from the most elemental perceptual level to the most complex cognitive or emotional level (see note 4).

Existential humanists also expressed the belief that in each person certain issues, called by Perls "unfinished business" (often emotional in nature), will be most pressing and need to be dealt with accordingly. Failure to do so, or failure in "closure" on old business, prevents the individual from attending fully to new experiences (Perls, 1969). Thus, the therapist attempts to ascertain with the individual what he experiences as priorities in therapy. Existential humanists placed emphasis on the "here and now" of an individual's life rather than on his past, but they did not discount the past. Rogers, for example, saw in early childhood experiences the basis for many distortions in the individual's self-awareness. The youngster, seeking to please his parents and gain their approval, was believed to behave according to their wishes, and by mimicking demonstrated that the "feelings" they communicated were valid. If this continued into maturity, the individual lost touch with his own perceptions and values. His parent's hopes for his career often became his hopes; their life style was reflected unthinkingly in his. Frequently he spent his adult life seeking an external approval that was never forthcoming or that never seemed quite sufficient. Moving away from the parent-child model, the therapist sought to help the individual realize that the locus of approval was in himself. The therapist did not see the individual as there to make her feel important, to follow her advice, or to mold himself after her expectations. One important function of the therapist was for her to relate to the individual perspectives and options that she perceived in the "here and now" and that the individual had blocked from his own awareness. This did not mean that the individual necessarily chose these options, but that with more information about tools, paths, and activities, his range of potential opportunities became greater.

Existential Anxiety. Anxiety was viewed by existential humanists as a key concern in therapy and was conceived as deriving from one or more of four essential conditions: (1) the individual recognized the need for a significant change in his life or was in the midst of change; (2) the individual recognized his own failure to live authentically, that is, consistently and in accordance with his own beliefs and values; (3) the individual could find no real meaning or purpose in his life; (4) the individual recognized that he had not developed his own unique skills and had failed to be "all he can be" (Corey, 1982). The therapist realized that the individual might be out of touch or unaware of his own values and skills, owing to his prior concern for acting as he believed others wanted him to. The occupational therapist supported his attempts to risk change, to try new roles, and to experience himself in new ways. She understood that such change may feel very "scary" to the patient.

Self-actualization. While Freud conceptualized a tension reduction model of behavior, existential humanists conceived of a fulfillment model — perceiving an innate striving in each individual to be all he can be. They termed the life-long striving towards this ultimate goal *self-actualization*. Self-actualization can include the kind of biologically rooted drives described by Freud, but goes much further. As described by Rogers, self-actualization is "the urge which is evident in all organic and human life — to expand, extend, become autonomous, develop, mature — the tendency to express and activate all the capacities of the organism" (Rogers, 1961, p. 35). One is reminded of Jung's conceptualization of transcendence — a state perhaps achieved by only a few — in which all aspects of the individual find expression during the course of his life.

If there appears to be a loftiness or esoteric quality to this goal of self-actualization, there is a humbleness and integrity inherent in existential humanism that should not go unnoticed, for basic to this ideology are the beliefs that all individuals have wisdom and worth and that one man's path to knowledge and purpose is no more or less valuable than another's, provided each is using his abilities as best he can and living according to his own beliefs. Thus, a simple task or basic skill has as much essential worth as intellectual prowess.

Parallels Between Existential Humanism and Occupational Therapy. The reader will discern many themes in existential humanism that are parallel to basic tenets of occupational therapy. The belief that individuals need to feel valuable and purposeful in their lives; the belief that the therapist must understand an individual's goal for therapy in terms of his priorities and in accordance with his perceptions; the belief that the individual has inner motivation to explore and to master — these tenets have been recounted in occupational therapy literature from the inception of the profession (Meyers) through to the present day (Yerxa, 1967, 1978; Gilfoyle, 1980; Baum, 1980). However, it may be useful to remind ourselves of some of these tenets. It was not so many years ago that occupational therapists believed that their professional obligation to the patient was to decide, without collaboration, what was best for him, and they sought to instill confidence through behavior designed to accentuate their difference from the patient rather than their relatedness to him.

The therapist comfortable with existential humanistic ideology within the object relations framework seeks to understand her patient's subjective experience and allows herself to share with him her own perceptions and feelings. She trusts that even in anxiety or confusion, the individual has much wisdom and information about what is "good" for himself. She strives to encourage his responsiveness to inner-directed motives rather than his overconcern for the approval of others. She realizes that personal growth occurs in the context of relatedness to others, and she seeks to help the individual gain a realistic understanding of how his behavior is received by others. Activities that have their origin in existential humanistic ideology include values clarification activities, body awareness experiences, gestalt art experiences (see Rhyne, 1973), and "new" less competitive games (see Fluegelman, 1976). However, the therapist realizes that all activities have the potential to provide meaning and facilitate growth.

Freudian Psychotherapy and Ideology Today

Mental health treatment and object relations practice continue to be affected by Freudian ideology albeit with modification. Today's psychosocial occupational therapist will likely be directly or indirectly influenced by this ideology in her practice, especially when her practice interfaces with a traditional medical or medical-model setting.

Current trends in psychotherapy and current trends in psychoanalysis (Freud's "method") are not duplicated in object relations occupational therapy, but there are clearly parallels that can be discerned. In the broader perspective, current trends in psychotherapy and psychoanalysis parallel many of the concerns and priorities of contemporary society as a whole. One cannot be certain where the mental health treatment community has led, and where it has followed or reacted in the response to these concerns.

The following brief overview is designed to assist the reader in recognizing significant changes in Freudian-based mental health treatment, as they influence object relations practice in occupational therapy. The reader acquainted with current mental health treatment will recognize many of these influences, and she may be practicing within treatment systems that have incorporated these changes. The student looking towards her anticipated career may find in some of the following trends an indication of potential directions her own practice might take.

For the sake of simplification, the therapist operating within an object relations framework will be referred to here as the Freudian therapist. When the discussion is specific for the occupational therapist, this will be noted.

Altered View of the Role of Past History

While Freud stood firmly by his belief that events in the past (through their retention in conscious and unconscious memory) caused events in the present, and that therapy should attempt to understand these causes, current Freudian thinking operates under a newer model. Today childhood experiences are not conceived as necessarily causing events to occur in adult life, and therapy is believed to be most productive when it focuses on the here-and-now interaction between the therapist and the patient (Michels, 1983, p. 69; see note 5).

New Conceptualization of the Development of Gender Identity: Altered View of Femininity

Freud's perspective on women has been especially criticized as patriarchal, biased, and totally inadequate (Lerner, 1983; Bernstein, 1983; Eichenbaum and Orbach, 1983; Blum, 1976; Person, 1983; Notman and Nadelson, 1982; Money and Ehrhardt, 1972). It was a view based on the belief that psychology was rooted in biology; that women wished (unconsciously) to be men; that appropriate female behavior was dependent, passive, and masochistic; and that the proper feminine role was that associated with nurturing and childbearing. It was an interpretation (or perhaps an absence of one) that was based on the belief that female or male gender was not established until about age four, with the advent of the early genital phase. Undoubtedly it represents Freud's own observations of the women of his times and represents his incorporation of the cultural bias and values of his day.

Today's Freudian therapist is knowledgeable about the information gained in the area of child development and the importance of cultural shaping in gender identity. *Gender identity* is "the knowledge and awareness, conscious or unconscious, that one belongs to one sex and not the other" (Stoller, R., 1968, as cited in Notman and Nadelson, 1982, p. 5). The child is now understood to be establishing gender identity upon his very birth (and quite possibly before his birth). Countless studies and simple observation have shown that males and females begin to diverge in interests, mannerisms, and conduct by one to one and one-half years (Person, 1983; Notman and Nadelson, 1982; Stoller, 1968; Money and Ehrhardt, 1972). The understanding of gender identity is one of many areas in which today's Freudian therapist views Freud's original premises as too rooted in biology, and as placing too much emphasis on the phallic period. Differences in gender role are now attributed to many antecedents, including biological differences, social learning, "scripting," and cultural myths (Person, 1983, p.43).

The 1970's and especially the "women's movement" challenged the Freudian bias that women needed to be passive and dependent to be "feminine" (and psychologically healthy). Cultural changes, the emerging role of women in positions of power and authority, and the increasingly diversified models for child-rearing and family role-taking have all affected the societal norms regarding appropriate female and male conduct. Today's Freudian therapist, looking beyond anatomy, has a much broader view of masculinity and feminity. This has special implication for the occupational therapist working to facilitate meaningful object involvement for her patients — both male and female. While she has incorporated a liberalized perspective about appropriate gender activity, she may encounter in her practice individuals who still grapple with sex stereotypes, as regards themselves and those they encounter. The occupational therapist need be aware that both in terms of the activities and media she makes available and in terms of her own function as a therapist (possibly a female in a position of authority), she may precipitate her patient's conflictive feelings concerning gender role.

Challenging the Supremacy of Biological Determination

The change in views regarding appropriate male and female behavior reflects a contemporary ability to see behavior as determined by more than "anatomy." Freud is described as never having been able to adequately interface between cultural injunction and individual psychology (Person, 1983).

Today object relations theory attempts to understand the significance of all aspects of the external world (environment and culture) as experienced by the individual and giving unique meaning to his existence. Even sexual objects (i.e., those related to genital sexuality) are considered in light of their cultural-societal association and not merely as appendages to an instinctive biological drive.

Such a broadened understanding of the individual, his object choices, and his means of relating to objects through activity is necessary, in the estimation of the authors and consistent with their conceptualization of a viable object relations framework for practice in occupational therapy.

Prephallic Experiencing

For a long time, the Freudian therapist thought the therapist-patient relationship was, at an affective level, a re-experiencing of the child-parent relationship of the early genital period; in other words, the therapist was the longed-for Oedipal parent (Eichenbaum and Orbach, 1983,

p. 71). Today the Freudian psychotherapist is aware of the special relationship of infant to mother, which is critical in terms of mother's physical and emotional nurturance. As the ego develops, the child is increasingly able to go off by himself, thus beginning the process of *separation-individuation*. Successful separation-individuation is dependent on the ability of the child to experience the mother as consistent and nurturing, to retain her in memory, and to trust that she will be there when he returns.

At the risk of overgeneralizing, the need for successful "separation-individuation" appears to be a major concern in the object relations practice of the 1980's, and its implications and meaning need to be thoughtfully considered by the occupational therapist working in a psychosocial setting.

With much more emphasis being given to early (prephallic) development, it is not surprising that current Freudian psychotherapists also perceive the development of the superego as beginning much earlier than as conceived by Freud. This would be more consistent with the work of such developmentalists as Piaget and Kohlberg. (See Brickman, 1983 for a more in-depth discussion of this shift.)

Geriatric Psychiatry

With the increased longevity of the average American, the last decade has seen major changes in public priorities regarding the elderly. Where Freud felt that change was not likely to occur in the older individual, Freudian psychotherapists have become increasingly involved (within their professional organization and as reflected in their practice) in better understanding the special problems of the elderly and making treatment available to them. (Busse, 1983).

In an associated shift in priorities, individuals with cognitive impairment (e.g., the organically impaired, those with senile and presenile dementias, the traumatically assaulted) have been "rediscovered by American psychiatry in the last decade" (Sloane, 1983, p. 106). The renewed interest by Freudian psychotherapists in the function and chemistry of the brain is reflected in the extensive attention paid this topic in the last volume of *Psychiatry Update* (Vol. IV, 1985). It remains to be seen whether the contemporary Freudian psychotherapist can retain his essential allegiance to Freudian constructs while accomodating to the special problems posed by neuropsychological dysfunction, or whether neuropsychiatry will emerge as a unique specialty, divested from the traditional constructs of conscious-unconscious, id-ego-superego, defense mechanisms, and the like.

Shortened Length of Treatment

The final trend emerging in Freudian literature and practice is the acknowledgment of a need for shortened psychotherapeutic treatment. (This trend does not extend to the traditional process of psychoanalysis, but certainly helps dictate whether psychoanalysis is a viable alternative for given individuals.)

Shortened treatment duration is in some cases a reflection of changing therapeutic directives. There are now, for example, more treatment programs directed toward crisis intervention and prevention. Shortened treatment must be viewed also as a response to the increasingly felt need to contain medical costs.

While the occupational therapist in the past has often had the luxury of an extended period in which to proceed with her assessment and treatment, even in the so-called traditional, medically oriented setting, this is changing. The therapist considering her career options might consider her potential involvement in such short-term oriented treatment settings, including those involved with spouse and child abuse, substance abuse, and stress management.

Current Practice in Occupational Therapy

The Person and Behavior

In current object relations practice there come together constructs that at times seem quite antithetical, in origin at least. The degree to which a therapist leans more toward contemporary Freudian ideology, Jung, or the existential humanists in her philosophy will help give her practice a unique flavor. The following can serve as only a generalized statement regarding the object relations view of man.

A person is a dynamic energy system, composed of parts known to himself (conscious) and parts of which he is unaware. He is composed of an id, ego, and superego, each with its own role in maintaining selfhood and continuous experiencing, but each a conceptualization of parts of the personality not to be confused with selfhood itself. The individual knows himself better than anyone else can. Early experiences tend to determine object choices and ways of relating to human and nonhuman objects, but objects have no meaning in and of themselves. Individuals give meaning to them via their unique perceptions and experiences. Understanding his own behavior and being given the opportunity to do so, a person may make deliberate choices to change the manner in which he relates to objects. A person needs to feel safe in his environment; he needs to love and feel loved and accepted. He needs to be himself and seeks to recognize his assets, limits, and potential. Thus, he strives toward self-actualization. While he may fear change or resist seeing himself in a new way, there exists in each person an innate striving to grow and mature and be all he can be. When he is mature, he accepts responsibility for his own actions; he is congruent, changes his perceptions according to real data, values himself, and values others (Rogers, 1961, p. 36).

Only the person can develop his own opportunities; no one can do it for him. Self-actualization is a process more than an outcome. A person moves toward self-actualization when he uses his thoughts, feelings, senses, and perceptions to increase self-awareness (that is subjective), to develop insight, and to open his vision in order that he might perceive and act on more opportunities while respecting his own limitations and the rights and boundaries of others.

The Role of the Occupational Therapist

The occupational therapist serves as a knowledgeable, empathetic guide who develops a collaborative relationship with the patient and maintains the framework of treatment. The therapist is not an authority who passively participates in evaluation and treatment as was done in the classic psychoanalytic approach. Neither does she foster a parent-child relationship. The occupational therapist takes a more neo-Freudian, humanistic approach in which she provides "unconditional positive regard" (Rogers, 1951) and a framework of concern and interaction.

In this collaborative relationship, the occupational therapist acknowledges that the patient has a will and responsibility for making decisions and choices. Patient and therapist mutually assume responsibility for evaluation, identification of treatment goals, and development of a treatment plan. They cooperatively work together during the treatment process. When the occupational therapist has an attitude of unconditional positive regard, she sees the patient as equal; she accepts his thoughts, feelings, and behavior without attaching a value to them (Benjamin, 1969, p. 42). When therapy occurs in a group context, the occupational therapist has a key role in establishing group norms that facilitate exploration and positive social interaction. This role as a group leader is further discussed later in the chapter.

The framework for interaction and decision-making defines the expectations for participation in occupational therapy and identifies the activities and resources available in occupational therapy from which the patient can choose. Within this framework the patient makes choices and shares his thoughts about the outcome and personal significance of activities. To help him understand his symbols and to help the patient achieve a dynamic understanding of behavior and problems as presented during the activity process, the occupational therapist uses her knowledge of personality, group process, and normal growth and development. Most often, the therapist functions as a participant-observer. As an observer, she may reflect her observations to the patient and check their validity. It is important to remember that the therapist is not there to "tell" a patient what his behavior "means," but rather to facilitate his own discovery of meaning. The therapist has a responsibility, with the patient, to keep the movement of therapy going, that is, to reassess as needed, the goals that have been established for treatment and to redefine these as the patient broadens his perceptions and becomes aware of more choices.

The Function of Activities

As each therapist looks at activities in relation to her patient, the following will be at the core: What activity can best provide this individual with an opportunity to learn more about himself and experience himself in a broader, more successful way? Closely akin to this, What are this person's most pressing needs now? These are the questions that the patient and therapist will look at, from the beginning to the end of therapy. The answers may be difficult to tease out, or may be quite apparent, and the activities may run the gamut, from trying on make-up to preparing a meal, from coping with an unbalanced checkbook to expressing oneself in art, from learning to give to learning to receive. Patients are seen as always changing; the process of growth is more important than the tangible end product.

Appropriate Expression of Feeling. If a patient is feeling confused, describing himself perhaps as "out of touch with feelings," as "sad" without knowing why, or "anxious" but uncertain of what, the therapist might suggest expressive media. These include art, poetry, clay modeling, drama, dance and movement, and the like. In this case the activity process rather than the end product is the primary focus of treatment. As Mosey states, "the therapist tells the patient that the 'purpose of using art media is to help him discover unknown aspects of the self, not to develop his skill as an artist'" (Mosey, 1970, p. 77). Further, the activity may serve as a catalyst in facilitating interaction between the patient and therapist, or among patients, and can be used to help the patient relate present experience to a past or future situations. Whatever activity or medium is chosen, when the patient is given some choices within the activity as to color, design, or other personal preference, we will always see some "projection" of the patient into the activity. In many cases, this projection is far from mysterious. We recollect a woman who came to an outpatient setting because of feelings of depression. When she was asked to draw herself, she depicted a small female stick figure hanging up the laundry. It was not difficult for her to verbalize her belief that not only did she have a housekeeping role, but this role encompassed all that she was. With children gone to college, and less housekeeping to do, her identity was severely assaulted. The kind of expressive activities suggested here tend to stimulate fantasizing, an id activity, and to tap into unconscious content.

Regaining a Sense of Control. In some persons, the most urgent need may be for them to regain or strengthen their sense of mastery and control. Thus, the occupational therapist is equally concerned about ego function as it is reflected in a patient's ability to problem-solve, to deal with frustration, to accomplish a task, to feel confidence in his own ability, and to integrate new insight into awareness and put it into action. To illustrate: A woman in her early thirties came into the occupational therapy setting during her brief hospitalization. She was attractive and articulate and very pleasant as she assured the therapist that there was "nothing" that occupational therapy could do for her. When asked what she might do for herself, the patient laughed and said, "Are you kidding? Everything I touch, I mess up. I'm a walking disaster area." Here the pressing need was for this woman to experience herself as successful, and it became clear, as she gradually did try some activities, that she was determined to fulfill her prophecies. Through her interaction with very structured media and tangible results, she was able to learn about her own need to "mess up" and could gradually make some choices that were far more positive.

Improving Ego Function. To assess and ultimately improve *ego function,* the occupational therapist might offer the patient a selection of activities that are more structured. By this we mean that the activity needs to be done in logical steps and that there may be a plan or design to follow; the patient will be required to organize and plan ahead in anticipation of each new step; gratification may not be immediate, or may be achieved in increments as each step in the activity process is completed. Think for a moment about the requisite demands in following a sewing pattern, or building a birdhouse, or repairing a broken clock, or baking a cake. By offering the patient a choice, perhaps from a selection of structured activities, the therapist communicates her belief that the patient is a competent human being, capable of making decisions, and ultimately responsible for the outcome of his own actions. Even when freedom of choice results in a less than perfect outcome, looking at one's own errors in an atmosphere of tolerance, acceptance, and patience can turn a "disaster" into an education and need not be an assault on one's self concept. By seeing his own successes and limitations, the patient can move toward improved yet realistic self-confidence.

Sometimes, when given free choice, a patient feeling emotionally empty may try to substitute nonhuman objects for persons and may verbalize the wish to do as many "projects" as possible in order to take home as many tangible goods as possible. At one community mental health center, it was not uncommon for many of the adolescent patients who were, not incidently, having many family problems, to attempt to carry away literally armfuls of material from the clinic, plants from the greenhouse, and cookies from the kitchen in order to fill the vacancies they experienced in people relationships.

Seeing Oneself in a New Way. For others, occupational therapy activities may be a vehicle to explore untapped skills and/or see themselves in new roles. We might think for a moment of what is probably a classic situation: A male patient, about age 55, is brought to the occupational therapy setting for the first time. He looks around and sees what appears to be a great deal of art and craft material, or perhaps a greenhouse, or even a woodshop. Red flags figuratively flash before him, and he announces in his own fashion something akin to "Get me out of here!" With appreciation of the roles and values this patient brings into the occupational therapy setting, this man can be helped to look at the ideas he has about himself and the kind of tolerance he has for others. Perhaps he has never allowed himself to enjoy play, or a hobby, or time for quiet thinking. The choices may be reaffirmed or disavowed. It will always be up to him to decide. When occupational therapy offers group activities, a patient may learn about himself and his concerns in a group. He has an opportunity to learn more about how others view him, or may have a chance to test out his ideas about others. He has a vehicle for developing trust, for trying out dependence or independence. He may have the chance to compete, or to try noncompetitive play; he may learn more about his feelings about sharing, about losing, about winning. He may try out a new role as a leader or as a follower.

Processing the Activity. Whatever the medium and the activity, any activity may be explored dynamically. In regard to the dynamics of the activity, the patient and the therapist together look at the end product, form, content and, process that occurred. Patients are encouraged to talk about the significance of the activity: How did it feel to have so many others compliment you on your work? Is this (product) for you or a gift for someone else? How did it feel to win, or lose? What did you learn about yourself? What did you learn about the others?

In their book, *Occupational Therapy: A Communication Process in Psychiatry,* Fidler and Fidler included a substantive discussion about the utilization of activities. As they state, the "extent to which a patient is encouraged to talk about feelings associated with the activity process" will depend partially on "the patient's readiness or ability to communicate certain associations verbally" (Fidler and Fidler, 1963, p. 82). We would add that the degree to which a patient is encouraged to talk about an activity will depend equally on the therapist's comfort in instigating and following through with such a dialogue. If we are not comfortable with ourselves, how can we expect our patient's to be comfortable with themselves? It is a frequent concern of students and beginning therapists that they not analyze or delve too much. If one can provide permission for a patient to explore his own activities and ultimately his own world rather than make demands that he do so, we suggest that there exists in most of us a healthy curiosity in wishing to know more about ourselves; we may well find a patient who is disappointed to have the discussion end.

In summary, occupational therapy activities in the object relations frame of reference and the discussion around them are seen as serving one or more of the following functions:

1. To provide an avenue for appropriate expression of feeling.

2. To provide an opportunity to improve ego function.

3. To provide a means to establish or re-establish a sense of self and control.

4. To provide a vehicle for learning new skills, improving skills, or gaining confidence in skills already held.

5. To provide an opportunity for trying out new roles or gaining confidence with already established roles.

6. To provide a vehicle for learning more about one's self and one's relationship to others.

7. To provide a means toward increased self-acceptance.

8. To facilitate movement towards flexibility in approaching life tasks.

Theoretical Assumptions

Prior to embarking upon the discussions of the evaluation and treatment processes in occupational therapy, the basic theoretical assumptions which provide a framework for practice based upon the principles of object relations theory will be outlined:

1. A patient is a valuable, unique individual.

2. A patient's perceptions of his reality and experience are more valid than any diagnosis.

3. A patient capable of logical thinking is capable of developing increased understanding of self and other, cause and effect, and the interplay of past, present, and future that we call insight.

4. A patient's most pressing needs will naturally emerge and need to be dealt with first.

5. The id, ego, and superego are useful constructs if they are understood to represent portions of the self, each serving to enhance the experiencing of the self while helping the self to respond and accomodate to the real needs of others. When the wholeness and integrity of the self is lost in focusing on these parts, these have ceased to be useful constructs.

6. A therapist who is comfortable with herself, able to communicate concern, and able to see her own responsibilities in the therapy process is most able to foster a helpful relationship and positive movement in therapy.

7. A patient is not likely to be open to increased insight when his sense of self is threatened.

8. Objects have no meaning in and of themselves. Persons give them meaning.

9. Objects and object relationships can stand for more than themselves and thus serve as symbols.

10. A patient can be assisted to understand himself in a new way when he can learn to understand the personal significance of his symbols, as they may be produced during an occupational therapy session.

11. The patient who can be more self-accepting and who has less need to keep "secrets" from himself has more energy to put toward establishing an abundance of satisfying object relationships.

12. A patient who can try out a new experience, as in the occupational therapy setting, has an opportunity to integrate verbalization, insight, and action that verbalization and hypothesizing alone cannot provide.

Evaluation

The purpose of the occupational therapy evaluation is to gather information that will increase the mutual understanding of the patient's difficulties, which will help in clarifying the thoughts, feelings, and experiences that are influencing behavior and identify the areas in which the patient wishes to grow and the means and resources available for achieving that growth. To gather this information, the occupational therapist uses activities in conjunction with an interview. Interview questions and activities are designed to gain an understanding of the following:

1. Does the patient have a well established sense of self? What are his thoughts and feelings about his physical image? What is his level of self-esteem? What are his social roles and responsibilities? Can he identify his strengths and weaknesses? Does he accept them? What does he perceive as his resources?

2. Does the patient have the ability to trust? Does he trust himself? Can he trust others? Does he feel free to share his thoughts and feelings with the therapist?

3. What is the patient's primary mode of communication? Verbal or nonverbal? Feeling oriented or intellectual? Spontaneous or controlled?

4. What is the patient's affect? Is his behavior consistent and congruent with his verbalization?

5. Does the patient have significant realationships? Family? Friends? Peers? Colleagues? Community? Can he establish and maintain these relationships? What are his relationships with other patients and staff?

6. Can the patient identify and meet his needs? How are his safety, physical, love, belonging, self-esteem, and self-actualization needs being met?

7. How does the patient respond to change?

8. How does the patient invest and use his energy?

9. What is the patient's cognitive level of function?

10. What does the patient value?

11. Does the patient want to participate in the evaluation and treatment process?

12. What does the patient hope to achieve in treatment? In occupational therapy?

13. Can the patient cope with the anxiety of self-discovery and change? (Fidler and Fidler, 1963; Mosey, 1970)

Assessment Instruments. The Azima test battery was one of the first occupational therapy evaluation instruments to be well documented. It consists of four tasks: (1) draw a picture using a pencil; (2) draw a whole person and draw a person of the opposite sex; (3) make an object out of clay; and (4) do a finger painting. The purposes of the test battery were to uncover the psychodynamics of behavior and to determine the level of function of psychosexual development through the interpretation of objects.

Following the development of the Azima battery, Fidler modified the battery and expanded the evaluation process through the identification of five general areas to be assessed. The battery has three activities: (1) draw a person; (2) do a finger painting; and (3) make an object from clay. After completion of the activities the occupational therapist assesses the patient's concept of himself, his concept of others, his ego organization, his unconscious conflicts, and his nature and manner of communication. Fidler and Fidler outline the method of interpreting patient behavior by considering the patient-therapist, patient-group, and patient-activity relationships. They also provide an outline for activity analysis which can be used with any activity as an assessment instrument. It is these outlines by the Fidlers which continue to influence the use of projective activities as assessment tools (Fidler and Fidler, 1963).

The test battery that Mosey suggests in the area of object relations is a modification of the ones developed by Azima and Fidler. It has the patient complete three tasks : (1) a drawing with colored pencils; (2) a finger painting; and (3) a clay object (Mosey, 1970).

Although not identified with a particular frame of reference, recent literature gives an extensive list and description of projective instruments which include the following: (1) The Azima Battery; (2) The Shoemyen Battery; (3) The Goodman Battery; (4) The BH (Barbara Hemphill) Battery; (5) The Magazine Picture Collage; (6) The Comprehensive Assessment Process: A Group Evaluation; (7) The Person Symbol as an Assessment Tool; and (8) The Activity Laboratory: A Structure for Observing and Assessing Perceptual, Integrative and Behavioral Strategies (Hemphill, 1982).

Since projective media and approaches are identified with the object relations frame of reference, they are listed and summarized here. For a thorough discussion of the evaluation process and protocol for each of the evaluation summarized, refer to Hemphill, *The Evaluation Process in Psychiatric Occupational Therapy* (1982).

The Azima Battery. The battery consists of three media that facilitate free association and exploration of personality dynamics. The patient is asked to do the following tasks: draw anything using a paper and pencil; draw a whole person and then draw a person of the opposite sex; make anything out of a clay ball; do a finger painting. The therapist then makes interpretations based upon the following: (1) organization of mood, (2) organization of drives,

(3) organization of the ego, and (4) organization of object relations (Hemphill, 1982).

The Shoemyen Battery. The therapist evaluates one to four patients at a time and requests the patients to complete four projects. They are: (1) construct a mosaic tile trivet; (2) using three primary colors, paint whatever finger painting you want; (3) carve an object from a four inch vermiculite-plaster cube; (4) model a human figure from clay. The therapist then completes a data form that summarizes the patient's responses to the task, media, and the discussion between therapist and patient (Hemphill, 1982).

The Goodman Battery. The battery consists of four tasks that begin with the most structured and become progressively less structured. First, the patient copies a mosaic tile design to reproduce a tile trivet. The second task is a spontaneous drawing; then the patient does a figure drawing, and finally he is asked to make an object from clay. The therapist then rates the patient's behavior, using a seven point scale (Hemphill, 1982).

The Barbara Hemphill (BH) Battery. The BH battery consists of a mosaic tile trivet and a finger painting. The therapist evaluates the patient's approach to the media, the manner in which he uses space, and his verbal responses. A rating form is used (Hemphill, 1982).

The Lerner Magazine Picture Collage. The patient is given colored construction paper and magazines and is asked to construct a collage. The therapist assesses cognitive-perceptual skills, the nature and quality of defenses, the patient's affect and sense of self, and the quality of object relations (Hemphill, 1982).

Ehrenberg Comprehensive Assessment Process: A Group Evaluation. During three one-hour group sessions patients are asked to complete a tile trivet, choose one of three projects (a collage, group drawing, or a problem solving task), and then complete one of the three chosen activities. The therapist evaluates general appearance, interaction skills, work skills, and activities of daily living skills. The assessment defines behaviors that need to be assessed (Hemphill, 1982).

King Person Symbol as an Assessment Tool. The patient is given a pencil and paper and asked to draw a person. There is no discussion of the drawing with the patient. The therapist uses the Goodenough-Harris Scale to interpret the drawing (Hemphill, 1982).

Fidler: Activity Laboratory, A Structure for Observing and Assessing Perceptual Integrative and Behavioral Strategies. Fidler states that this is an assessment used to establish a tentative behavioral profile. Five activities are used: (1) the patient traces one of two pictures and cuts it out and (2) does a finger painting and (3) a collage; (4) then the patient performs through an obstacle course and (5) participates in a ball tag game. The patient then completes a questionnaire (Hemphill, 1982).

All the previous assessments have been categorized as projective assessments. The authors feel that this categorization is based upon a broad interpretation of projective testing, perhaps somewhat broader than that used by the psychology community. Do activities of daily living, ball games, and obstacle courses provide stimuli that are open to interpretation? Might these also be "amorphous, somewhat unstructured situations" onto which the patient projects his needs? (Kaplan and Sadock, 1983, p. 209).

The Evaluation Process . . . Opening the Evaluation. During the evaluation interview, the therapist allows time to establish rapport with the patient. Rapport is enhanced by the therapist's attitude of warmth, openness, and regard, as discussed; also, confidentiality may be discussed and the therapist is open in stating why she has asked the patient to engage in the specified evaluation activities. When giving instructions for evaluation tasks, the therapist gives clear, specific instructions but does not give suggestions for methods of task accomplishment. As the patient works, the therapist observes and notes verbal and nonverbal behaviors. She allows the patient to complete each task and then discusses the activity process and behaviors that she observed. Discussion during the activity may be too distracting for the patient and can affect patient performance.

The atmosphere during the evaluation should be one of mutual sharing and learning, not interrogation. The patient learns about himself, and the therapist learns about the patient's thoughts, feelings, and concerns as well as his manner of approaching certain tasks. She is open in sharing her views with the patient. It may be that during this interview the therapist will orient the patient to occupational therapy, its purposes, and how the patient might benefit from the activities available.

The Figure Drawing as an Evalution Task. The projective assessments previously summarized seek the reflection of unconscious content and as such are quite traditionally analytic in their assumptions. Additionally, these batteries provide a means to assess the ability of the person in regard to (ego-directed) problem solving. With the moderating input of human existential theory into the object relations frame, the object relations therapist would be less concerned about "analyzing" patient productions, because she would be seeking to use the evaluation activities as a springboard for helping the patient become more aware of his own approach to activity, his strengths and limitations, his feelings about himself, his interests, and his relationship to others. Since the person drawing is used in several of the aforementioned batteries and is a therapeutic task seen as very useful by the authors (whether practice is in psychosocial dysfunction or physical medicine), we will illustrate how a "person drawing" might be presented and followed up as part of the evaluation process.

It should be noted that in the classic projective presentation of the person drawing, the patient is asked to draw a "person." Whatever gender is depicted, the request is then made for a second drawing depicting the opposite gender. Most often the individual will draw first a figure that is the same sex as himself; projectively speaking, both drawings relate to aspects of the self (Hammer, 1968). The authors prefer to request one "self drawing," which can then be discussed without confusion as a reflection of the "self." The method which follows is not a cut-and-dried one but serves as an example. The use of other evaluation media, such as collage and structured tasks, could be presented and discussed in much the same way.

The request for a person drawing might be as part of a given projective battery or singly with an interview. Although person drawings are viewed as projective and thereby consonant with object relations theory, they can be adapted and used effectively with any frame of reference discussed in the text.

The drawing requested might be of a "person," the "self," the "self engaged in an activity," the "self as a member of a family," the "self three, five, and 10 years hence," or the "idealized self." These are just a few examples of how the drawing has been used.

The therapist should have available several pieces of white paper (at least 8 X 11 inches; larger pieces can bring more expressive results), two or more pencils and functioning erasers, and crayons or colored marking pens or pencils (if the therapist wishes to allow color to be an aspect of the drawing and increase the opportunity for expressiveness). The patient is typically seated with the therapist and asked, "Please draw a picture of yourself" (or "yourself with your family"). The patient may express the concern that he "can't draw" or "can't do this." The therapist will communicate her understanding, and assure him that she is not concerned about his artistic ability and that she would like him to "try." She can also assure him that when he is finished, they will together look at the drawing. Letting the patient know that she will not be interpreting the drawing but, rather, that he will have the opportunity to look and see what he thinks, frequently lessens the resistance to what can be a very anxiety-laden task. If possible, there should be no limitation on the time allowed for the drawing. Individuals frequently feel a strong need to get the drawing "right." However, when there is a time limit, the patient is told in advance how much time he will have. The therapist pays attention to the following: (1) the manner in which the patient selects and uses the media; (2) comments he makes while engaged in the task; (3) the parts or aspects of the body or drawing into which he puts special time or care, or which he tends to gloss over; (4) his general affect while doing the drawing; (5) peripheral drawings or scribbles on the page and when, in the process, they were done; and (6) the person figure itself. Once the drawing is complete, the authors would frequently ask the patient to pause, look at the drawing, and then give it a "title."

Since the authors favor talking about the drawing immediately upon its completion, when the drawing is done as part of a battery of evaluation tasks, the drawing is the last task presented in the sequence. This task sequence also allows time for the therapist to establish rapport with the patient and for him to gain comfort with the evaluation process as he completes the other tasks. Thus, there is usually less resistance when it is time to draw.

Upon completion of the drawing, the therapist communicates her wish to look at the drawing with the patient in order that they might both "learn more about" the patient. The process might be started with the statement, "I am hoping that together we can look at this drawing and learn more about you, and get a better understanding of what you want to accomplish for yourself while you are here in treatment. What can you tell me about the person in this drawing?" or "Please tell me about the person in this drawing."

When a patient is reluctant or unable to respond to an initial request to "tell about" the drawing, the therapist might facilitate the process by making an observation about the drawing or the manner in which it was approached — always with a note of tentativeness in her voice, in order that the patient feel invited to expand upon or "correct" her observation. For example, the therapist might say, "I noticed that you drew a very light figure, almost as if it wasn't supposed to be seen. How do you feel in looking at it?" Or "I noticed that you erased your drawing several times, and I wondered how you felt while doing the drawing?" Some patients are unable to talk about their figure drawing even with support and assistance, and their limitations must be respected. Occasionally such a patient is able to structure his thoughts in writing, and the therapist might ask him to respond to one or more issues in writing (see note 6).

Some issues that might be discussed in regards to the figure drawing include the following:

What is the figure doing?

Is the figure male or female (if that is not evident)?

What does the figure in the drawing like about himself?

What would he like to change?

What are his roles? And to whom is he responsible? If the person in the drawing is engaged in a task, why was this task chosen?

If it is a family drawing, whom is the patient placed near?

Who is close to whom in the family? Who is isolated?

What is the significance of the title (if one was requested)?

What is the person in the drawing thinking about?

What is the person in the drawing feeling?

What does the patient feel in looking at the drawing?

What has he learned about himself from doing the drawing?

If a physical change and/or disability is reflected, what does the person feel about these? Are physical changes accurately depicted?

While there are several manuals available for the projective interpretation of person drawings (see references), the therapist is encouraged to respond to the feeling tone of the drawing and to the organization of the task as well as the approach as a whole. For example:

1. Small, lightly drawn and/or frequently erased drawings tend to appear "apologetic"; they do not communicate confidence or comfort.

2. Large, bright drawings may exude confidence and a sense of importance, but one needs to be aware of how this fits with the fact that the patient is in treatment.

3. Body parts may be missing or covered, scribbled, and/or erased when there is discomfort with their function.

4. Drawings tend to appear masculine, feminine, or asexual or bisexual. What does the drawing communicate about the individual's comfort with his own sexuality?

5. A figure's expression, posture, and use of color communicate an affect or feeling tone. Is it sorrow, confusion, "flatness" (lack of affect), or joy?

6. If there is loss of integration in the figure, e.g., body parts disconnected, distorted, or missing, or the use of excess symbolism, it often reflects a loss of integration in the individual himself.

7. The inability to complete the task or a highly symbolic rendering may reflect an inability to deal with the self as a real and meaningful entity.

8. Background objects placed with the figure in the drawing may provide emotional support and/or help define the individual's roles.

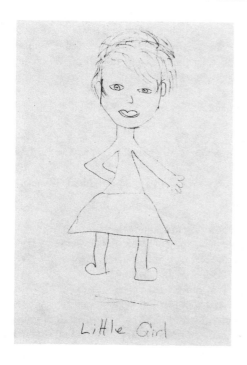

Figure 3-1.

Little Girl

9. Drawings may be internally congruent or incongruent. For example, the title of the drawing might be "I'm me and I'm OK," but the figure in the drawing is frowning. The drawing may also be congruent or incongruent in relation to the patient doing the drawing. For example, the patient may appear sad and states that he is in treatment because of depression, but the figure in the drawing is smiling.

10. The amount of time and energy spent on the figure drawing and on specific figure parts may relate to their importance to the individual. Figures F1 through F18 in Appendix F, "person drawings", are self-drawings completed by patients with whom the authors worked. Some pertinent biographical data are included. They will illustrate, we believe, the manner in which figure drawings can reflect vividly an individual's sense of self and his concerns.

For Figure 3-1 we have included the beginning patient-therapist dialogue, to further illustrate how communication around a task can be developed. This figure was drawn by a 19 year old Caucasian female. She sought outpatient treatment because of feelings of depression, but was then hospitalized because of her physician's concern regarding her suicidal potential. Her parents were recently divorced.

In the interview she is seen to be a bit heavy, wears a very short dress, and is well groomed. When asked to "please draw a picture of yourself," she uses the pencil to draw a figure about 6 ½ inches tall in the middle of a 12 × 16 inch piece of paper and titles it "Little Girl." When the task is completed, the therapist initiates the following interview:

Th.: "What can you tell me about this drawing?"

Pt.: "I like my eyes. I think they're my best feature."

Th.: "And the rest of you. . . ?"

Pt.: "I'm too fat (pause). I don't like my body."

Th.: "I'm struck by the title that you gave this picture. Can you tell me how you came to use this title?"

Pt.: "Sometimes I feel like a little girl (pause). I wish I were a little girl again. It was so much easier."

Th.: "Easier than being a woman?"

Pt.: "I know my parents don't approve of me, especially my father. They don't like the way I dress. . . or the guys I date. I'm dating a guy right now. Sometimes he calls me at 11 o'clock and wants me to come over (pause, looking down). You know what I mean. He doesn't even ask me out on regular dates. When I come home, I feel really crummy."

Th.: "It sounds like you disapprove of yourself as much as your parents do."

Pt.: "That's right — I really hate myself. I wish I could be little again; then my parents would love me, and they'd be together and I wouldn't have to feel so crummy. I don't even know what I want to be, and I have a crummy job as a . . . I'm a big flop. Do you know what I mean?"

Th.: "Well, I think I'm starting to understand why being little again could seem so appealing."

Summary. The evaluation process is designed to help clarify the problem or pressing need(s) as perceived by the patient and to help identify the patient's strengths and resources available. The person drawing was discussed to illustrate the development of an evaluation task in the evaluation process. Both structured and unstructured evaluation tasks as well as patient-therapist dialogue are used to help identify the patient's perceptions of himself, his goals for treatment, and the ways in which these goals might be accomplished. During the evaluation the patient is helped to focus on and identify specifics regarding his goals for treatment and for occupational therapy. A patient unfamiliar with occupational therapy may need assistance from the therapist in understanding what resources are available to him and how these might be used effectively by him. Once the initial evaluation is complete, the therapist turns the process to goal setting and program planning. The evaluation process is really an on-going process of reassessing patient participation and change, and of helping to identify new areas in which growth is desired.

Treatment Goals

In the early days of psychiatric occupational therapy an analytically oriented approach was used under the close supervision of the physician who prescribed treatment. Knowledge of psychodynamics and activities were used to identify personality structures, object relationships, defenses, and conscious and unconscious meanings of behavior. The occupational therapist used projective activities to develop object relationships, ego function, and defenses and to increase the conscious awareness of the dynamic reason for symptoms (Fidler and Fidler, 1963).

Since this time the philosophy of treatment based upon object relations and the communication process has evolved so that now the occupational therapist is expected to function more independently in evaluation and treatment planning, and to assume more responsibility for decision making. The physician or primary therapist refers the patient to occupational therapy and expects the therapist to evaluate the patient and design a treatment program that effectively responds to the patient's needs. Setting treatment goals encompasses (1) stating what the patient would like to accomplish and (2) planning a program that will provide the patient a means to this accomplishment. The occupational therapist may continue to use projective or expressive media to achieve traditional analytic goals, as discussed. In addition she will strive to increase the patient's ability to identify and satisfy personal needs, achieve greater insight, and be able to use this insight to interact more effectively with the world around him. Within the broad goals of increasing self-awareness, developing insight, and improving problem solving, the occupational therapist will set specific, individualized treatment goals for each patient. Ten years ago one might have found occupational therapy goals to be lofty but vague. Such goals might have stated that the therapist would seek to "increase self-esteem" or "decrease depression" or "improve problem solving." The contemporary occupational therapist will write more specific objectives which will be clearly understood, be in terms of patient outcome, and probably be behaviorally identified by the patient, treatment team, and third party payer.

Sample treatment goals include the following:

1. The patient will describe his feelings of inadequacy and identify sources of these feelings.

2. The patient will increase his self-esteem through the completion of a (specified) occupational therapy activity.

3. The patient will identify and explore through occupational therapy media his feelings of loss and grief.

4. The patient will identify his strengths and weaknesses within the context of the occupational therapy activity.

The treatment goals are discussed jointly by the patient and the therapist and a treatment plan is developed. Treatment goals are then re-evaluated periodically, typically weekly or bimonthly, and modified as needed.

Treatment Process

The application of the object relations frame of reference in the treatment process occurs in individual and group situations in occupational therapy with patients who are reality oriented and capable of logical thinking. To facilitate a dynamic understanding of behavior and problems, the occupational therapist uses creative media or semistructured experiences to help the patient project his thoughts, feelings, needs, fantasies, desires, and frustrations onto the end product (activity), or she uses structured activities to assist the patient in increasing organizational and problem-solving skills.

Creating a Climate. Individual treatment sessions usually last 40 to 60 minutes and group sessions are one to one and one-half hours in length. The optimum group size is five to eight patients. During the treatment sessions the therapist is an observer and participant-observer. The therapist participates in the activity when she wishes to process the activity or influence the treatment outcome. Her participation can also ease patient anxiety or the initial resistance due to the threat posed by the activity. When participating in treatment groups, she can influence the focus of the group. For example, when a patient refuses to experiment with drawing media, the occupational therapist might suggest that she and the patient experiment with colors, or each can do "scribbles" and then share their view of the identifiable images in the scribbles. Sharing in this manner can help establish rapport. Or perhaps the occupational therapist is aware of much anger in the patient group and senses that the group is threatened by the expression of this feeling. The therapist could request that each patient pantomime a feeling and then have the group discuss what they saw. During this, the therapist might mime "anger" and depict how she handles anger. This is one way of role modeling and is a way of giving the group permission to express angry feelings. However, should the group resist this permission, the therapist would be sensitive to this resistance and would not try to force anyone to go beyond his present need or capacity. The process of change may be both inviting and threatening and thus tends to occur slowly.

Increasing Self-knowledge. As an observer during the treatment process the occupational therapist notes significant behaviors which occur during the activity process. These behaviors as well as the significance or symbolic meaning of the activity are discussed when the activity is completed. During the discussion the occupational therapist tries to do the following:

1. Help the patient explore his thoughts and feelings and memories aroused by the activity.

2. Help the patient make conscious associations between the activity experience and past, present, and future experiences and/or difficulties.

3. Using conscious associations, help the patient increase his self-understanding and broaden his perspective on current behavior and problems and possible solutions.

4. Help the patient to interpret the meaning of symbols and integrate this new knowledge (Mosey, 1970).

When an activity, process, or medium is seen to hold special symbolic content, the occupational therapist may seek to help the patient understand the latent as well as obvious significance therein. We would suggest that symbols are expressed not only in art form but in all our actions and interactions. To give a popular example: When I jog, I may do so because I really enjoy jogging or perhaps because it symbolizes to me health and well-being or prosperity or independence. When I draw myself jogging, I may be symbolizing my quest for health, or prosperity, or I may wear jogging shoes as a symbol of my having attained prosperity. When interpreting symbols, the occupational therapist focuses on the function of the symbol. When looking with a patient at a person drawing, she does not ask him to defend his symbols. That is, she does not ask, "Why did you draw this man wearing jogging shoes?" Rather she asks, "I wonder how this man feels jogging?"

The therapist may give her view of the meaning of a symbol, but it must always be validated by the patient. The ultimate purpose of looking at symbols is to help the patient understand, for himself, the unique purpose of his symbols. Even when Freudian and Jungian symbolism is of special interest to the therapist, it would seem to us a great disservice to overgeneralize these interpretations if in so doing the unique personal context is lost.

A brief illustration from practice can show this: It is not uncommon for patients working with clay to rather absent-mindedly make snakelike coils. On one occasion, a young man did this and then presented this "snake" to the therapist. He smiled and asked, "How do you like your present?" The therapist asked, "Is this a snake?" He responded, "Yes," and again asked, "Do you like it?" The therapist then asked, "How do you expect me to react?" He smiled and explained, "When I was a lot younger, I brought home a small garter snake. My Mom freaked out! You should have seen her. It was so fun to scare her." Neither the Freudian tendency to see snakes as a phallic symbol nor the Jungian tendency to see the snake as a symbol of power (as in the physicians' caduceus) is discounted in this example; but the personal experience of the young man with his mother gives this symbol a personal touch.

Guidelines for Exploring Symbols. The therapist wishing to explore symbol production is reminded of the guidelines suggested by Mosey in *Three Frames of Reference,* which are summarized here:

1. Symbols have no fixed meaning.

2. Symbols have individual significance.

3. Symbols are given reality through reproduction, such as art work, speech, and behavior.

4. Explore the content of symbols — their size, shape, form, placement on the page, the method of production, and the use of materials.

5. Identify themes or commonalities that relate to past, present, and future life situations.

6. Relate in the "here and now."

7. The process of symbol production should be noted.

8. Interpretations should be used sparingly. Too many interpretations are confusing and may be difficult to integrate (Mosey, 1970, pp.71-81). It cannot be overemphasized that in looking at symbol production, the therapist does not simply look at a list of Freudian, Jungian, or other symbol discussions and apply them to the patient's symbols. The symbol serves as a nonverbal expression of personal meaning. When the patient has the ability for much insight and verbal exchange, looking at his own symbol production may be a means for him to become better acquainted with his own intent.

The Impact of the Group Process in Treatment. As stated, occupational therapy in the object relations framework frequently is carried out in a group context. When this occurs, there are special considerations regarding group influence and group process that need be considered by the therapist.

The patient, especially one new to treatment, is usually quite uncertain regarding the expectations of him in a patient group. He may be frightened that the patient group will see him as "sick" or a "mental case," and he may be equally concerned regarding "them." The therapist needs to respect these concerns, while setting a tone of mutual regard. The therapist also needs to be certain that the patient is introduced to the other group members, and that he is given a chance to become more comfortable before a lot of demands for interaction are made of him. Depending on the format within a clinical setting, and on the therapist's goals, the following degrees of interaction may be in evidence, and are reminiscent of the development of play interaction among children:

1. Individuals are working by themselves on their own projects, with little interaction, but in the same work space as other patients.

2. Several patients are sitting together, sharing materials and talking, but each is working on his own activity.

3. Several patients or the entire group is working together, cooperating to the end of accomplishing an agreed upon task; interaction and sharing are high and occur around the task as well as personal feelings. Even when the level of patient interaction is minimal, the therapist has a "gatekeeping" responsibility to see that safety needs (physical and emotional) are met, disruptions (subgrouping, scapegoating, abusive behavior) are dealt with, materials and equipment are shared and used appropriately, and patient and clinic scheduling needs are met.

When the therapist wishes individuals to function cooperatively as a group, her concerns become much broader. Materials and seating may be arranged to facilitate sharing and interaction; group tasks, activities, or games may be introduced that will depend for their vitality on patients' interdependence.

To illustrate, in one community health center outpatient group, there was a frequent change in the patient population, the average length of patient treatment being one month. To encourage interaction and to build specific skills, the occupational therapist had the patient group, which varied in size from five to 10, plan and carry out the preparation of a noon or evening meal. Purchasing supplies, if necessary, was done by the patients as was all food preparation and clean up. The occupational therapist served as a resource person only. On some occasions, the patient group would vote to invite one guest each to share their meal. It was useful for the group to look at their own feelings about having guests.

When the group had achieved a strong sense of unity and when each patient felt accepted by the group, the issue of having guests was not a volatile one. When there was less ease and cohesion, the prospect of having guests made many patients anxious. When potential guests included persons not in psychiatric treatment, many patients were led to confront the personal struggle they were experiencing regarding their own feelings about being in treatment. This group had many tasks and subtasks that necessitated good organization and problem solving. Equally significant, patients had the opportunity to experience themselves in a social setting that was quite similar to an everyday social situation.

This "cooking group," as it was called by the patients, was a popular patient activity. It should be noted that food and "feeding" play important symbolic functions in our culture. In "breaking bread" together the patients could give to themselves and to each other in a significant way.

Another group commonly used at this treatment center, for both inpatients and outpatients, was a gardening group. The group size varied from five to 12 patients. A portion of land was designated for planting. Each patient was given responsibility for either a part of maintaining the whole area (i.e., for weeding, watering) or full responsibility for a specific portion of the garden within the whole; that is, he could plant whatever he wished and then had responsibility for its maintainance. This group offered a great deal of opportunity for independent functioning within the patient group and for a patient to achieve a sense of "personal ownership" as well as opportunity to build a sense of community. Again, the symbolic nature of planting and nurturing were important in influencing the degree of personal investment many patients felt in regard to the garden.

The Group as a Social Microcosm. It has been suggested that whenever people get together in this way, there exists a *social microcosm*. In each group of which he is a member, an individual will tend to replicate the patterns or ways of behaving that typify his everyday social dealings. Thus, the occupational therapy group experience is a vehicle for learning about and possibly enhancing social skill. When it provides a chance for intimacy and mature interaction (that may be lacking or minimal in his everyday dealings), the patient in the group has an opportunity for what Alexander called a *corrective emotional experience* (Alexander, 1963, as discussed in Patterson, 1973, pp. 270-271).

Feedback. If the group is open in its verbal sharing, the patient can be given feedback regarding his behavior (that is, he is told how he is perceived by others) from not just the therapist but the entire group. Yalom suggests that in a group context, the patient may gain insight at several levels. Those most applicable to an occupational therapy group are:

1. Insight as to how I am perceived by others: Am I tense? Warm? Aloof?

2. Insight as regards how I interact with others: Do I tend to exploit them? Reject them? Overdepend? Do I behave differently towards men and women?

3. Insight regarding why I behave the way I do: How does my behavior make me feel? (Yalom, 1975, p. 32).

By receiving this kind of feedback, the patient can engage in *consensual validation*; that is, he can compare his thoughts about himself to the statements that others make about him, and perhaps he can reassess his thinking when he becomes aware of discrepencies. Studies suggest that whether the patient receives so-called "superficial" or "deep" insight appears not to influence the degree to which the patient finds feedback to be helpful. Any accurate feedback is considered useful (Yalom, 1975, p. 33).

With dynamics similar to those of the therapeutic one-to-one realtionship, if group feedback is to be really "heard" by a patient, he must perceive the group as accepting and supportive of him. Otherwise he will feel too strong a need to defend against perceived assaults on his self-esteem. To ensure that the group is one in which patients feel a sense of acceptance and trust, and one in which feedback is effectively given, the therapist must be cognizant of her important role in helping set the norms of behavior. These norms would include free interaction among members, nonjudgemental acceptance, respect for individual boundaries, honest expression of affection, displeasure, and other feelings, and confidentiality (Yalom, 1975, p. 84).

One way that a therapist can effectively do this is to be a model-setting participant, as we have discussed. However, she cannot get so involved as a participant that she loses her perspective and ability to stand back and process the group interaction. Therapist openness has its place, but the therapist is not in the group to solve her problems!

Processing the Activity Group. Group activity sessions may be viewed in much the same way as individual activities, with the added dimension of group interaction. The occupational therapist continues to focus on the process of the activity, rather than the end product. The therapist notes the following:

1. The choice of the activity and how this choice is made.

2. The individual skills demonstrated when manipulating material: motor coordination, workmanship, ability to follow instructions.

3. The satisfaction of each group member with the end product or the activity outcome.

4. The attitude of the group members toward each other and toward the therapist.

5. How each patient evaluates the activity and the group experience.

6. The role that each group member assumes.

7. The feelings of each group member about the group.

8. How the group members respond to feelings or situations that arise during the activity process.

9. The type, quality, and system of communication that occurs during the group sessions.

10. Overt behavior of the individual or the group during the activity (Fidler and Fidler, 1963; Mosey, 1970).

The ultimate aim is to assist each patient to better understand his social and task behavior, and thereby allow him to make conscious efforts to change or expand the way(s) in which he relates interpersonally and approaches activities. Further, when the patient has the chance to try out new more successful behaviors within the group, he may have the added advantage of having the group express their approval and appreciation of his new manner of relating. He thereby increases his self-esteem and the confidence he carries into future situations.

Chapter Summary

"Physical concepts are free creations of the human mind, and not, however it may seem, uniquely determined by the external world. In our endeavor to understand reality we are somewhat like a man trying to understand the mechanism of a closed watch. He sees the face and the moving hands, even hears its ticking, but has no way of opening the case. If he is ingenious he may form some picture of the mechanism which could be responsible for all the things he observes, but he may never be quite sure his picture is the only one which could explain his observations. He will never be able to compare his picture with the real mechanism and he cannot even imagine the possibility of the meaning of such a comparison" (Albert Einstein, cited in Zukav's *The Dancing Wuli Masters: An Overview of the New Physics,* 1980, p. 8).

The object relations framework for understanding man and his endeavors is, without question, one that depends on the therapist's belief in the integrity of subjective experiencing. While it draws its philosophical base from a diversity of sources — Freud, Jung, contemporary Freudians, the humanist-existentialists — these beliefs are key:

1. The belief that as a man sees his world, so is his world.

2. The belief that a man's feelings and perceptions about his endeavors have a significant impact on his actions.

3. The belief that persons are interested in learning more about the obvious as well as "hidden" parts of themselves.

4. The belief that the more a person is aware of his own needs, beliefs, and values and feelings, the more real freedom he has in making choices.

5. The belief that understanding a patient's personal and social history can assist the therapist in understanding the patient's current approach to life.

6. The belief that the patient-therapist relationship significantly affects the therapeutic process and its outcome.

7. The belief that there exists in each individual an internal drive to love and be loved, to use unique skills, to feel purposeful and significant — and that this is achieved throught active interrelatedness with persons and nonhuman objects.

8. The belief that human endeavor is influenced by conscious and unconscious intent.

9. The belief that the person who is more self-accepting has more means available to interact positively with others and to develop his potential.

While consideration is given to the social context and the quality and function of activity, the locus for looking at activity is from the view of the individual himself. While not discussed in this text with other developmental theories, the object-relations approach is, in fact, developmental in its ascribing to the person a sequential development in self-perception, relatedness to others, relatedness to objects, and ability to successfully engage in activity.

Before considering the contributions and limitations of the object-relations framework for occupational therapy, we need make some precursory comments.

Disenchantment with Freud

First, there is a growing tendency in occupational therapy literature and in the field of psychology to discard Freudian ideology. Since the object-relations theory has much basis in Freudian theory, the therapist needs to evaluate her stance in regard to incorporating Freudian concepts. As the scientific community and helping community look with hindsight on

Freudian theory, there are obvious limitations, limitations acknowledged by Freud himself. As Corey comments, it is easier to discern the need for change and reach out to build new theories when one "stands on the giant's shoulders" (Corey, 1982, p. 30). Freud was a product of his times and own biases, much as we are of ours. In each frame of reference in this text and in each discipline, we encounter "leaders" whose ideas have at one time been accepted with authority, ideas which eventually have succumbed to selection and adaptation. If one chooses to discard, nonselectively, all constructs that are Freudian in origin, one may discard constructs that address aspects of human thought and activity not as thoroughly or adeptly handled by other theoretical frameworks. The final judgment lies with each reader.

Occupational Therapy — Not Psychoanalysis

The occupational therapist who is knowledgeable in object relations theory and applies it appropriately in practice is not doing psychoanalysis; the method suggested by Freud is not that of the occupational therapist — nor is the goal extensive reworking of unconscious content and major personality change. It should be added that most contemporary psychotherapists cognizant of Freudian ideology are not engaged in psychoanalysis. Nor need the occupational therapist carry out verbal psychotherapy to use Freudian constructs. Contemporary object relations theory speaks to the function of activity in the development of personhood, and one can accept certain aspects of the Freudian ideology and approach and use this understanding to enrich one's own practice. If psychotherapists rely almost exclusively on verbal exchange, it may be to our advantage that occupational therapy provides in addition a "living laboratory" for active engagement.

Second, subjectivity is held with great disdain by the scientific community, and occupational therapy is being pressed to objectify its data, along with other health professionals. As a profession whose personnel have been historically better at considering feelings than clarifying fact, the need to objectify may seem clear and unquestionable. However, before we become overly zealous in discarding subjective data, we need to recognize that we can never really separate ourselves from our own goals and interests in our research, and we must realize that our science can only discover what its tools and tests accomodate. If we choose, we can determine that thoughts and feelings are irrelevant as indices of change. If we do this, will we move forward or backward in our understanding of the human condition and the therapeutic process?

Contributions of the Object Relations Frame of Reference

1. As has been stated, the object relations framework provides a vocabulary and hypothetical constructs for talking about and understanding feelings (or the subjective self), and proponents of this framework emphasize that subjective experience is a valid and integral part of the human condition. In our experience, patients who have the opportunity to express their feelings and trust that they are "heard" have more ability to attend to objective tasks. Further,

patients who have both a limited and a broad range of ability for insight have demonstrated an interest in increasing their understanding of why events — within and outside themselves — occur. While insight cannot be achieved by all of us to the same degree, the desire to understand "why" is evident in most of us.

2. The object relations framework provides a context for approaching and understanding an individual's history or previous experience. This has been considered by many to be a detriment, rather than a contribution, to the extent that traditional Freudian ideology is seen to have placed too much emphasis on patient history. However, with the moderating input of humanistic-existential theory, the patient is given an opportunity to reflect upon and better understand his past experience while being encouraged to recognize that it is his "today" that offers the opportunity for change. Each of us might pause to reflect on our own feelings about our personal past. How often do we, upon making new friends, wish to share with them information about "where we come from" — our family upbringing, meaningful events and relationships in our lives? How often do our children ask us to tell them about ourselves when we were children? It does not seem that understanding and reflecting upon our roots need keep us forever looking back.

The therapist conceptualizing life as a process of continuing development (much as Jung and humanist-existentialists do) would be encouraged to explore the recent work in the study of the adult life span as a developmental, task-related process. (See Chapter VII, Developmental Frame of Reference, for a discussion of contemporary work in this area.)

3. The humanistic-existential influence has moderated the deterministic analytic view of man, providing a positive posture regarding man and his potential for change. It is an optimistic posture and one that puts an emphasis on the possibilities, not fallibilities, of the individual.

4. Humanistic-existential input has emphasized the importance of the human element and the therapeutic relationship in treatment. It has encouraged the therapist to be more conscious of her role and responsibilities in the therapeutic relationship, requiring active participation and not a passive neutrality. For those new therapists who may be especially concerned that they will harm a patient by saying or doing the "wrong" thing, the emphasis on listening to the patient and respecting his pace and choices might serve to lessen that concern.

5. In encouraging a patient to be independent and emphasizing the responsibility he has for his own welfare, the object relations framework strives to facilitate carryover of treatment benefits to home, when the patient is no longer in treatment. Also, by looking to internal, naturally evolving rewards rather than rewards designed by staff members, behavioral change is viewed as more stable.

6. An important contribution of humanistic-existential and contemporary Freudian input into object relations theory is that it encourages the therapist to consider each person as unique, the implication being that there is no one best approach or technique and, further, that the therapist would profit from being cognizant of a diversity of philosophical and treatment principles.

Limitations of the Object Relations Frame of Reference

1. When subjective-reality forms a basis for treatment, there exists the issue of proving, via research and verifiable outcomes, the veracity of one's conclusions about therapy and the efficacy of treatment intervention. Both the Freudian use of case studies to exemplify the outcomes of treatment and the humanistic reliance on feeling barometers have been criticized as too subjective. Freudian, Jungian, and existential-humanistic constructs (i.e., libido, ego, unconscious, collective unconscious, unconditional positive regard) have been described as "picturesque" but not useful for scientific inquiry. Further, there is no comprehensive research in occupational therapy (beyond descriptive case studies) in support of an object relations treatment approach. In contrast, cognitive theorists, to be discussed later in the text, have sought to objectify "thoughts" and demonstrate the outcome of therapeutic intervention through objective (or behavioral) means. Eventually the theorist and practitioner within this framework must ask, "Does feeling-oriented therapeutic intervention improve the quality of individuals' lives? If so, how can this improvement be demonstrated?" Indeed, are both the objective and subjective worlds of experience available for scientific inquiry?

2. The contemporary Freudian, humanistic-existential, and Jungian understanding of the development of object cathexes in early childhood, while much more concerned with social and cultural influences upon early personality development, has not rejected much traditional Freudian conceptualization of early object choice. Thus, the object relations framework, as presented, may be accused of placing a lopsided emphasis on the role of anatomy and the significance of the parent-child relationship in the development of object choice.

It would be the authors' stance, in this text's formulation of an object relations framework, to view early, anatomically related drives as one influence — neither most important nor insignificant — in the early characterization of object relationships. The germinal as well as continued impact of interaction with significant others as well as the influence of the broadest range of environmental "offerings" and demands would be especially significant in both the beginning of object choice and the inevitable changes in object choice throughout life.

3. As with any body of knowledge, there exists the danger in knowing just enough to be conversant as regards a theory and subsequently being led to believe that we know all that we need. We have been acquainted with students and long-time therapists who became quite fascinated with their encounter with elements of the "unconscious." However, haphazard dabbling with unconscious accoutrements, misguided efforts to analyze symbols, and the like lends itself to a great deal of useless interpretation and much misinterpretation and little in the way of helpful intervention. Further, there exists the danger that the therapist may get the notion that she somehow knows more about the patient than he knows about himself.

4. When humanistic principles are applied, there can be a tendency to view therapy as overly simplistic. Being warm and concerned about our patients is important, but just because this is achieved it does not mean that therapy has occurred. Unconditional positive regard is not viewed as desirable by all therapists, and it may be one of the most difficult postures to

achieve — yet it wears the guise of simplicity. Finding one's own place within this construct depends on experience and a maturing into the therapist role. Phony acceptance by the therapist of behaviors that she finds unacceptable confuses the patient and confounds the relationship.

5. The object relations use of interpretation and insight is most successful with patients who have a good functioning ego and a capacity for logical thinking. However, we must remember that even patients who present as more confused often have times when they are quite lucid, and they may well have more ability for insight than the treatment staff gives them credit for. Further, when insight is not the goal per se, the therapist's ability to understand conceptually the behavior she is seeing may make the behavior more meaningful and manageable for her and thereby may facilitate her ability to respond constructively. Attempts at empathic understanding and the communication of positive regard we feel are important with all patients.

The object relations framework as presented is an eclectic framework. As such, it is open to attack on a variety of grounds. As Patterson notes, eclecticism has been considered as undesirable because of its lack of direction, the inevitable "inconsistencies" in practice, and the difficulties in its examination through research (Patterson, 1973, p. 459). However, if one accepts that no one current theory or technique best fits each individual treated or each situation, one can seek to synthesize common compatible and workable constructs from a range of therapy approaches. Patterson cites the definition of eclecticism given by English and English in *A Comprehensive Dictionary of Psychological and Psychoanalytic Terms*:

"Eclecticism . . . in theoretical system building, the selection and orderly combination of compatible features from diverse sources, sometimes from incompatible theories and systems; the effort to find valid elements in all doctrines or theories and to combine them into a harmonious whole. The resulting system is open to constant revision even in its major outlines. . . . Eclecticism is to be distinguished from unsystematic and uncritical combinations, for which the name is syncretism. The eclectic seeks as much consistency as is currently possible, but he is unwilling to sacrifice conceptualizations that put meaning into a wide range of facts for the sake of what he is apt to think of as an unworkable overall systematization. The formalist finds the eclectic's position too loose and uncritical. For his part the ecelctic finds formalism and schools too dogmatic and rigid, too much inclined to reject if not facts, at least helpful conceptualizations of facts" (Patterson, 1973, p. 460).

The object relations framework for understanding man and his activity is an attempt at the kind of integration of which English and English speak. As we leave this model and move to the next, we will be confronted again and again with trends toward eclecticism in other theoretical frameworks. The reader is encouraged to be open-minded and journey with us.

End Notes

1. It is interesting to compare Freud's constructs of id-ego and conscious-unconscious to more recent studies of the lateralization of brain function. For the right-handed person, the left hemisphere is considered primarily (but not solely) responsible for the ability to verbalize, do

mathematics, think logically (that is, in terms of cause preceding an effect), and deal in ordinary time-space constructs. The right, or nondominant, hemisphere has more responsibility for the ability to intuit, to visualize, and to deal with affect. The right hemisphere lives in "timelessness," does not see events proceeding logically one before another, and is therefore "acausal." The reader is referred to *Psychology of Consciousness* by Robert E. Ornstein and *Left Brain, Right Brain* by Springer and Deutsch.

2. Freud saw the intrusive, sexual action of the male as prototypic of masculine activity: outgoing, aggressive, commanding. The female, whose sexual role or function was seen as "receptive," was, by extension, viewed as "feminine" when her behavior was "passive" and subservient to the male.

It is this conceptualization of social role as derived from sexual function — and a Victorian interpretation of function at that — that has led to some of the most severe criticism of Freud's psychology. Clearly, this belief that women needed to be passive if they were to be feminine influenced the field of psychology for decades and has since been challenged as an incomplete, biased understanding of the female (Dowling, 1981; Eichenbaum and Orbach, 1983).

3. The dualities discussed by Jung also correspond to the dualities suggested by split-brain studies. In the right handed person, the left or dominant hemisphere is seen to correspond to feelings of "light" and to a sense of masculinity, as well as the verbal-intellectual function, as was mentioned earlier. The right, nondominant hemisphere corresponds to a sense of "dark" or night, to feelings of feminity, as well as the acausal-intuitive function of perceiving and problem solving. Orstein makes the observation that various occupations tend to depend more on the function of one or the other hemisphere: "Many different occupations and disciplines involve one of the major modes of consciousness. Science and law are highly involved in linearity, duration and verbal logic. Crafts, the "mystical" disciplines, and music are more present-centered, aconceptual, intuitive" (Ornstein, 1972, p. 83).

4. The foundation for such "holism" may be found in the early works of the Gestalt psychologists, Wertheimer, Koffka, and Kohler, whose studies were focused on the study of visual perception and learning, and on the "organismic" theory of Kurt Goldstein (Goldstein, 1939, 1940). This is not to be confused with the writing of Perls and his "Gestalt therapy" (Perls, 1969).

5. While focusing on the "here and now" of the patient-therapist relationship may be reminiscent of the existential-humanistic mandates, the nature of the here-and-now interaction in the psychoanalytic process is quite different from that in the humanistic interaction. The psychoanalytic exchange is not the give and take, mutual sharing and disclosure by therapist and patient. Rather, it is a unidirectional interpretation by the analyst of the patient's behavior.

6. The manner in which a person drawing is handled is a reflection of the integrity of the concept of self as well as, more broadly, the development and integration of a "person" concept as applied to all persons. The ability to depict visually as well as talk about a

"person" advances predictably in a developmental sequence. The reader is referred to *Person Perception in Childhood and Adolescence* by W.J. Livesley and D.B. Bromley (1973).

References

Alexander F: Fundamentals of Psychoanalysis. New York, Norton, 1963.

Azima H, Azima F: Outline of a dynamic theory of occupational therapy. AJOT 8(5):215, 1959.

Baum C. Occupational therapists put care in the health system. AJOT 34(8):505-516, 1980.

Benjamin A: The Helping Interview. Boston, Houghton Mifflin Co., 1969.

Bernstein D: The female superego. Int J Psychoanal 64(2):187-201, 1983.

Blum H: Masochism, the ego ideal and the psychoanalysis of women.FI J Am Psychoanal Assoc 24:157-191, 1976.

Brickman A: Pre-oedipal development of the superego. Int J Psychoanal 64:83-91, 1983.

Busse E: Introduction to Part II, Geriatric Psychiatry. Psychiatry Update: The American Psychiatric Association Annual Review, Vol. II. Washington, DC, American Psychiatry Press, 1983, pp 83-87.

Campbell J (Ed): The Portable Jung. New York, Viking Press, 1971.

Cohn R: The Person Symbol in Clinical Medicine. Springfield, IL, Charles C Thomas, 1960.

Corey G: Theory and Practice of Counseling and Psychotherapy. Ed 2. Monterey, CA, Brooks/Cole, 1982.

Dowling C: The Cinderella Complex. New York, Simon and Schuster, 1981.

Eichenbaum L, Orbach S: Understanding Women — A Feminine Psychoanalytic Approach. New York, Basic Books, 1983.

Fidler G, Fidler J: Occupational Therapy — A Communication Process in Psychiatry. New York, Macmillan Co., 1963.

Fluegelman A (Ed): The New Games Book. New York, Dolphin Books/Doubleday and Co., 1976.

Freud S: Interpretation of Dreams (1900). (Translated by Brill AA) New York, Random House, 1950.

Freud S: Three essays on sexuality (1905). In Standard Edition of the Complete Psychological Works of Sigmund Freud. Vol. XII. (Translated under the general editorship of J. Strachey, in collaboration with Anna Freud, assisted by Starchey A, Tyson A). London, The Hogart Press, 1953, pp 135-243.

Gilfoyle E: Caring: A philosophy for practice. AJOT 34(8):517-521, 1980.

Goldstein K: The Organism. New York, American Book Co., 1939.

Goldstein K: Human Nature in the Light of Psychopathology. Cambridge, Harvard University Press, 1940.

Grinspoon L (Ed): Psychiatry Update: The American Psychiatric Association Annual

Review, Vol.III. Washington, DC, American Psychiatric Press, 1984.

Gruenbaum H, Glick I: The basics of family treatment. In Grinspoon L (Ed): Psychiatry Update: The American Psychiatric Association Annual Review, Vol. II. Washington, DC, American Psychiatric Press, 1983, pp 185-203.

Hales R, Frances A (Eds): Psychiatry Update: The American Psychiatric Association Annual Review, Vol.IV. Washington, DC, American Psychiatry Press, 1985.

Hall CS, Nordby V: Primer of Jungian Psychology. New York, New American Library, 1973.

Hall CS: Primer of Freudian Psychology. New York, New American Library, 1954.

Hammer E: The clinical application of projective drawings. In Rabin A: Projective Technique in Personality Assessment. New York, Springer Publishing Co., 1968.

Hemphill B: The Evaluative Process in Psychiatric Occupational Therapy. Thorofare, NJ, Charles B. Slack Inc., 1982.

Jourard S: The Transparent Self. Rev ed. New York, Van Nostrand Reinhold, 1971.

Jung C (Ed): Man and His Symbols. Garden City, NY, Doubleday and Co., Inc., 1979.

Jung C: The Portable Jung. Campbell J (Ed), New York, Penguin Books, 1971.

Kaplan H, Sadock B: Modern Synopsis of Psychiatry III. Baltimore, Williams and Wilkins, 1981.

Lerner H: Female dependency in context. Am J Orthopsychiatry 53(4):697-705, 1983.

Livesley W, Bromley DB: Person Perception in Childhood and Adolescence. London, John Wiley and Sons, Ltd., 1973.

Malone C: Family therapy and childhood disorders. In Grinspoon L (Ed): Psychiatry Update: The American Psychiatric Association Annual Review, Vol.II. Washington DC, American Psychiatric Press, 1983, pp 228-241.

Maslow A: Toward a Psychology of Being. Rev ed. New York, Van Nostrand, 1968.

Maslow A: The Farther Reaches of Human Nature: An Esalen Book. New York, Viking Press Inc., 1971.

May R: The Meaning of Anxiety. New York, Ronald Press, 1950.

May R: Man's Search for Himself. New York, Norton, 1953 (Also New York, New American Library, 1967).

May R: Love and Will. New York, Norton, 1969 (Also New York, Delta Books, 1973).

McFarlane W, et al.: New developments in the family treatment of psychotic disorders. In Grinspoon L (Ed): Psychiatry Update: The American Psychiatric Association Annual Review, Vol. II. Washington, DC, American Psychiatric Press, 1983, pp 242-256.

Michels R: Contemporary psychoanalytic views of interpretation. In Grinspoon L (Ed): Psychiatry Update: The American Psychiatric Association Annual Review, Vol. II. Washington, DC, American Psychiatric Press, 1983.

Money J, Ehrhardt A: Man and Woman, Boy and Girl. Baltimore, John Hopkins University Press, 1972.

Mosey A: Three Frames of Reference in Mental Health. Thorofare, NJ, Charles B. Slack Inc., 1970.

Moustakas C: The Self: Exploration in Personal Growth. New York, Harper, 1956.

Moustakas C: Loneliness. Englewood Cliffs, NJ, Prentice-Hall, 1961.

Notman M, Nadelson C (Eds): The Woman Patient: Aggression, Adaptations and Psychotherapy, Vol. 3. New York, Plenum Press, 1982.

Ornstein R: Psychology of Consciousness. New York, Penguin Books, 1973.

Patterson CH: Theories of Counseling and Psychotherapy. New York, Harper and Row, 1973.

Perls F: Gestalt Therapy Verbatum. Moab, UT, Real People Press, 1969.

Person E: The influence of values in psychoanalysis: The case of female psychology. In Grinspoon L (Ed): Psychiatry Update, The American Psychiatric Association Annual Review, Vol. II. Washington DC, American Psychiatric Press, 1983, pp 36-50.

Rhyne J: The Gestalt Art Experience. Monterey, CA, Brooks/Cole, 1973.

Rogers C: Client-Centered Therapy. Boston, Houghton-Mifflin, 1951.

Rogers C: On Becoming a Person. Boston, Houghton-Mifflin, 1961.

Sadler A: Psychoanalysis in later life: Problems in the psychoanalysis of an aging narcissistic patient. J Geriatr Psychiatry 11(1):5, 1978.

Sheehy G: Passages: Predictable Crises of Adult Life. New York, E. P. Dutton and Co., 1976.

Sloane R: Organic mental disorders. In Grinspoon L (Ed): Psychiatry Update: The American Psychiatric Association Annual Review, Vol. II. Washington, DC, American Psychiatric Press, 1983.

Springer S, Deutsch D: Left Brain, Right Brain. San Francisco, W .H. Freeman and Co., 1981.

Stafford-Clark D: What Freud Really Said. Excerpt from Freud S: An Outline of Psychoanalysis, Vol. 23 (1939), New York, Schocken Books, 1966.

Stoller R: Sex and Gender. New York, Science House, 1968.

Yalom I: The Theory and Practice of Group Psychotherapy. Ed 2. New York, Basic Books, 1975.

Yerxa E: Authentic occupational therapy. AJOT 21(1):1-9, 1967.

Yerxa E: The philosophical base of occupational therapy. In Occupational Therapy: 2001 A.D. Rockville, MD, American Occupational Therapy Association, 1978.

Zukav G: The Dancing Wu Li Masters: An Overview of the New Physics. New York, Bantam Books, 1980.

Chapter 4

The Behavioral Frame of Reference

The behavioral frame of reference is based upon experimental inquiry and principles of cognitive, social, and conditioned learning theories. Within the context of a therapeutic relationship these principles are systematically applied to develop behavioral techniques and procedures that bring about behavior change. Therapy within the behavioral frame is concerned with behavioral problems, and is not concerned primarily with feelings, past history, or the development of insight. Human maladjustment is seen as the result of faulty learning; no disease process is implied. The techniques and procedures utilize "action oriented" experiences to teach, model, shape, and/or reinforce adaptive behavior during the therapeutic-learning process. The therapist and patient actively participate in a learning process that develops the adaptive behaviors necessary for activities of daily living, work, and leisure. Through patient-environment-therapist interactions, activities of daily living, work, and leisure skills are learned and are evident through overt behaviors which can be observed and measured in occupational therapy and in the patient's natural environment.

Theoretical Development

Since the late 1960's occupational therapists who work in mental health (Ogburn et al., 1972; Christiansen et al., 1974; Jodrell et al. 1975; Watts et al., 1976), physical medicine (Kuhulka et al., 1975; Greenberg and Fowler, 1980; Agnew and Shannon, 1981; Talbot and Junkala, 1981), and developmental delay (Lemke and Mitchell, 1972; Leibowitz et al., 1974; Mann and Sobsey, 1975; Ford, 1975; Clark et al., 1978; Wehman and Marchant, 1978; Weber,

1978) have documented the efficacy of the behavioral approach in occupational therapy. There is also literature that is not applied to any specialty area of practice (Stein, 1982; Sieg, 1974; Wanderer, 1974; Norman, 1976). Originally the approaches used in occupational therapy were derived from principles of conditioned learning. Now the behavioral approach in occupational therapy incorporates cognitive, social, and operant learning theory, although cognitive-behaviorists tend to view themselves as being in a "different camp" from traditional behaviorists (discussed in Chapter VI, Cognitive-Behavioral Frame of Reference).

Therapists who have written about the theoretical basis for behavioral occupational therapy include Karen Diasio (1968), Ann Mosey (1970, 1973, 1981), and Trombly and Scott (1984). Additionally, there are many psychologists, counselors, and scientists who have contributed to the theory and development of behavioral therapy. Those most frequently cited in the occupational therapy literature include Robert White, Thomas Clayton, Hilgard, Bower, Hartmann, Rapaport, Tolman, Alexander, Bandura, Skinner, Wolpe, Dollard and Miller, Goldfried and Davidson, Lieberman and Spiegler, Azigan, Bakker, and Armstrong. While each behaviorist offers a differing explanation of learning and the application of learning theory to therapy, the student would be advised to view each interpretation as differing mainly in emphasis. There exist many elements of behavioral theory that are held in common, and it is those that we will synthesize and summarize. Such a summary lacks the individual flavor of behaviorism given by individual contributors. The interested reader is referred to works by Hilgard and Bower (1975) and Kafner and Phillips (1970) for comprehensive reviews of a broad range of behavioral theory. For a straightforward discussion of the application of behavior theory in practice, we recommend G.L. Martin's *Behavior Modification* (1978).

How Learning Occurs

All behavior, both adaptive and maladaptive, not attributable to physical maturation or "accident," is learned, and behavioral therapy rests upon the assumptions of learning theory (see note 1). When an organism "learns," certain factors come into play: the organism (for our discussion we will use the word "person"), his capacity, intelligence, and bodily functions; the drive or motives that impel him to act; the thoughts, perceptions, and feelings of the person; the situation or setting in which the person finds himself; and the response or behavior that is present, as well as the behavior that is desired. Of the foregoing, much is internal and must be inferred (i.e., intelligence, motives, feelings, thoughts, and tolerance of change) . Even when these can be described or verbalized, they are not external and measurable as such. The setting and the existent and desired behavior or response(s) can be seen and measured, and it is these that define learning (see note 2). Although a setting typically consists of many sights and sounds, we will here speak of setting in its most basic sense, a single *stimulus*. Similarly, most behavior is very complex, but we will refer for a moment to the most elemental behavior, a single *response*. When a new stimulus brings about or elicits a given response (one that already has been demonstrated), or when a given stimulus brings about a new response, learning is said to occur. For example, yesterday a child could climb only the stairs from his basement; today he was able to climb the stairs to his attic. Or yesterday, confronted with any of the stairs in his home, the child could only crawl up them. Today, confronted with these stairs, he walked up them for the first time. In both cases, learning took place. When a given stimulus consistently evokes a given response, we say that an association has been made between them; in every day behavior, such an asssociation may also be termed a habit.

Classical Conditioning

According to behavioral inquiry there are several ways in which learning occurs. The first to be discussed is called *classical* (or *respondent*) *conditioning*. In classical conditioning a new stimulus becomes capable of evoking a given response because the new stimulus is presented together with a stimulus that already evokes the response. For example, eating a bit of lemon will cause a person's mouth to pucker. This puckering is a natural autonomic response and does not need to be learned. Most often, a person tasting a lemon will also be seeing the lemon, and in very short time just the sight of a lemon, without any necessity for tasting, will elicit the puckering response. In order for this kind of learning to occur, the two stimuli (taste of lemon, sight of lemon) need to be presented at virtually the same time, or in what is termed *close temporal contiguity*. If the lemon were shown visually over an extended period of time but not tasted, the tendency of the sight of the lemon to elicit puckering would diminish until it had become eliminated or extinguished, via a process called *spontaneous recovery*.

Classical conditioning most often has been carried out in relationship to autonomic body functions. As such, its application to therapy might seem limited. However, there are further apsects of classical conditioning that have important implications in learning. Learning occurs in classical conditioning (and in operant conditioning, which will be discussed) in part because of stimulus and response generalization. For example, if the sight of an actual lemon makes your mouth pucker, a photograph of a lemon or perhaps a plastic facsimile may also. This is the result of *stimulus generalization*. Stimuli that look (or sound, or taste) alike become capable of eliciting a given response. For instance, most newborn and young infants attach quickly to the mother and have a positive response (e.g., body relaxation) when the mother holds them. It is quite typical for young infants to respond more positively to other women than to males because females are more like the mother; this is due to a series of stimulus generalizations. Similarly, a patient may respond to you, as a therapist, much as he does to "Mom" because of stimulus generalization. In *response generalization,* two or more responses are evoked by the same stimulus, because these responses occur in close temporal contiguity, or because the two responses are perceived as similar. For example, we may learn to say "thank you" upon being given a present, or we may, upon being given a gift, shorten our response to "thanks." Or, as may occur in treatment, when an individual builds specified social skills in the clinic setting (learning to say "please," waiting to take his turn), frequently other social skills that were not targeted for improvement end up improving also. This type of response generalization is often complex and therefore difficult to specify, yet plays a significant role in everyday learning (G.L. Martin, 1978, p. 173).

Stimulus and response generalizations are most likely to occur when the stimuli look or act similarly, and when the responses are very similar or occur in close temporal contiguity. Through an infinite number of response and stimulus generalizations, the stimuli that become capable of evoking a given response may become very different, and the repertoire of responses that may be elicited by a given stimulus becomes vast. It is because of this generalization in learning that we do not need to relearn how to drive a car every time we purchase a new automobile, nor do we have to relearn how to button our clothes every time we change our shirts.

The ability to generalize learning depends on the ability of the person to recognize the similarities in a variety of situations and behaviors and to respond to those similarities. The occupational therapist will use this principle when she plans learning experiences. The more similarities that exist between two or more environments, the more likely it becomes that the individual can perceive and respond to these similarities, and the more vivid the similarities, the greater the likelihood of generalization. Therefore, the therapist often creates a learning structure in which multisensory stimuli are used, and in which similarities between the learning and natural environment are amplified.

Operant Conditioning

B. F. Skinner focused his attention on the role of reward or *reinforcement* in learning and described the process known as *operant (or instrumental) conditioning* (1938, 1953, 1968, 1971). Skinner looked first at the behavior or response that was in evidence. When the reponse was a desirable one, it was rewarded, or reinforced.

When the response was reinforced in the presence of one stimulus but not in the presence of another, the response tended to occur in the presence of the former and not the latter. The former stimulus, called a *discriminating stimulus,* was said to act as a *cue*, telling the person when to emit the response. If the stimulus and response were paired repeatedly, but without the reward, the response ceased, and *extinction* was said to have occurred.

To illustrate, a patient might have difficulty in asking for help and making his needs known to others. As a goal of treatment, he might agree to come to your desk and ask for assistance when needed. You would wait for the patient to come and ask for help; when he succeeds, you might smile and say, "I'll be glad to help you" (reinforcement). If the patient approached you while you were away from your desk, helping someone else in the clinic, you would ignore his evocation (no reinforcement). Seeing you at your desk is his cue that he should come and ask for help. In this case, the cue has two parts (you are alone and you are at your desk), and two responses are desired (approaching you and asking for help). Being able to perceive the difference between your being at your desk and your being elsewhere in the clinic is the basis for *discrimination*. Discriminatory behavior is the opposite of generalization. It depends on being able to see the differences between situations or settings, thereby enabling the individual to determine when a behavior is appropriate and when it is not. It is because of many stimulus and response discriminations that we know that it is appropriate to act differently in a movie theater and during church prayer.

It is easier to discriminate between gross or obvious differences in stimuli than between subtle differences. For example, the junctions of most busy streets utilize discriminating stimuli designed to be noticed; these are the red and green traffic signals that cue our traffic behaviors. However, discriminating among subtle differences in stimuli makes possible the execution of highly skilled motor and social acts. If, for instance, an individual is adept at perceiving slight changes in the voice or nonverbal behaviors of his peers (and he can respond accordingly), we might tend to say that this individual is "sensitive" or "gracious." If he fails to take notice of such changes, he might be considered to be "insensitive," "crude," or a "boor." Or we might say that this individual needs to be "hit over the head before he gets the message."

In the object-relations framework, the power of discrimination would be considered an ego function. From the behavioral stance, in order for effective and adaptive discrimination to be learned, there must be appropriate giving and withholding of reinforcement according to the situation, and the individual must be able to perceive differences in stimuli and cues.

The occupational therapist would be aware of her role in the therapeutic milieu in relation to (1) seeing to it that only properly discriminated behavior is supported and (2) making certain that the individual perceives the differences between given stimuli. In regard to this second aim she might direct the patient's attention to the discriminating features of a setting and/or amplify the differences between settings.

Kinds of Reinforcement

Skinner defined reinforcement as anything that increased the likelihood that a behavior would recur. (For our discussion in this chapter we will speak primarily of "positive" reinforcement, although some behavior therapists utilize also what they refer to as "negative" reinforcement; see note 3.) A significant role of the therapist in planning to use operant conditioning is to identify what in the environment serves to reinforce, and therefore maintain, specific patient behaviors, both adaptive and maladaptive.

While one tends to hear of certain types of reinforcers quite frequently (e.g., attention, hugs, tokens, material goods), there are five categories of reinforcement suggested by G.L. Martin (1978, p. 22) that seem especially helpful to consider in planning a behavioral occupational therapy program. Combined by us into three broad categories, these are consumable reinforcers, social reinforcers, and activity reinforcers. *Consumable reinforcers* are those such as candy, cigarettes, fruit snacks, and coffee. *Social reinforcers* include any signs of attention, hugs, smiles, pats on the back, verbal praise, and so on. *Activity reinforcers* cover a broad range and may require some diligence on the part of the therapist and patient to identify. These include the opportunity to engage in a favored activity, e.g., to tinker with one's car, to ride a bike, to read a book, to spend time alone, to engage with media in an art or craft form, to go shopping. Activity reinforcers, as we conceive them, also include the ability to wear one's favorite shirt, to hold a favored toy, or to sit in one's favorite chair. (These activities are referred to as possessional reinforcers by Martin.)

Schedules of Reinforcement

In actual day to day living, environmental goods and opportunities are reinforcing to the individual, in part because they are not constantly available. For instance, food is rewarding because we have times of abstinence, and our hunger ensues. Reading a book may be reinforcing because it represents a diversion from a more exacting or work related task. We function in a world where we are not flooded with reinforcement yet where we are reinforced often enough that given behaviors are encouraged.

In therapy, reinforcement is supplied according to what is termed a *schedule* of reinforcement. If behavior is reinforced every time it occurs, there exists *continuous reinforcement*. If it occurs following a given number of correct responses (as in every third or fourth time the behavior is exhibited), there exists a *fixed ratio* of reinforcement. If behavior is reinforced at a consistent interval of time (as every 10 minutes), there exists a *fixed interval* of reinforcement. There exist also variable (unpredictable) ratios and intervals of reinforcement and complex combinations of ratios and intervals. When a new behavior is being learned, the individual may need continuous reinforcement. This is exemplified in occupational therapy when the therapist acknowledges the patient's achievement of splinter skills or performance of the desired behavior by giving verbal praise or attention, or candy or tokens.

Over a period of time in therapy the patient is usually weaned to less frequent reinforcement. *Intermittent reinforcement* is that in which behavior is reinforced only occasionally. If a behavior is maintained by reinforcement that is both intermittent and unpredictable, this behavior is the most difficult to extinguish, and therefore most stable.

We can illustrate this, for example, by the behavior some may exhibit when hoping for a phone call from a new "romantic" interest. If we expect a call from our would-be date, we may stay near the phone for many nights, hoping for a call. If he or she calls only once in a week's time, that may be enough to keep us at home waiting for many more days, since there exists the chance that this person will call again. If, however, no such call has ever been received (no reinforcement), we would typically stop waiting around for the call within a relatively short time.

It is difficult to determine how often an individual will need to be rewarded in order for a specified desired behavior to occur. For instance, one employee may require a great deal of recognition and "pats on the back" from his employer to maintain a higher level of output; another might find only a yearly brief "Thanks for a good job" adequate reinforcement. The extent to which each of us needs external and/or carefully planned reinforcement from outside sources, of course, is related to the extent that we achieve self-satisfaction from our own behavior.

In addition to what has already been discussed, behavioral scientists have learned the following about reinforcement, which may be especially useful to the therapist planning to use operant conditioning:

1. An agent or event will be particularly reinforcing if one has been deprived of it, at least for a brief time. Therefore, food will be more rewarding in the clinic setting if the patient has not just finished lunch; being able to work on a fine-motor craft will be more satisfying if the patient has not been working a similar task prior to occupational therapy. Even smiles and praise, when available in excess, tend to lose their capacity to be rewarding. (When an agent or activity is no longer experienced as reinforcing because the patient has "had enough," *satiation* is said to have occurred, and an alternative reinforcement must be utilized.)

2. An individual should be reinforced immediately following a desired behavior in order for the correct response-reinforcement association to be made.

3. By providing verbalization along with the reinforcement, we can through the principle of stimulus generalization make the verbalization alone a reinforcement. For instance, when a patient is on time for his therapy five days in succession, he may "earn" the right to take a walk to a local shopping mall, unattended. If, when informing him of his "reward," the therapist adds enthusiastically, "I'm really proud of you, and I'll bet you feel good too!" her praise has been coupled with the earned walk. If this association is repeated many times, her praise alone may eventually be adequate reinforcement for the patient to maintain promptness.

4. The thoughts or internal statements that an individual tells himself may act as stimuli for action, as cues telling him when to act, as drives impelling actions, as responses, and as reinforcement.

5. Behavior that depends solely on external reward for its maintenance is precarious behavior, for reinforcement may be removed by others, without recourse by the individual. The most stable behavior is that in which personal satisfaction (e.g., living up to one's standards) is the most durable reinforcement.

Reinforcement is the term used most typically to describe the positive consequences that follow a given behavior. When an individual consistently demonstrates a behavior (regardless of whether it is behavior he has consciously thought about) as a consequence of a specified reinforcement, learning is said to have occurred. Behavior may also be followed by a consequence that is not positive. One instance of this is referred to as punishment.

Punishment

Punishment occurs when a given behavior is followed by an adverse stimulus that cannot be escaped or avoided. Punishment has been shown to suppress behavior but not to extinguish it. There is no change in learning. For example, if the therapist criticizes a patient for interrupting a conversation, she may, for the time being, stop the behavior. However, no new response has been associated with the situation. There is instead a behavioral vacuum. It has been shown that behavior stopped in this fashion is likely to reappear. Further, the therapist has to deal with the possibility that she has fostered negative feelings from the patient about the therapy setting and/or the therapist. If instead, an undesirable response is ignored (neither positive nor negative reinforcement follows) and positive reinforcement is withheld until the desired response occurs, a pattern of desired behavior is more likely to be achieved. Punishment may be useful insofar as it interrupts an undesirable behavior, thereby providing an opportunity for some alternative (desirable) behavior to be exhibited. The key is that the undesirable behavior is not merely suppressed, but that an adaptive behavior takes its place and is rewarded.

Both reinforcement and punishment can be used when an individual has shown that he is capable of a specified behavior. When a desired, adaptive response appears not to be in the patient's behavior repertoire, other behavioral techniques may be used. They include shaping, building chains of behavior, and modeling.

Shaping

If, as in a previous illustration, the desired behavior of asking the therapist's assistance is not demonstrated, shaping techniques could be used. In *shaping,* any action that is similar to or preliminary to the desired behavior is reinforced, as are successive actions that more closely approximate or lead to the desired response. If, for example, our patient did not succeed initially in approaching your desk and asking for help, you might watch to see whether he arose from his seat or even just looked your way. Then you might choose to reinforce this anticipatory behavior, and continue to reinforce subsequent behavior (e.g., with smiles) that brought him closer to you. While utilizing the principle of shaping, the therapist would also be careful to not reinforce any maladaptive responses.

When using shaping as part of her behavior program, the therapist must begin with a behavior of which the patient is capable, and be prepared to reinforce rather small steps toward the final, desired goal. G.L. Martin (1978, pp. 58-59) suggests that the therapist begin by making her own list of the approximate steps that will lead from the beginning to the final behavior. It should be understood that each step in the sequence might have to be repeated and reinforced many times before the therapist can expect the next step in the sequence to be exhibited. In other instances, however, several steps might follow in quick succession.

Building Chains of Behavior

Skinner believed that most complex behavior can be understood as chains of stimulus-response connections, links in which a completed response acts as a stimulus signaling that it is time for the next in the series of responses. One might consider the steps in the process of planting a flower garden. We see the seedlings at the store, which signals us that it is time for a planting, which cues us to collect our tools (and other paraphernalia), which leads us to select a potential site for planting, which when chosen cues us to begin digging a hole, and so on. In fact, each of these primary steps in itself consists of even smaller, discrete stimulus-response links.

When we think about learning, we tend to conceive of developing learning chains in a forward order. Frequently in therapy, however, *backward chaining* is used. The term backward chaining might seem to imply that the individual is taught to do a procedure backwards, but that is not the case (G.L. Martin, 1978, p. 149). If we return to the example of planting a seedling, backward chaining, and its potential advantage, can be illustrated.

Suppose for a moment that you are teaching a young child (or someone who has a short attention span) the procedures just indicated. By the time you have helped him select tools, choose a planting site, and dig a hole, he may have lost interest in completing the process. The most rewarding part of planting is, for most, seeing the young plant standing upright firmly in the ground. If, as one often does with a young child, we prepare the ground and call the child over to put the plant in the hole, or just ask him to cover the roots of the plant with dirt, the child begins with the final step and immediately gains the reward of seeing the plant in the ground. After helping us with several plants in this manner, the child may express the wish to help "dig the holes." In that case, we might start the hole for the child so that not too much digging is needed and then let him finish the digging, insert the plant, and cover its roots with soil. As the child becomes more interested and better able to persevere, we continue to add steps in a backward chain, always allowing him to move from the chosen step through the subsequent steps he has already learned, to the last step — and the reinforcement. Thus, the final reward comes to sustain a long series of stimulus-response links.

As with shaping, the therapist may find it useful to make a list of the approximate steps taken from start to finish in a given process. She then starts with the last step and upon its completion provides a suitable reinforcement. Then she proceeds backward down the chain, giving the patient ample opportunity to practice each step or series of steps, as needed, before trying to add a new stimulus-response link.

Modeling

One hears a great deal about the significance of the therapist as a "role model." In terms of learning theory, modeling has been better understood largely as a result of the investigation of Albert Bandura (Bandura, 1963, 1971). Bandura, along with such others as Mischel (1973, 1968) and Rotter (1954), has proposed a social learning theory that attempts not only to incorporate the traditional reinforcement and contiguity elements of behavioral theory, but to add to these the significance of imitation in learning. Bandura and his associates believe that when a person observes the actions of another, he can learn "vicariously" a new behavior which he can later demonstrate through imitation. Much learning appears to be accomplished more easily by imitation than through the development of stimulus-response chains or the shaping of behavior.

For example, when an individual wishes to learn to swing a golf club correctly, he often imitates his teacher. Learning new words, learning to drive a car, learning to play baseball — all these can be viewed as highly imitative forms of learning. There is nothing in this concept that is new to most occupational therapists, who have long known the value of demonstration and imitation when trying to teach new skills. However, modeling needs to be understood as being quite different conceptually from other aspects of learning theory, for the modeled behavior is conceived of as having been "learned" internally and vicariously before any actual response has been demonstrated or rewarded. There are significant aspects of modeling highlighted by the study of Bandura that can be considered by the occupational therapist who seeks to be more cognizant of the impact she may have as a model (condensed from Hilgard and Bower, 1975, pp. 601-605):

1. A person is more likely to be imitated if he is perceived as having high status; thus a therapist (typically viewed by patients as having status) has a potentially significant impact as a social model.

2. A person is more likely to be imitated if the observor can see the similarities between himself and the model.

3. An individual will more likely imitate behavior he perceives as leading to reward (this may occur when he sees the model receiving a reward); likewise, he is more likely to inhibit a response he perceives as leading to a punishment (as when the model is seen being punished).

4. Hostility, aggression, and moral behavior have all been shown to be highly accessible in learning through modeling.

5. In order to be successfully imitated, the model behavior must be well attended to. Distraction in the learning setting can be expected to decrease imitative learning.

6. Many skilled acts, especially those involving fine-motor coordination, can be learned only in part through modeling; participation and practice are necessary adjuncts to learning.

7. When the individual can give verbal labels or descriptions to the behavior he is observing, that behavior is more successfully remembered and imitated.

Bandura and other social learning proponents differ from traditional behaviorists with their inclusion of such concepts as *vicarious learning*, *symbolic representation*, *imagery*, and *cognitive problem solving*. Social learning has become an increasingly significant part of behavioral theory, and also with cognitive-behaviorism appears to represent the direction of much recent behavioral inquiry. More of Bandura's theory and cognitive-behavioral approaches will be discussed in Chapter VI, Cognitive-Behavioral Frame of Reference.

Token Economies

Token economies are systems of operant conditioning designed to alter behavior with several or more individuals, especially when internal and/or intangible reinforcements (e.g., social approval) have not proven effective. Tokens, which can be metal washers, plastic discs, credit cards that can be punched, and the like, are tangible rewards, given for appropriate designated behavior. They can be exchanged for privileges, cigarettes, candy, involvment in desired activities, and other desired outcomes. For example, if a hospitalized patient makes his bed, he might receive three tokens; if he completes an occupational therapy project, he receives five tokens. A candy bar might "cost" three tokens; a pass home might cost 20 tokens. While some token economies use only positive reinforcement, others use negative procedures as well; e.g., "fines" (tokens given back) are assessed when a patient fails to meet a requirement. As noted by Corey, tokens can have several advantages, some of which include:

1. Tokens reduce the delay between appropriate behavior and its reward.

2. Tokens can be used as a concrete measure of motivation.

3. There is an element of choice in that the person has an opportunity to decide how he wishes to spend his tokens (Corey, 1982, p. 135).

During the 1960's and 1970's there was a proliferation of token economies, especially to deal with the long term "chronic" patient, the developmentally delayed person, and the person in a forensic setting. Some major and positive outcomes were seen in the ability to affect behavior, teach new skills to those who up until then had seemed "unteachable," and manage large populations more effectively. As journals cited cases in which bizarre behavior was improved dramatically (Overbaugh and Bucher, 1970; Ogburn, 1972), token economies and the concomitant strict observance of operant behaviorism were tauted as breakthroughs in mental health care. However, since this time, many difficulties have come to light. The Overbaugh and Bucher article is cited to exemplify an area of concern. In their article, Overbaugh and Bucher describe a patient who had been in treatment for 45 years, yet continued to respond with little in the way of appropriate behavior. The decision was made by the treatment team to apply a rigorous token system. As the authors state: "Throughout the therapy, the patient was on a deprivation schedule. He received no breakfast at any time during the study and received cigarettes only from the therapist. Receipt of tokens redeemable for the noon and evening meals was contingent on meeting each day's global performance criterion (quality and quantity)" (Overbaugh and Bucher, 1970, p. 424).

The authors go on to say that in a short time the patient exhibited markedly improved behavior and was more manageable within the institution.

The ethics of depriving an individual of such a basic need as food is at issue — even for what is described as a "short period" and for positive intent. In 1962, President Kennedy outlined a Consumer's Bill of Rights, which provided for the consumer's right to safety, right to be informed, right to choose, and right to be heard. Since that time, patients and clients have been viewed increasingly as "consumers," and certainly these rights extend to them also. However, persons in institutions, especially those involuntarily committed, often have not received treatment sensitive to patients' rights. In 1972, the court decision of *Wyatt vs. Stickney* represented a significant move toward increased specificity as regards patient rights. As part of the resolution of this case, the court (assisted by the American Civil Liberties Union, the American Orthopsychiatric Association, the American Psychological Association, and the American Association of Mental Deficiency) specified in detail rights for those individuals who were under involuntary commitment, to include: the right to privacy, the right to wear one's own clothes, the right to have personal possessions, the right to regular physical exercise, the right to be outdoors from time to time, the right to nutritionally adequate meals, and the right to the "least restrictive conditions necessary to achieve the purposes of treatment" (Geiser, 1976, p. 42). These are absolute rights and cannot be made contingent on a token economy or other treatment system. Certainly one can operate a token economy without depriving individuals of their basic rights, but the kind of things spelled out in the *Wyatt* decision tended to be in the areas in which reinforcement was identified in many of the token systems until that time.

Finding effective reinforcements for very regressed and uncommunicative or uncooperative patients can be very difficult. This problem has been addressed by Lorna Jean King (1974), who noted that many institutionalized patients suffered from *anhedonia*, or the inability to experience pleasure from the kinds of everyday events most of us find pleasurable. There is no way of knowing the degree to which *Wyatt vs. Stickney* has moderated treatment in token economies, especially given that the involuntarily committed individual's rights tend not to be championed. However, with concern for human dignity, we need always to be concerned with the rights of all whom we encounter.

There have been other factors considered as token economies are followed up through time. There has been no clear evidence that the gains made within a token system are sustained once the individual returns home (or to a nontreatment setting) (Martin, M., 1972, p. 292.). While token economies do seem capable of managing behavior within an institution, they are not the panacea for behavioral change that they were once conceived to be.

Desensitization

Since the late 1950's systematic desensitization has been used as a behavioral strategy to reduce anxiety. Although the reasons for its effectiveness are not entirely understood, persons with test anxiety, speech anxiety, interpersonal-social anxiety, stuttering, and phobias have been successfully treated by desensitization (Cormier and Cormier, 1979, p. 430). After identifying the source of fear or anxiety, the patient participates in experiences which help him to gradually get comfortable with the situation. The anxiety provoking stimulus is presented in a series of graded experiences which proceed from low intensity to high intensity. The graded experience may incorporate imagery, role playing, simulated activities, homework, or real situations (inside or outside the treatment setting) which stimulate fear and anxiety (Cormier and Cormier, 1979).

Biofeedback

Biofeedback emerged from behavior-learning theory, which seeks to shape and control behavior in a controlled environment with immediate rewards, and from advances in technology, which promote the use of electronic equipment during the evaluation and treatment process. Biofeedback is "a process of using equipment (usually electronic) to reveal to human beings some of their internal physiological events, normal and abnormal, in the form of visual and auditory signals to teach them to influence these otherwise involuntary or unfelt events by manipulating the displayed signals" (Abildness, 1982, p. 8). The signals that the patient receives may act as stimuli (or cues) and as reinforcement.

Biofeedback has been applied by occupational therapists and other professionals in physical medicine and mental health treatment settings. In rehabilitation settings biofeedback can be used for physical reconditioning, muscle re-education, increasing motor control and coordination, and strengthening muscles. Also in physical medicine settings it is used to monitor heart rate, visceral activities, blood pressure, and skin temperature. It has been used in pain management programs and with psychosomatic conditions such as tension and migraine headaches and fecal incontinence (Albildness, 1982).

In mental health practice biofeedback more frequently is applied to promote relaxation and manage stress. It has also been successful in helping patients manage symptoms that are an outcome of neurotic disorders, phobic reactions, depression, drug addiction, schizophrenia, and character disorder (Albildness, 1982).

In occupational therapy, biofeedback is used in conjunction with activities and is integrated with the application of other major theoretical treatment approaches such as biomechanical, neurodevelopmental, rehabilitation, psychodynamic, and sensory integrative approaches. During evaluation and treatment, biofeedback is given regarding the effects of the occupational therapy activity on the individual . Patients have been monitored during group projects, home activities, social experiences, work projects, and community outings. This feedback is used to teach the patient self-control, to change intervention strategies, and to document progress (Albildness, 1982).

Difference Between Feeling-Oriented and Behavioral Approaches

Before proceeding, we will pause to illustrate the difference between a feeling-oriented approach to understanding and treating psychosocial difficulties, and a behavioral approach.

One can take as an example the common difficulty of "sadness" or depression. The feeling-oriented therapist might note that the individual who identifies himself as "depressed" has poor self-esteem; that he feels "helpless"; that he has poor social relationships, lacks confidence in tasks, and feels that others do not approve of him; and that he does not approve of himself. The feeling-oriented therapist might try to understand and help the person understand when these feelings began and how they were experienced. The therapist might help the patient become aware of the ways in which significant relationships influenced his feelings about himself and others. The therapist would provide a relationship in which the patient felt warmly and positively regarded, without condition, and she would seek to understand the internal experiences of this patient. She would want her patient to know that he could express sadness without reprisal, and frequently the expression of sadness would be encouraged, based upon the belief that such expression was a pressing need and would result in therapeutic gain. The therapist would try to make available experiences in which the person could try out a variety of new ways of relating, without fear of failure. The patient would be encouraged to understand and explore his own interests, beliefs, and values and to behave in a manner that was not only socially acceptable but in which he was consistent, "real," and in tune with his inner voice.

The behavioral therapist would not be primarily concerned about how the depression began, historically, but would identify those behaviors that were associated with the individual's depression. These might include the inability to carry out everyday tasks, a reduction in social interaction, crying and/or fatigue, concerns expressed regarding health, self-deprecating statements, and changes in grooming, eating, sleeping, and other aspects of self-care. The therapist would try to identify current environmental factors that tended to sustain the sad behaviors, e.g., attention from a concerned spouse or other patients. She might note that the more depressed the patient became, the more his behavior(s) tended to reaffirm the negative feelings he had about himself; i.e., the more he withdrew from social contact, the fewer positive interactions he had with others, thus affirming his belief that "no one likes me."

The therapist would seek to reverse this process. She would be concerned about encouraging expressions of sadness, because the attention to sadness would be a positive reinforcement for an undesired behavior. Rather, she would try to help the patient identify some activity in which he received pleasure and/or felt positive about himself; concurrently, she would identify what in the environment would reinforce positive behaviors. She would try to elicit from him a commitment to engage in a specified activity in which he could learn new skills that would ultimately be more successful for him.

For example, she might involve him in a patient group in which he would be positively reinforced for assertive behaviors. Or she might seek to engage him in an activity that he found pleasurable. To help ensure a successful outcome, she would (when necessary) break the activity into discrete, achievable units in which success was discernable by him, and which would lead to accomplishment of the larger goal. When the patient's depression tended to cause him to withdraw or be minimally communicative, the therapist would attend to and reinforce any behavior, however slight, that represented a step toward appropriate involvment while simultaneously assuring that withdrawal behavior was not reinforced. Achievement of treatment goals would be measured by the increase in patient participation, the reduction of depressive behaviors, and the increase in behaviors identified as pleasurable, socially acceptable, and indicative of increased competency.

Current Practice in Occupational Therapy

The Person and Behavior

From 1940 through the 1960'S the deterministic view of behavior predominated. This view was seen as "radical" (Corey, 1978, p. ll9) because it saw man as limited in the ability to actively choose and learn. The early behaviorists, operating on Skinner's behavioral theory, believed that virtually all behavior was determined and therefore controlled by the introduction and maintenance of reinforcement (Skinner, 1971). The persons who controlled reinforcement were viewed as those in charge, and the concept of "free will" was challenged. Since the late 1960's and up to the present, the behavioral view has incorporated cognitive and social learning theories, which consider man to be both the product and the producer of his environment.

Man's essence is neither good nor bad. Whether behavior is considered *adaptive* or *maladaptive* depends on the degree to which it conforms to societal norms. Man is believed to be motivated by basic biologic drives, i.e., the need for food, sex, and the avoidance of pain, as well as the secondary needs for love and approval and other social needs. Fear and anxiety are considered important learned motivators. Thoughts, words, and memory are believed to become associated with and therefore to mediate between motive, stimulus, and response and may act as cues, helping to define where, when, and how behavior should occur. Thoughts and words may also become associated with and act as rewards or reinforcement (Dollard and Miller, in Patterson, 1973, p. 94).

An important influence of behavioral therapy has been to challenge the supposition that deviant behavior is an illness. Deviant or maladaptive behaviors are seen as the result of faulty learning and/or previous learning in which undesirable behavior has been intentionally or inadvertently reinforced. Behavior therapy also challenges many of the accepted constructs in "care giving"; for example, it sees "tender loving care" as given too unconditionally and uses it as an appropriate response to the demonstration of desired behavior.

Man is an active and choosing agent who interacts with and acts upon his environment. The environment responds to man and selectively reinforces his behavior. Those behaviors which are reinforced will most likely recur. As a result of environmental interaction and selective reinforcement the individual becomes socialized and develops a repertoire of behaviors which are used for adaptation through work, activities of daily living, and leisure. All behavior may be broken down into observable, measurable actions or discrete skills. These discrete skills plus the larger behavior of which they are a part will be viewed as adaptive if they enable the individual to satisfy his needs, live according to his values, achieve independence, achieve pleasure, and live in harmony with others in his society.

The Role of the Occupational Therapist

The behavioral frame of reference identifies the occupational therapist as a motivator, a reinforcing agent, a teacher, a social role model, and a consultant. She assumes one or more of these roles in the therapeutic learning environment, which is where she and the patient work in collaboration to identify and accomplish specific goals through identified learning experiences. Contrary to common belief, the occupational therapist is not an "expert" who assumes total responsibility and authority for treatment. Rather she recognizes the patient's ability to contribute to the therapeutic process and the benefits of the patient's assuming mutual responsibility for the treatment outcome.

The Therapist as Motivator and Reinforcing Agent. Therapy may involve motivating the patient to try new behaviors that are anxiety-producing. Techniques for motivating include giving explanations to the patient about his "condition," providing explanations and assurance regarding the function of activities, and offering support and affirmation that the patient can succeed (Patterson, 1973, p. 150).

Treatment teams (the occupational therapist included) frequently use the awarding of "privileges" as the motivator for participation in therapy. The patient who refuses to participate in occupational therapy or other therapy programs in the therapeutic milieu may be refused passes home, free time away from the nursing unit, passes for community visits, or time free of staff supervision. The existence of rapport between patient and therapist is important as it enables therapist attention and approval to serve as an effective reinforcement.

The patient who might otherwise avoid participation in an occupational therapy activity may participate in order to gain this approval, or the patient who enjoys occupational therapy may be given extra time in the clinic as a reward for his appropriate participation in other therapeutic activities. How and when this interdependent relationship between therapy participation and the privilege system are presented to the patient and how it is enforced determine whether motivation, reinforcement, or punishment is occurring.

The Therapist as Teacher. In the role of teacher the occupational therapist provides new learning or relearning experiences . When teaching new skills, the therapist uses activities that help the patient learn to cook, apply for a job, or use community resources, for example. These skills are most frequently taught to the patient with a history of chronic problems who has had limited life experiences, or to the younger patient who needs these experiences as a part of the process of normal development.

The patient who has come through a trauma or one of life's natural changes which occur in the process of normal development may also need to learn new adaptive responses. For example, when children leave home or a spouse is lost through death or divorce, the patient must adjust to a new life style. Part of this adjustment may be facilitated in occupational therapy through the process of learning to be more independent in home management, financial planning, and socialization, to name just a few areas. During treatment sessions the occupational therapist will target skills needed for independence and not focus on the feelings that the patient experiences due to the loss and changes that have occurred. It is assumed that if the patient's skill level improves, his feelings will change also, even though feelings are not the primary focus.

Another form of teaching occurs when relearning is required. For example, the patient may have the basic knowledge and skills but for some reason is not utilizing them to function independently. The patient knows how to cook, has had a job, has gone to the store, library, or bank but has failed to do so for an extended period of time. Perhaps the patient has not had the opportunity to assume these responsibilities, is depressed, or needs support to gain the confidence needed for independent functioning in activities of daily living, work, or leisure. The reasons that skills have not been exercised is not the concern. Eliciting and reinforcing the desired skill or behavior are the focus of the learning experience (treatment).

In the psychiatric learning setting the occupational therapist may also provide corrective learning experiences through social skills groups in which the patient can acquire verbal and behavioral skills which enhance his ability to function within his social network. For example, a child who was abused by a parent often re-enacts these abusive behaviors with his own children when he becomes an adult. The therapist may teach the patient to recognize internal signals that he is loosing control and then educate the patient in alternative means of handling feelings, or she may choose to improve his parent effectiveness by teaching him specific "child rearing" skills.

Regardless of the learning focus, it is assumed that as a teacher the therapist has specific skills and expertise which are shared with the patient as she designs and implements learning activities. These activities are based upon the patient's interests and goals, and are selected for their ability to develop the skills needed for adaptation and independent functioning in the patient's natural environment.

Occupational Therapist as Role Model. As a social role model the therapist exhibits behaviors from which the patient can learn. Here the learning process occurs as the patient identifies with and imitates the therapist (see note 4). The patient can learn verbal behavior as well as other specific skills, particularly social skills. This may occur quite naturally as the patient observes the therapist in a variety of interactions about the clinic. The identification process in interactions is also apparent as we see one patient teach another the activity process, just as he has seen the therapist do.

The occupational therapist may use activities which incorporate role playing (also called *behavioral rehearsal*). During role plays the therapist demonstrates desirable verbal and nonverbal behaviors which can later be mimicked by the patient when he role plays a situation. Individual and group role play experiences are used to teach new behaviors or to provide support to patients in allowing them to explore multiple responses to problem situations.

Role playing can involve both practicing an expected social role and learning more about the roles of others through role reversals. The authors recall situations in psychodrama sessions in which the patients and staff were asked to reverse roles. The modeling and identification process was readily apparent. Both patients and staff benefited from the humor as well as the serious implications of the role play situation. These role plays frequently resulted in meaningful discussions between the two groups, eased the tensions that existed in the patient unit, and facilitated the resolution of ward problems. (Note: these sessions were led by a trained psychodramatist.)

Role playing is frequently used in occupational therapy to practice such skills as applying for a job, asking for a date, saying "no" to a friend or spouse, or talking with parents about a concern. These scenarios allow the patient to experiment with introducing himself to a potential employer or new acquaintance and to decide how he will respond to the situations that he encounters. For example, patients often worry about "What will I do if someone knows I've been in a psychiatric hospital? What should I say or do? Should I lie?" The occupational therapist can help the patient group experiment with different verbal and nonverbal behaviors and help the patient become aware of his options and their likely consequences in addition to gaining confidence in the option he chooses.

The Occupational Therapist as Consultant. In the consultant role the occupational therapist designs the behavior program that best responds to the patient's goals and problems and trains an aide to cooperatively work with the patient or with the family or staff to implement the intervention plan. The occupational therapist teaches methods of providing reinforcement and documenting behavior change.

Whatever her role, the occupational therapist is always aware that her interest and approval and disapproval have an important effect as reinforcers of behavior and that through reinforcement she facilitates the learning of specific skills that lead to an adaptive or maladaptive response.

Function of Activities

Building Skills. The behavioral occupational therapist uses activities to teach specific skills, to provide simulated learning experiences, and to serve as a reinforcement. The therapist breaks down activities into their component parts and is aware of the level of challenge presented to the patient and the skills required of the patient when completing each activity component. Activities are graded from simple to complex and used in evaluation and treatment. Activities are selected according to their interest to the patient and the degree to which they are consonant with sociocultural expectations. When operant conditioning is to be used, the activity must begin at the level of behavior the patient is currently capable of. When modeling and imitative behavior are incorporated, activities may be selected which begin with novel (not previously emitted) behavior. Frequently, during evaluation, the therapist observes the patient performing tasks in simulated experiences in the occupational therapy clinic or in the patient's natural (post-treatment) environment to determine the extent of adaptive and maladaptive behavior.

Treatment activities are the concrete specific tasks that the occupational therapist uses to develop specific skills for independence in activities of daily living, work, and leisure. Activities are identified which are consistent with the interests and expectations of the adult patient. These activities are broken down into specific tasks and skill components (which may be called *splinter skills*). A splinter skill is "a specific motor or mental skill that is performed only under specific circumstances and not integrated into a person's total behavior" (Banus, p. 260, 1979). A splinter skill is nonstage specific and may be performed without the development of subskills (or enabling skills) which are acquired in a chronological developmental sequence. Splinter skills are skills needed in the present situation; they may be lost if not practiced continually and usually are not generalized (Nuse-Clark and Allen, 1985, p. 271). For example, a child can memorize the alphabet song without understanding the concept and function of letters. He will forget the alphabet if he does not practice the song frequently.

Activities are graded, and specific tasks are presented to provide progressively more difficult learning challenges which develop splinter skills and shape the adaptive behavior needed in the patient's roles and responsibilities in his community environment. The skills must be practiced repeatedly in order to be maintained.

The Components of the Activity. Activities can be broken down into almost endless behavioral components. A simplified example is provided here:

Meal planning and preparation require knowledge of nutrition and knowledge of and skills in budgeting, food purchase, meal preparation, serving, and clean-up. These major components can then be further delineated and used to form behavioral objectives for the intervention program. Food purchasing can be further broken down into the following skill components: (1) Make a shopping list which would include items from the four major food groups and which would be sufficient in quantity to feed a given number of persons. (2) Use public transportation in order to get to the supermarket. (3) Use interpersonal skills which enable appropriate discourse to be carried out in the community setting. (4) Use financial skills necessary for purchasing the food (making change, for example).

The End Product. Activities frequently utilized when applying this frame of reference include craft activities, task groups, prevocational or work experiences, relaxation experiences, assertiveness groups, social skills training, desensitization experiences, and activities related to the use of token economies.

The therapist uses activities to achieve an end, that is, to produce an end product and not to give primary attention to the activity process that occurs during the activity. The focus is on the outcome, as one asks, "Can the patient initiate a conversation? Can the patient cook a meal? Can the patient go to the bank and set up a new account? Did the group finish the task and accomplish its goal?" The focus is not on "What does it feel like to be in this group? What did you learn about yourself from this experience?" These feelings and "process" concerns are the primary focus of treatment in the object-relations frame of reference.

The Activity as a Reinforcer. Activities can also serve to reinforce behavior. For many (but not everyone) mastery of activities and one's environment becomes an internal reinforcer. Although she will not focus discussion on how the patient feels about a task experience, the occupational therapist recognizes that successful task experience and the sense of accomplishment that comes from the task completion can be a source of reinforcement. The therapist can further reinforce the patient's behavior by commenting on the quality of the end product and give "strokes," saying, "I like your breadboard; you did a good job sanding and smoothing the surface" or "I know that you have worked hard in order to finish this project and carry through with your choice." The therapist may also ask the patient to confirm his accomplishment by asking him to identify the skills that were acquired during the activity process. The therapist might, for example, say, "Tell me what you learned about yourself — about how to work with others, about how to approach a work problem."

Theoretical Assumptions

When applying the behavioral frame of reference in occupational therapy, the therapist bases evaluation and treatment upon the following assumptions, which have been derived from behavioral theory and are summarized here:

1. Behavior is predictable, measurable, and objective.

2. A person's verbalization and self-descriptions are behaviors.

3. The patient has a repertoire of behaviors (adaptive and maladaptive) that have been learned through selective reinforcement from the environment. The therapist is concerned both with extinguishing maladaptive behaviors and with establishing adaptive behavior.

4. The patient's repertoire of behavior determines his ability to function in activities of daily living, work, and leisure.

5. Through positive and differential reinforcement and the systematic application of learning techinques, the patient can learn to modify and control his behavior.

6. Only behavior that is demonstrated can be reinforced.

7. New behavior may be established through the use of continuous or frequent and

predictable reinforcement; however, the most stable behavior (the most difficult to extinguish) is that maintained by intermittent reinforcement.

8. If maladaptive behavior is only occassionally reinforced, it is strengthened.

9. The strength of the patient's response is influenced by bodily conditions such as those related to emotions, drives, and the use of drugs.

10. In occupational therapy the patient can learn new skills or refine present skills, or learn to manipulate his environment to problem solve and improve his functioning in his community.

11. The skills for adaptive functioning in the natural environment are independent and nonstage specific.

12. In occupational therapy the therapist seeks to increase the patient's ability to transfer (or generalize) the behaviors learned during treatment to a broad range of appropriate situations.

13. Clear, concrete goals increase the patient's understanding of the focus of treatment which in turn expedites the treatment process and facilitates the evaluation of the treatment outcome.

Evaluation

During the evaluation the occupational therapist uses activities to determine (a) what behaviors are required for adequate function in the patient's expected environment, (b) which of these behaviors are currently demonstrated by the patient, and (c) what skills need to be learned or strengthened. It is common to group these behaviors according to skills of daily living, work, and leisure. However, the therapist must specify the behaviors to be built, and not merely note that a category of skills is deficient. When assessing skill level, the therapist determines the existence and strength of age appropriate, culturally acceptable behavior. She does not apply developmental "ages" to the behavior that is demonstrated, nor does she design her evaluation to determine the interrelationship of skills. Rather she determines that a specific needed skill does or does not exist (and to what quantifiable extent). In each of the areas of concern, the therapist (with the patient) typically will identify the following:

1. Behaviors that contribute to adaptive function.
2. Behaviors that interfere with adaptive function.
3. Behaviors necessary for adequate function in the patient's natural environment.
4. The frequency of specific adaptive and maladaptive behavior.
5. The stimuli that are acting as cues.
6. The reinforcers for specific behaviors and, when appropriate, the person who supplies reinforcement.
7. The sources of motivation for the patient's behavior.
8. The ability of the patient to discriminate among stimuli and to generalize learning effectively.
9. Priorities in treatment.

From the preceding, the occupational therapist establishes a data base, or baseline in which she notes the frequency and strength of specified responses during a limited period of time. Often this baseline information is depicted in a chart or graph. She then targets skills that will be learned or extinguished, formulates possible methods of motivation, and selects possible reinforcers that could be utilized during the treatment-learning process (Mosey, 1970)

A characteristic of the behavioral evaluation is the specificity sought in designating the strength of behavior. For example, rather than making a general evaluative statement indicating that the patient "fails to ask for assistance in the clinic as needed" or "tends not to clean up his work area," the therapist may indicate as part of her data base that (the patient) "asked for assistance one time during a 50 minute session" and (the patient) "cleaned his work areas one time during a five session week."

The Method of Assessment. The method of assessment is typically a combination of observation and rating of task performance along with an interview. When an interview is used, the behavioral interview is different from the "traditional" interview in that it is not designed to help the patient develop insight (see note 5). It is not designed to establish a medical "diagnosis" (see note 6), nor is it designed to help the patient understand more about his feelings or past history. It does aim to elicit the required information about current targeted problems, and is concerned with history only to the extent that history influences current reinforcers. The therapist may also use questionnaires or behavior check lists in order to structure the interview situation.

One example of behavioral evaluation and goal setting was given by Kaye, Mackie, and Hitzing in their article, Continency Management in a Workshop Setting . . . Innovation in Occupational Therapy (1970). In describing their work with eight male "chronic patients," they noted that all the patients exhibited minimal social skills, "bizarre motor and verbal behavior, tardiness and inattention" (Kaye et al., 1970, p. 414). The patients participated for an hour each weekday in a workshop occupational therapy setting. During the "baseline" period the patients were observed for "several weeks" and then a list of undesired behaviors (at least six per patient) was made up and resulted in terms of a positive behavioral objective. For example, the following behavioral goals were among those listed by the authors: "on time; cleaned up assigned work area; told the truth; stayed at the job with no pausing or pacing longer than . . . minutes per session; initiated relevant, appropriate conversation at least . . . times" (Kaye et al., 1970, p. 414). The six behavioral goals for each patient were tallied by the therapist on a survey sheet. The authors included a sample behavioral survey sheet to illustrate the vehicle for weekly tallying (Table 4-1, Figure 4-1). pg. 106-107.

The progress of each patient was then made visible via a graph. This concluded the establishing of behavior baselines. Baseline data surveys and graphs were then displayed prominently, and the therapist spoke to each patient about the goals of treatment and the responsibility of each for filling out his own behavior objectives survey and for being able to verbalize his own behavioral goals from memory and to cite criteria for appropriate behavior. Reinforcement revolved around the accumulation of token points as well as social reinforce-

Table 4-1

**TYPICAL BEHAVIORAL OBJECTIVES SURVEY SHEET
OBTAINED DURING BASELINE**

NAME Joe Smith   **WEEK OF 5/19-23/69**

DAYS

BEHAVIOR	M	T	W	TH	F	WEEKLY TOTAL
1. On time: Present before 10:03			X	X	X	3
2. Stayed at job with no pausing or pacing longer than 5 minutes per session		X			X	2
3. Cleaned up assigned area(s)		X		X		2
4. Well-groomed; Shaven hair combed, clothes properly secured	X		X	X		3
5. Initiated relevant, appropriate conversation 2 times			X			1
6. Smiled (at least 3 times)	X				X	2
TOTALS	2	2	3	3	3	13

Kaye J, Mackie V, Hitzing EW Contingency Management in a Workshop Setting . . . Innovating in Occupational Therapy. *AJOT* 24(6):415, 1970. Reproduced with permission.

ments (e.g., smiles, pats on the back; Kaye, et al., 1970, p. 415).

Another example follows. It is an adapted behavior evaluation format that incorporates the use of a behavioral check list and an interview:

During the evaluation interview the patient is asked to complete a self-inventory (Table 4-2). The one from which this excerpt was taken had 50 "self statements." The patient, a 21 year old female, came to the interview somewhat carelessly dressed, appeared overweight, and had facial acne. She was asked to rate her performance as described by each of the 50 statements. The patient indicated her performance by checking one of the following: always (A), frequently (F), sometimes (S), or never (N). The patient was also asked to indicate

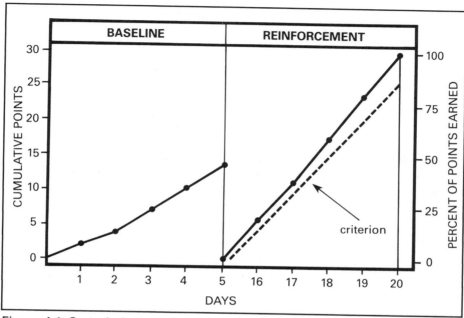

Figure 4-1. Cumulative graph points earned by Patient D during last week of baseline and third week of reinforcement. Kaye J, Mackie V, Hetzing EW Contingency Management in a Workshop Setting . . . Innovation in Occupational Therapy *AJOT* 24(6):415, 1970. Reproduced with permission.

whether she was satisfied with her performance or whether she wished to change her behavior. The statements related to the patient's behavior in interpersonal, self-care, task, community, and communication activities. The responses on the form were then discussed by the patient and the therapist in order to target behaviors for change, set treatment goals, and discuss the resources available for learning experiences in occupational therapy.

Note: It would not be unusual for a patient to rate himself low on many areas of such a check list and to desire to make multiple changes. This can be a huge blow to the patient's self-esteem as well as an overwhelming experience. Therefore the occupational therapist should use questionnaires judiciously and help the patient organize the information in a manner that helps the patient to identify desired changes as well as his own strengths (adaptive behaviors), to prioritize the desired changes, and to identify resources that will culminate in a successful learning experience and one that will enhance the patient's sense of accomplishment.

Discussion of Patient Questionnaire. The following is an excerpt from the patient-therapist dialogue following completion of the inventory. The reader will see the contrast between this dialogue and that in Chapter III, Object Relations Frame of Reference, even when there are similarities in the patients' concerns regarding physical appearance:

Table 4-2

Excerpt from Completed Questionnaire

Behavioral Statement	Rating*	Satisfaction
I am satisfied with my physical self (Body weight and shape, muscle strength).	N	Want to Change
I can find clothes that fit well and that are attractive and comfortable.	S	Want to Change
I am satisfied with my general appearance (Hair style, skin condition, etc).	S	Want to Change
I am satisfied with my physical coordination (e.g., the way I walk, my ability to use my hands).	S	Want to Change

*N=Never, S= Seldom.

OTR: "On your list you have indicated that you'd like to change your appearance and your clothes and improve your physical coordination and skin condition."

Pt.: "I'm heavy and clumsy . . . I'd like new clothes . . . I need new makeup."

OTR: "I can't buy you new clothes or makeup, but in occupational therapy I can help you to improve your physical coordination so that you're less clumsy, and I can help you plan a weight reduction program. You also can experiment with skin care and makeup and clothing selection in occupational therapy. (Pause) Where would you like to begin?"

PT" "I can't decide."

OTR: "Let's talk about the first statement that you made about yourself, and I will help you begin. You first mentioned that you're 'heavy.' Are you interested in working toward a weight loss while you're in the hospital?"

Pt.: "I've tried. It's hard."

OTR: "Yes, it's difficult. . . and I think we have some supports here that can help you. We could look at both your eating habits and your level of physical activity. Have you spoken to your doctor about your weight concerns? He can order special weight reduction meals for you."

Pt.: "No. I don't like many foods. I thrive on junk food."

OTR: "If you decide that you want to work toward losing weight, you will need to speak to your doctor when you see him. Perhaps too you'll have to work on changing your eating habits."

Pt.: "I love the snacks here in the hospital, and my parents always bring me my favorite treat when they come to visit."

OTR: "Do you think that you could ask them not to bring food when they come to visit? You might find it useful to give them a suggestion of something else you'd like, since visitors frequently express concern and care for you through a gift."

Pt.: "I'll ask for my makeup!"

OTR: "To help you avoid the snacks here in the hospital, we could write a contract. A contract is a written statement of your goals, such as 'I want to lose five pounds.' Then you write down how you intend to reach your goal, and what your reward will be for doing it. You might contract to limit your in-between snacks to one or two a day and reward yourself at the end of the week."

Pt.: "I'm not in the mood to write today. I'm tired."

OTR: "I think that we have done enough for today, and it is almost time to stop. Tomorrow in occupational therapy we will talk more about your specific goals and work on your contract for occupational therapy."

During this interview the therapist summarized one area of the questionnaire and worked with the patient to identify specific problems and prioritize desired changes rather than pursue the patient's feelings about herself. Although the patient was not ready to complete her contract, the therapist established that there would be an emphasis on "action."

Simulated Experience. Assessment may also occur in the context of simulated experiences in the hospital or occupational therapy setting. Simulated experiences are situations designed by the therapist to replicate the patient's natural environment. While it would be ideal to evaluate the patient in his everyday environment, because of the limits imposed by short hospitalizations and the lack of funds for home visits, the therapist may be unable to do this. For some information she will more than likely depend on verbal reports from family members or significant others with whom the patient lives. In some hospitals the living unit or ward is structured as much as possible to simulate an "extended family" home environment. Therefore the occupational therpist can gain evaluation data from the informal interaction that occurs between patients and staff as well as from observations of the patient's room (e.g., organization, neatness) and his daily routines that indicate daily living skills.

Another simulated experience that occurs in occupational therapy evaluation or treatment is in the area of financial management. Financial management includes the ability to make money transactions in the community, make banking transactions, pay one's bills, plan a budget, and identify and use sources of income (community and personal). To determine the ability to make banking transactions, the therapist uses bank deposit or withdrawal forms for savings and checking accounts to detemine whether the patient is capable of managing banking responsibilities that are a part of personal financial management. To complete these forms, the patient needs also to be able to read, write, and make mathematical computations. Simulated experiences are designed in accordance with the principle that although every situation or setting contains a slightly different set of stimuli and cues and calls for a slightly different response, learning is most likely to be generalized when the patient can recognize the similarities between given settings.

Assessment Instruments. The occupational therapy literature identifies the following as behavioral assessments: the Kohlman Evaluation of Living Skills, the Bay Area Functional Performance Evaluation (BaFPE), the Comprehensive Occupational Therapy Evaluation (COTE; Hemphill, 1982), and the Scorable Self Care Evaluation (Clark and Peters, 1984). These evaluations are summarized here. Details and specific protocols are available from the identified sources.

The Kohlman Evaluation of Living Skills. The Kohlman evaluation was developed in an acute psychiatric setting. Interviews and tasks are used to determine the patient's ability to function in everyday living situations. Administered in 30 minutes, this battery identifies 18 living skills that are categorized under the broad headings of self-care, safety and health, money management, transportation and telephone, work, and leisure. Forms and problem solving tasks are used to identify skills within these broad categories (e.g., reading and writing ability, self-care and appearance, knowledge of danger, use of the telephone, money management, work, and leisure interests and abilities). The test manual is available from Linda Kohlman McGourty, KELS Research, Box 33201, Seattle, Washington 98113.

The Comprehensive Occupational Therapy Evaluation (COTE). This assessment was developed in an acute psychiatric setting in order to identify behaviors relevant to occupational therapy, to improve communication with staff, and to improve the system of data formation and retrieval. It identifies 25 behaviors that can be seen in occupational therapy. They are organized under three major categories: general behavior, interpersonal behavior, and task behavior. The behaviors are rated on a 0 to 4 scale. A format for evaluation and reporting is provided. The assessment is described in detail in Hemphill's *The Evaluation Process in Psychiatric Occupational Therapy* (1982).

The Bay Area Functional Performance Evaluation (BaFPE). The BaFPE has two subtests — the Task Oriented Assessment (TOA) and the Social Interaction Scale (SIS). The TOA consists of five time limited tasks that are both structured and nonstructured: sorting shells, completing a bank deposit slip, drawing a house floor plan, duplicating a block design, and drawing a person. The therapist then rates 10 functional behaviors: the ability to paraphrase instructions, productive decision making, organization of time and materials, those related to mastery and self-esteem, frustration tolerance, attention span, ability to abstract, verbal or behavioral evidence of thought or mood disorder, and ability to follow instructions leading to correct task completion.

The SIS is a behavior rating scale, not a behavior check list. It is used to assess seven categories of social interaction: response to authority figures, verbal communication, psychomotor behavior, dependency versus independency, socially appropriate behavior, ability to work with peers, and participation in group activities.

The test manual and materials are available from Consulting Psychologist Press.

Scorable Self Care Evaluation. A standardized self-care evaluation instrument designed by Nelson Clark and Mary Peters, this evaluation is used to identify baseline performance in basic living skills (personal care, housekeeping, work and leisure, and financial management). The authors provide subtasks for each of the basic living skill areas, a format for administering subtasks, a format for scoring performance during subtasks, reliability studies and standard scores to assist in the interpretation of patient scores, and forms for communicating evaluation and progress data (Clark and Peters, 1984). The Scorable Self Care Evaluation is available from Charles B. Slack, Inc.

Treatment Goals

An important contribution of the behavioral frame of reference comes from the guidelines it has established for writing treatment goals. Owing to the desire to establish efficacy of treatment and the requirements of third party payers, most clinicians have been influenced by the behavioral goal setting system. In general, goals must be observable and measurable.

Originally the behavioral occupational therapist identified problems, determined the goals for treatment, and designed the intervention plan. (This continues to occur in situations in which the patient is believed to be incapable of contributing to the process.) Today the patient participates more actively in the decision making process and works cooperatively with the therapist to target the patient's problems and to determine the specific changes that need to occur.

The targeted problems must be defined in observable terms and as measurable outcomes and must be individualized for the specific patient. There are multiple resources to serve as guides that can aid the therapist in the goal setting process (Mager, 1962). This process is summarized as follows: After the completion of the evaluation, the therapist and the patient identify the changes that need to occur in order to improve the patient's functioning within his natural environment. These changes may be stated in terms of the patient's feelings, desires, interests, or concerns and are usually general statements.

Next the therapist takes the patient's general statements and works to identify the specific behaviors that would indicate that the patient has learned a new skill or has changed his behavior to satisfy his desires, develop his interests, or alleviate his concerns. These behavioral statements, which are derived from an analysis of the tasks that relate to the patient's broad concerns, must be understood by the patient and agreed upon as subskills of behaviors to be learned or modified and as indicators that change has occurred.

After targeting behaviors, observable goals are established. The therapist and the patient establish behavioral expectations within a framework that may identify the context, the time and place of behavior, and the significant persons involved or affected by the behavior.

Having identified the observable behavioral goal, the patient and therapist then discuss the frequency of behaviors expected and the criteria that indicate success or failure to accomplish the goal. Thus the observable behaviors become measurable goals.

The goal setting process is exemplified as follows: Let us take a frequent situation that occurs in psychiatric settings with the patient having chronic problems and frequent outbursts of disruptive behavior. The patient's family members decide that they can no longer cope with the "problematic childlike adult" and inform the patient that he may not return home. The patient's problem and concern are: "Where am I going to live? How am I going to care for myself?" As the patient and therapist discuss the concern, the following issues and adaptive behaviors emerge as necessary issues for focus:

Concern: Where am I going to live?

Issues: What is important to me about where I live? How will I pay for the setting (apartment, boarding home, house)? What are my alternatives and choices? What supports are available (financial, interpersonal)?

Necessary skills: Identify alternatives by scanning the classified advertisements and contacting community agencies. Clarify values and identify personal needs. Speak to personal and community resources regarding financial support.

Behavioral goal statements:

Patient will identify two possible settings in which he could live.

Patient will speak to his parents regarding possible financial support.

Patient will participate in values clarification group and identify what type of setting he wants to live in, whom he wishes to live with, and what kind of support group or social network he desires.

Patient will gain employment capable of meeting financial responsibilities.

In the process of determining treatment goals, the patient and therapist will often identify behaviors that are not adaptive and that interfere with goal attainment. Typically the therapist will take note of these and seek to remove reinforcement for these maladaptive behaviors. Unless she and the staff have complete control of the patient's environment, eliminating such reinforcement is very difficult, and at times not possible.

Goals are most often (but not always) written in terms of what will be attained, and not what will be eliminated. For example, the "problematic childlike" behavior in our example might include excessive time spent by the patient "brooding" in isolation in his room. Positive actions taken toward exploring community resources and gaining employment would be seen as the adaptive behavior opposite of brooding and isolative behaviors, and these positive actions would serve as treatment goals.

Usually there are multiple issues, problems, and behavioral goals, as can be easily seen in the example above. Therefore the therapist helps the patient to set priorities for treatment in order to set realistic expectations and to avoid overwhelming the patient. Whenever possible, the patient will choose where he wishes to begin. This process also is indicative of the humanistic influence in behaviorally based occupational therapy.

As treatment progresses, the measurable statements are reviewed frequently to determine progress. Measurable goals and the review process allow the patient to clearly see his progress and enable the staff to evaluate the success and limitations of the intervention plan.

Sometimes the treatment goals and intervention strategies are written in the form of a *"contract."* A contract is a verbal or written agreement between the patient and the therapist that defines the roles of each during treatment, the behavioral goals, reinforcements and their schedules, the treatment procedures, and other related negotiations. Written contracts are signed by both the therapist and the patient, the contracts are time limited and are, at agreed intervals, reviewed, renegotiated, and/or terminated.

Problem Oriented Record. Simultaneous with behavioral movement, the increased support for specific, observable, and if possible measurable treatment goals and the growing interest in data processing came the desire for specific formats of documentation. One of these formats was the *problem oriented record*, described by Weed in 1969. This format was not specifically designed for occupational therapy or for psychiatry. It was first used in general medicine settings, but has influenced documentation in many medical and occupational therapy treatment programs. The problem oriented record has four major components: The *data base* includes demographics; medical and social history; medical, laboratory, and psychological test results and/or related clinical reports; and a statement of the patient's chief complaint. The *subjective data* include the views expressed by the patient and his family. The *objective data* include staff observations and laboratory reports. Finally, the *problem list* includes past and present psychiatric and medical problems identified from information in the other three components of the problem oriented record.

For each problem listed by number and title, a diagnostic plan and a treatment plan are listed. Progress notes are then keyed to a particular numbered problem and are written according to the "SOAP" format. "SOAP" is an acronym for the following: "S," the patient's subjective response to treatment and patient observations; "O," objective data from laboratory studies, diagnostic reports, and so forth; "A," the assessment and analysis of the subjective and objective data; "P," the diagnostic, therapeutic, and patient education plan (Weed, 1969).

The influence of the problem oriented record system or adaptations of the system are evident in the records and documentation that exists today in many mental health settings. The problem oriented record is reflected in goal oriented treatment in which there is a problem list, specific goals (long and short term), and treatment strategies for each problem on the list.

The authors are also familiar with a system which uses a "NAP" note ("N," narrative which combines the subjective and objective data; "A," assessment which identifies the problems and states how they were determined; "P," plan with the goals and intervention strategies used to identify problems.

Treatment Process

Behaviorally based occupational therapy is concerned with building skills that contribute to adaptive function while eliminating those that interfere. The straightforward nature of this intent should not suggest that behavioral treatment is "simple" or necessarily similar across various treatment programs. While behavioral therapists hold in common the concern for observable measurable behavior, the techniques employed to modify and build specific behaviors vary. We wish to dispel the notion that merely acknowledging a patient's success in occupational therapy (as through smiles or "privileges"), ignoring maladaptive behaviors, and writing measurable treatment goals suffice as behavioral treatment. The complexity of the human being is such that identifying and isolating the (literally) thousands upon thousands of stimulus-response-reinforcement associations that compose one individual's learning are virtually impossible, at least in the practical sense. The behavioral therapist must be very diligent in her application of behavioral techniques if she is to avoid being suprised by the outcome of a treatment experience that failed to take into account the complex interrelationship of stimuli, responses, and reinforcements in even the most circumscribed learning setting.

Given this, the therapist endeavors to collect objective data and with the patient's cooperation takes charge of the learning milieu. Together she and the patient:

1. Identify and prioritize learning needs.

2. State learning needs as specific, observable behaviors.

3. Determine what learning techniques will be employed (operant conditioning, modeling, building response chains).

4. Specify one or more individual or group learning experiences in which (a) the learning experience is compatible with the patient's age, interests, values, societal expectations, and the expected duration of his treatment; (b) there will be an opportunity for the desired behavior to be demonstrated (and/or modeled, shaped, chained); (c) there is, when needed, an opportunity for trial and error problem solving and sufficient opportunity for repetition of adaptive responses (practice); (d) the therapist (and designated others) can ensure that positive reinforcement be given (per schedule) for adaptive responses, and reinforcement is withheld in response to maladaptive behavior; (e) there is opportunity within the experience to move from continuous or frequent external reinforcement to more everyday (intermittent, patient-maintained) kinds of reinforcement; (f) the patient can recognize the similarities between the utilization of the behavior in the therapeutic environment and its utilization in the natural environment (the therapist may amplify salient features of both the therapeutic and natural environment to make these similarities clearer); and (g) the patient can perceive the differences between the utilization of the learned behavior in appropriate versus inappropriate settings (the therapist may help the patient identify these differences).

5. Specify criteria for periodic reassessment of treatment.

Behavioral Interaction. Regardless of the activity or "techniques" employed, throughout the treatment process the patient is made aware of what is expected of him and the goal of each learning experience. In accordance, the therapist uses a vocabulary and manner of explaining that are understandable to the patient. For example, the therapist may state to the patient, "I would like you to work on this leather key case so that you can learn to follow the written instructions. I will be available for assistance if you need help; but I want you to try this on your own first, so that you can become more accustomed to working independently."

The therapist uses her dialogue with the patient to assist him to recognize the relationship of his behavior to the consequences that result. She dos not attempt to deny or overlook the patient's thoughts and feelings, but she responds to these in terms of the behavior that ensues. Rather than telling a patient that he looks sad, angry, or depressed, for example, she may say, "The way you're throwing that clay arounds looks angry" or "You've spent most of the hour sitting by yourself, and it appears that you feel discouraged."

When relating to the patient, the therapist tries to respond to behaviors in a positive manner and makes sure to specify behaviors she expects. During a community outing the therapist may say, "Please stay with the group when we leave the van and walk to the entrance of the YMCA. Enter the lobby, be seated, and wait for the 'Y' program director to join us" rather than just saying, "Don't stray from the group."

To cite another example, when a patient in her cooking group is using a knife carelessly, the therapist will not only say, "Be careful." She will also say, "Be careful; your hand is too far down on the knife blade. Here, let me show you." Then she proceeds to demonstrate the correct procedure. Even when giving criticism, the therapist avoids using blanket remarks that suggest that something is bad, wrong, or ugly. Rather she demonstrates how to use a tool or do a process correctly, suggests how a process might be improved, or identifies which characteristics of a task or project have been done successfully and which may need work.

The therapist uses her dialogue with the patient to help him to perceive the relationship between his behavior and its consequence and to generalize his learning to his natural environment. She encourages him to assume responsibility for his behavior and strives to build his sense of self-control.

Three Behavioral Occupational Therapy Groups. We have selected three examples of behavioral group learning experiences that we feel are representative of the current application of behavioral theory in occupational therapy. Although not all behavioral occupational therapy occurs in a group context, it frequently does in adult care; thus each of the group learning experiences that we discuss represents or is a "composite" of behavioral groups that have often been encountered by us and by many of the fieldwork students we have supervised.

In behavioral group treatment, the therapist must structure the group and learning environment in order to insure that specific target behaviors for each group member are facilitated and reinforced. She has the same "gatekeeping" functions described in the previous chapter. Additionally, she must see to it that there is a means to monitor specific behaviors and to supply (or withhold) reinforcement. At times this necessitates having other staff or aides present, all of whom coordinate their efforts.

Group I. A Prevocational Activity Group. One type of behavioral group is typified by the prevocational activity group in which each participant works on an individual project, but the patients have in common a need to learn general task skills that will enable each to ultimately succeed at a job after discharge.

For example, in an in-hospital clinic in a Veterans Administration psychiatric wing, all the patients are working in the wood shop, which has available both hand and power tools. The number of group members varies from six to eight and represents a stable group, with an occasional new admission or discharge changing group membership. The group meets twice daily during the week for one and one-half hour sessions.

The general work behaviors that the therapist tries to promote include:

1. The ability to initiate productive work.
2. The ability to pursue a task to completion.
3. The ability to work well alone.

4. The ability to cooperate with others.

5. Social skills related to sharing space, materials, and so forth.

6. The ability to make timely decisions based on available data.

7. The ability to anticipate consequences.

8. The acquisition of habits related to punctuality, safety, and cleanliness.

9. The ability to identify and use available resources (see note 7).

Before coming into the group, each patient has met individually with the therapist and developed a written contract which specifies what his project will be, what behaviors will be learned, the reinforcement and its criteria, and criteria for reassessing goals. The therapist shares with the other staff a copy or the contents of the agreement between herself and each of the patients. The clinic environment is designed to maximize the opportunity for all patients in the group to achieve their personal goals. In such an activity group a diversity of individual treatment goals can be accomodated. In some instances the clinic is structured to encourage sharing and social behavior (e.g., by limiting materials and tools available for use). In other instances, when many of the patients in the group are highly distractable and have difficulty attending to tasks, the work area is structured to minimize socialization. In order to maximize the transfer or generalization of learning, the therapist structures the work setting in a manner that will closely approximate key aspects of the work setting in which the patients will be headed after therapy. Toward this end the therapist has included a "point" system as part of the reinforcement, and each patient in this group has been assigned his own work area. Points are given when a patient completes designated steps on his project and when his work area is neat at the conclusion of the session. Points are also given for promptness. Points are deducted for specified misuse of tools. Socialization is encouraged during a designated "coffee break" during each work session. The occupational therapist and often auxiliary staff are primarily responsible for providing reinforcement; the occupational therapist, staff, and each patient are involved in determining whether target behaviors have been achieved. In this activity group the therapist is primarily an observer and not a participant.

Group II. Resocialization Group. In a second kind of behavioral group, the process of treatment may begin in much the same way. Each patient may meet individually with the therapist to target initial behavioral goals, or the patients may have been placed in a group to be observed, significant behaviors being targeted and baselined by the therapist; then each patient and the therapist mutually set treatment goals. In this case, several patients with similar social learning needs are placed in a resocialization group. For example, at a local mental health facility, outpatients are periodically selected into the FAC (Friday Afternoon Club).

On Wednesday of each week, all group members and the occupational therapist meet. The group typically but not necessarily consists of five to eight younger unmarried adults. Members come and go from the "club" as their treatment stay dictates. Thus the group must constantly respond to changes in its membership. All the patients in the group are unable to initiate or sustain social conversation, lack familiarity with community resources, have a low confidence level (especially in situations involving the opposite sex), exhibit poor grooming and dressing habits, and exhibit poor habits in regard to keeping appointments and arriving on time for appointments.

At the Wednesday meeting, each patient reports to the entire group on his progress regarding his weekly goals. Many weekly goals involve specific social behaviors that each patient is to exhibit while at home. For example, one participant may have agreed to check a book out from the local library, to call a designated friend on the phone, or to obtain a brochure describing extension classes at the community college. As an additional function of the Wednesday meeting, the group plans a Friday social outing at which the therapist is to be a participant-observer. Arrangements are made to meet at a specified locale (restaurant, skating-rink, bowling alley) on Friday afternoon. Each patient is to select one short term goal for the Friday engagement, e.g., to be on time, to order dinner independently, or to initiate a conversation with a group member or nongroup member. Further, one or two short term goals to be accomplished at home during the following week are verbalized by each patient and recorded by the therapist.

At the social outing, "therapy talk" is kept at a minimum. This outing is intended as much as possible to simulate a natural social event. While a participant, the therapist models appropriate social behavior and helps stimulate casual conversation. Group members and the therapist provide reinforcement in the natural sense, responding to the social overtures made by various patients. However, there is not the stringent kind of provision of reward as might occur in a prevocational activity group. Since patients have a large responsibility in reinforcing each other, the success of this group depends in part on the ability of patients to respond to other patients in terms of their positive and not negative behaviors. Again, the therapist, who is often mimicked, has a key role via her modeling, in helping the patient group attend to the positive behavior of its members. The therapist notes significant behaviors during the social outing that need to be addressed by the group at the following Wednesday meeting, and is responsible for communicating with the other treatment staff about the status of individual patients regarding their goal attainment.

Group III. Assertiveness Training Group. A third type of behavioral group is typified by the assertiveness training group (see note 8). As in the FAC group, patients are selected for the group according to similar needs and similar targeted behavioral goals. The kinds of patients who might benefit from such a group include those who cannot ask for what they need, those who cannot say "no," those who feel that they are "pushed around" or taken advantage of by others, those who are overly apologetic in their dealing with others, and those who feel guilty when they are angry. An assertiveness-training group is structured as follows:

1. All patients begin the group at the same time. The group is designated to last a given number of sessions, e.g., two times per week, one to one and one-half hours per session, for four weeks.

2. At the first meeting, the therapist describes the function and purposes of the group, the expectations of each group member, and what her role as "director" will entail. Each patient

is asked to describe briefly in writing five social situations in which he feels unable to make his needs known. Having written down the five situations, he is asked to order these from least to most difficult.

3. The therapist collects all the data provided by each patient, becoming cognizant of the common features in which the patients experience difficulty. Though the situations will vary for each patient and the order of difficulty will vary even when the situations are common, the therapist can establish a working hierarchy of situations that can be simulated and role played in each meeting. The kinds of situations frequently simulated, in a hierarchal order include dealing with a stranger who pushes ahead of you in a grocery line, asking for a refund at a store, saying "no" when asked to be on a committee, saying "no" to a sexual advance, and asking for a raise. However, while these are quite general, the therapist has the option of individualizing role plays as she deems necessary.

4. In each subsequent group meeting, one or more situations are constructed by the therapist for practice in role playing. She may start the meeting by giving some didactic information regarding what constitutes appropriate assertiveness, the contrast between assertiveness and aggressiveness, and so on. The group may, in some instances, proceed to a brief muscle relaxation exercise. The therapist then describes the hypothetical situation. For example, "You have been waiting for five minutes at the checkout line at your local grocery store. Suddenly you find that a newcomer has squeezed his way ahead of you. Everyone in line with you appears to notice, but no one has chosen to say anything. How might you handle this situation?"

5. Patients take turns playing a variety of roles in the simulations in order that they may be both the giver and the recipient of appropriate assertive responses. The therapist may ask for "volunteers" but seeks always to insure that all patients have opportunities to try out new behaviors. When appropriate, the therapist might interrupt the process to model an effective assertive response; she may "coach" and encourage as needed. The group members learn not only by their active participation but by observation of others. In this kind of group, modeling, as conceived by Bandura, plays a significant learning function.

6. In each meeting, after simulations are complete, verbal feedback by participants to each other is given regarding the effectiveness of others' responses; feelings, while they may be expressed, are not the focus of the interaction. The therapist, through enthusiastic praise, reinforces the effective playing out of assertive behaviors. The therapist helps patients to identify other situations that would be quite similar to the one just role played in order to facilitate the generalization of learning. The principle of desensitization plays an important role, as patients have the chance to try new behaviors in a setting which is typically less anxiety producing than those outside of treatment. Further, each patient is given the opportunity to build on past learning as each week he encounters increasingly problematic situations in role playing.

7. As the group meeting nears its completion, each patient targets one specific assertive behavior he will endeavor to accomplish before the next meeting. Time is allowed at the end of every subsequent meeting for members to relate in brief whether they attained their weekly

goal. The therapist records, as needed, changes in individual goals and progress made toward their attainment.

Chapter Summary

Behavioral therapy is the application of a collection of techniques that have been found empirically to affect behavior. As Franks notes, while individual therapists select from these behavioral techniques to create their own "brand" of behavioral therapy, all behavior therapies are "predicated upon the common, explicit, systematic, and a priori usage of learning principles to achieve well-defined and pre-determined goals" (Franks, in Patterson, 1973, p. 84). While it acknowledges the existence of biologic, cultural, cognitive, and emotional influence, it is not primarily concerned with these.

One can look at the behavioral approach historically and see it as a response in part to the medical, analytic approach to psychosocial problems that preceded it in the 1940's and 1950's, a stance seen by many as too vague, aloof, even "mystical" in its reliance on such constructs as id and ego that could not be seen, and tending in practice to promote a concept of mental illness. The behavioral approach offered an alternative explanation that pointed to the less menacing and seemingly more manageable concept of "faulty learning." Practitioners who continued to struggle with readmissions in the field of acute psychiatry and had little to offer the chronically, emotionally disabled other than medication now had some specific tools that seemed to offer the opportunity for real behavior change. Occupational therapists followed with other health practitioners, leaving the analytic approach and addressing such issues as "behavior change," behavioral goal setting, documentation, and the like. However, as tends to occur when any new treatment approach is embraced, or an old one re-engaged, there followed a period of overidentification and some inevitable disenchantment and, finally, the ability to look with perspective on the strengths and limitation of behavioral therapy.

Many practitioners and lay persons have reacted strongly to the implicit suggestions (made explicit by Skinner) that in the application of behavioral principles, the persons dispensing reinforcement are ultimately controlling human behavior. Occupational therapists, believing in the importance of internal motivation, striving to allow their patients and clients maximum choice, and seeing the holistic relationship of attitude to the healing process, were left to consider the possibility that freedom of choice was an illusion, and that healing could be reduced to a specifiable biochemical whole. Those believing in the value of human pleasure in discovery and competence found themselves unable to address these except perhaps tangentially in reference to external reward. Although it is not addressed in the literature, it was evident in much of the occupational therapy practice of the 1960's and early 1970's that therapists working in behavioral settings scribed in behavioral rhetoric but continued to function with the same values, purposes, and general direction that they had before. More recently occupational therapists have spoken out against the dogma of a strongly Skinnerian behaviorism, and are including principles of humanism, cognition, and social and developmental theory in their study, dialogue, practice, and research. What has resulted might be

119

termed an eclectic behaviorism as once again we confront the probability that no one explanation for the human condition — as presently exists — best describes it.

Contributions

Behavior therapists have selected and followed through with behavior change that can be studied and verified in the scientific sense. The behavioral approach to psychotherapy and specifically in occupational therapy can be credited for increasing the scrutiny given to treatment goals and the efficacy of treatment alternatives. Many therapists who felt, perhaps intuitively, that their treatment approach was helpful have been forced to look carefully and re-evaluate their treatment outcomes systematically. Further, many patients who have sought psychiatric or emotional aid have been given a concrete way to measure their own progress. While being accused of taking too much control of patient behavior, one might counter that, in discarding the use of psychiatric jargon and labels that tended to overpower the average lay person and perhaps obfuscated much of what was actually occurring in treatment, the behavioral approach gave back to the patient the ability to make understandable choices about his own treatment.

Behavioral techniques appear to work with patients with specific problems in daily functioning and can be used successfully for skill building. The improvements in grooming, appropriate speech, work skills, and social skills have all been addressed repeatedly in the literature. This has been especially significant in the treatment of patients who have been seen as requiring long term, habitual, and or institutional care. As such, behavioral therapy has been credited for "humanizing" the conditions of many persons whose lives have been otherwise void of success or joy.

The thrust of traditional behaviorism can be credited for spotlighting the importance of attention and approval as reinforcement, and for the significant role of modeling in the learning process. Behaviorism has acted as a springboard for those investigators who have since sought to understand better the probable intervening process of cognitive structuring and the heretofore undeveloped understanding of social learning.

Limitations

The behavioral approach does not appear to work as well when there is a lack of specific deviant behavior. For example, if a young man is doing well in school and fulfilling his societal obligations yet expresses the sentiment, "What is life all about?" the behavioral approach has to strain to address the issue and may, many feel, address it tangentially. This leads to the conclusion by many that behavioral therapy does not work well with persons functioning at a "high level." Strictly speaking, the behaviorist can address even these "high functioning" issues behaviorally, but it is worth noting that in the occupational therapy literature, there is no elucidation of treatment with higher functioning individuals or groups. This leads to a second suggestion of limitation.

The behavioral approach appears to work best in a closed or self-contained environment, and gains made in the closed system do not necessarily translate to long term gains at home.

In a closed therapy system, as in an institution, patients are more likely to be influenced by treatment staff injunctions and reinforcements. Further, there is more likelihood that reinforcement will be judiciously given, modeling carefully provided, and progress nurtured. While any behavioral therapist acknowledges that internal motivation and self-reward must at some point take over if a patient is to make a successful transition to an unsystemized community, this intervening step frequently does not occur. In the "real world" our fellow human beings may again reward our aberrant behavior or fail to notice our accomplishments, and many behaviors will revert to pretreatment levels. The occupational therapy literature again provides evidence of success within a highly structured setting, but has less to point to in terms of carryover to nontreatment environments, or to cases of behavioral therapy in which the patient was receiving intermittent therapy on an outpatient basis.

Designing and implementing an effective behavioral program for one or many patients are not necessarily as simple as they might appear. While targeting inappropriate behaviors may not be difficult, isolating these and rewarding just the appropriate responses can be difficult, especially when many patients are working together at one time. Identifying appropriate rewards may also be a difficult task. If all patients desired candy and cigarettes, the old standbys along with hugs and smiles, there would be no dilemna. However, for many depressed and/or regressed individuals the secondary (and at times unclear) gains that they received from maintaining their regressed behavior seem to be more rewarding than anything the staff has to offer. The therapist finds herself offering time alone as a reinforcement to a patient whose goal is to spend less time alone, or food to an adolescent with eating problems whose goal is to spend less time involved with food. Further, it is difficult to achieve the kind of generalization desired while not promoting undesirable response generalization. For example, a specific therapist might achieve increased verbalization from a patient, but this social gain may not be generalized to other staff or to significant others who await the patient's return to home.

Finally, the behavioral position that complex behaviors can be broken down into smaller discrete units may be true, but in practice the effort to do so can become unwieldy. If one is to define the exact circumstances under which a problem such as depression or diffuse anxiety occurs, there is a tendency to respond to the most obvious of the issues — the tip of the iceberg, so to speak. To do otherwise requires the kind of lengthy extensive therapy that behaviorism has sought to replace.

There are many variables that traditional behaviorism has not addressed. It has spoken little, for example, to the importance of internal motivation in human behavior — the motivation to excel when simple competence might have otherwise sufficed, the motivation to practice until perfect, the pleasure of activity for the activity's sake — and in failing to do so, traditional behavioral concepts seem self-limiting. The role of curiosity, e.g., the pleasure of a child in discovery and the joy of learning to speak a first word, is not the concern of behaviorists, yet it seems so integral to our understanding of "purpose" when as occupational therapists we use the term "purposeful activity."

Neither does the traditional behaviorist address the issue of cognitive structuring as an intervening variable in learning and in problem solving. With much of the early impetus coming from those who studied the function of language (Chomsky, 1967, 1972), scientists and practitioners have increasingly felt that such cognitive processing is necessarily conceived and is an activity separate and meaningful in itself.

In summary, one might see many of the oppositions to behavioral thinking as philosophic in essence. Behaviorism is a reductionist approach to understanding the human being. If one describes all the pieces, all the behaviors of a person, has he really described him? Or are behaviors the external display of a far more complex internal process that cannot as yet be as easily discerned? Does behaviorism "trivialize" the human condition, or is it an honest, practical approach to complex problems? After a person's conduct is broken down into discrete behaviors, do we know him? Are discrete behaviors necessary to know him better? With these questions in mind, we turn our attention to the cognitive behaviorists and others who are concerned with the role of cognitive structuring in learning and in treatment.

End Notes

1. "Learning theory" as used here refers to behavioral learning theory. There exists also a wealth of theory that address the question, "How does the individual learn?" from the perspective of psychoanalytic, developmental, humanistic-existential, cognitive, neurologic, and other frameworks.

2. Beginning with the pioneer work of Tolman (*Purposive Behavior in Animals and Man,* 1932), behaviorists began to grapple with the possibility that internal processes, as mediated by the central nervous system, also need to be considered when looking at behavior. Tolman conceived of the "cognitive map," or internal integration of data by the organism. He suggested that the individual, rather than responding in an automatic stimulus-response habit, is capable of holding a cognitive awareness of several means to achieve a desired goal. Tolman theorized that in the development of these cognitive maps, the organism is learning not just movement patterns but also meaning (Hilgard and Bower, 1975, p. 136). The attention given to the cognitive process was to be especially significant in the work of behaviorists who were interested in the development of language, and has ultimately led to a "division" between traditional behaviorists and those known as cognitive behaviorists.

3. Negative reinforcement, the use of *adverse stimuli*, when removed, increases the tendency for the desired behavior to occur. The behavior acts on the environment so as to remove the adverse stimuli or to remove or keep the individual from the situation. Adverse stimuli cause escape or avoidance behavior. For instance, in the winter we put on a coat to avoid getting cold; the cold weather outside negatively reinforces the behavior of putting a coat. One might also consider that getting warmer is a rewarding result of putting on a coat. Thus, as some suggest, negative reinforcement may be somewhat of a misleading term for adverse stimuli.

4. Although coined in slightly different terms, the process of imitation and modeling as described by Bandura is quite similar to the process of identification and the development of superego as conceived by Freud.

5. It is not that behavioral therapists are opposed to insight. They tend to emphasize, however, that knowing what one wants to do or should do does not necessarily translate into the ability to take the desired action. Similarly, seeing where one has made a mistake in the past does not necessarily prevent one from repeating similar mistakes in the future. The word "insight" is used when the behavioral therapist tries to increase the patient's recognition that a particular behavior has brought about a specific predictable result.

6. When the behavioral model is applied in a medical setting or when reimbursement is sought from the government or an insurance carrier, it may be required that the patient be given a medical, psychiatric diagnosis.

7. Specialized job task skills are taught by the occupational therapist in vocational rehabilitation centers, sheltered workshops, or simulated work experiences (such as assembly line work) that can occur in an occupational therapy setting. Occupational therapists have been known to contract with local agencies for simple jobs that patients could complete in short periods of time or to assume responsibility for jobs inside the hospital. Sample jobs include assembling cardboard boxes, packing machine or electronic parts in a container, collating printed materials, stuffing envelopes, folding linen, and sorting tasks.

8. An assertiveness group is also identified with the cognitive-behavioral framework. Depending upon the therapeutic approach of the occupational therapist and the needs of patients in the group, the therapist may give more emphasis to changing the patient's thoughts about himself as well as changing his behavior in an assertiveness group.

Additional Readings

Ellsworth P, Colman A: The application of operant conditioning principles to work group experience. AJOT 24(6):495-501, 1969.

Patterson CH: Relationship Counseling and Psychotherapy. New York, Harper and Row, 1974.

References

Abildness A: Biofeedback Strategies. Rockville, Maryland, The American Occupational Therapy Association, 1982.

Agnew P, Shannon G: Training program for a myo-electrically controlled prosthesis with sensory feedback system. AJOT 35(11):722-727, 1981.

Bandura A: Psychological Modeling: Conflicting Theories. New York, Adine-Atherton, 1971.

Bandura A: Social Learning and Personality Development. New York, Holt, Rinehart and Winston, 1963.

Bandura A: Social Learning Theory. New York, General Learning Press, 1971.

Banus B (Ed): The Developmental Therapist. Ed 2. Thorofare, NJ, Charles B. Slack Inc., 1979.

Becker M, Banus B: Sensory-perceptual dysfunction and its management. In Banus B, et al (Eds): The Developmental Therapist. Thorofare, NJ, Slack, Inc., 1979, pp 239-273.

Christiansen C, Davidson D: Community health program with low achieving adolescents. AJOT 28(6):346-350, 1974.

Chomsky N: Review of Skinner's verbal behavior. In Jakobovits L, Miron M (Eds): Readings in the Philosophy of Language. Englewood Cliffs, NJ, Prentice-Hall, 1967.

Chomsky N: Language and Mind (Enlarged Edition). New York, Harcourt Brace Jovanovich, 1972.

Clark F, et al.: Comparison of operant and sensory integrative methods on developmental parameters in profoundly retarded adults. AJOT 32(2):86-92, 1978.

Clark E, Peters M: Scorable Self Care Evaluation. Thorofare, NJ, Charles B. Slack Inc., 1984.

Cormier W, Cormier S: Interviewing Strategies for Helpers. Belmont, CA, Wadsworth, Inc., 1979.

Corey G: Theory and Practice of Counseling and Psychotherapy. Monterey, CA, Brooks/Cole, 1982.

Diasio K: Psychiatric occupational therapy: Search for a conceptual framework in the light of psychoanalytic ego psychology and learning theory. AJOT 22(5):400-414, 1968.

Dollard J, Miller N: Reinforcement theory and psychoanalytic therapy. In Patterson CH: Theories of Counseling and Psychotherapy. New York, Harper and Row, 1973, pp 89-124.

Ford AL: Teaching dressing skills to a severely retarded child. AJOT 29(2):87-92, 1975.

Franks CM: Introduction: Behavior therapy and its Pavlovian origins: Review and perspectives. In Franks CM (Ed): Behavior Therapy: Appraisal and Status. New York, McGraw-Hill Book Co., 1969, p 22.

Geiser R: Behavior Mode and the Managed Society. Boston, Beacon Press, 1976.

Greenberg S, Fowler R: Kinesthetic biofeedback: A treatment modality for elbow range of motion. AJOT 34(11):738-743, 1980.

Hilgard E, Bower G: Theories of Learning. Ed 3. Englewood Cliffs, NJ, Prentice-Hall, 1974.

Hilgard E, Bower G: Theories of Learning. Ed 4. Englewood Cliffs, NJ, Prentice-Hall, 1975.

Jodrell R, Sanson-Fisher R: Basic concepts of behavior therapy: An experiment involving disturbed adolescent girls. AJOT 29(10):620-624, 1975.

Kanfer FH, Phillips J: Learning Foundations of Behavior Therapy. New York, Wiley, 1970.

Kaye J, Mackie V, and Hitzing EW: Contingency management in a workshop setting: Innovation in occupational therapy. AJOT 24(6):413-417, 1970.

King L: A Sensory integrative approach to schizophrenia. AJOT 28(9):529-536, 1974.

King L: Information from author's notes on Sensory Integration Workshop, Colorado State University, May 19, 1974.

Kulkulka CG, Brown DM, Basmajian JV: A preliminary report: Biofeedback training for early finger joint mobilization. AJOT 29(8):469, 1975.

Leibowitz J, Holcer P: Building and maintaining self-feeding skills in a retarded child. AJOT 28(9):545-548, 1974.

Lemke H, Mitchell RD: A self-feeding program; controlling the behavior of a profoundly retarded child. AJOT 26(5):261-264, 1972.

Mager R: Preparing Instructional Objectives. Palo Alto, CA, Fearon Publishers Inc., 1962.

Mann W, Sobsey R: Feeding program for the institutionalized mentally retarded. AJOT 29(8):471-474, 1975.

Martin GL: Behavior Modification. Englewood Cliffs, NJ, Prentice-Hall, 1978.

Martin M: Behavior modification in the mental hospital: Assumptions and criticisms. Hosp Community Psychiatry September 1972, p. 292.

Mischel W: Toward a cognitive social learning reconceptualization of personality. Psychol Rev 80:252-283, 1973.

Mischel W: Personality and Assessment. New York, Wiley, 1968.

Mosey A: Three Frames of Reference in Mental Health. Thorofare, NJ: Charles B. Slack Inc., 1970.

Mosey A: Activities Therapy. New York, Raven Press, 1973.

Norman C: Behavior modification: A perspective. AJOT 30(8):491-497, 1976.

Nuse-Clark P, Allen A (Eds): Occupational Therapy for Children. St. Louis, Mosby, 1985.

Ogburn K, Fast D, Tiffany D: The effects of reinforcing working behavior. AJOT 26(1):32-35, 1972.

Overbaugh T, Bradley Bucher M: Use of operant conditioning to improve behavior of a severely deteriorated psychotic. AJOT 24(6):423-427, 1970.

Rotter JB: Social Learning and Clinical Psychology. Englewood Cliffs, NJ, Prentice-Hall, 1954.

Sieg K: Applying the behavioral model to the occupational therapy model. AJOT 28(7):421-428, 1974.

Skinner BF: The Behavior of Organisms: An Experimental Analysis. Englewood Cliffs, NJ, Prentice-Hall, 1938.

Skinner BF: Science and Human Behavior. New York, Macmillan, 1953.

Skinner BF: The Technology of Teaching. Englewood Cliffs, NJ, Prentice-Hall, 1968.

Skinner BF: Beyond Freedom and Dignity. New York, Knopf, 1971.

Stein F: A current review of the behavioral frame of reference and its application to occupational therapy. Occup Ther Ment Health 2(4):35-62, 1982.

Talbot M, Junkala J: The effects of auditorally augmented feedback on the eye-hand coordination of students with cerebral palsy. AJOT 35(8):525-528, 1981.

Trombley C, Scott A: Occupational Therapy for Physical Dysfunction. Baltimore, Williams & Wilkins, 1977.

Wanderer Z: Therapy as learning: Behavior therapy. AJOT 28(4):207-208, 1974.

Watts F: Modification of the employment handicaps of psychiatric patients by behavioral methods. AJOT 30(8):487-490, 1976.

Weber N: Chaining strategies for teaching sequenced motor tasks to mentally retarded adults. AJOT 32(6):385-389, 1978.

Weed L: Medical Records, Medical Education and Patient Care. Cleveland, Case Western Reserve University Press, 1969.

Wehman P, Marchant J: Improving free play skills of severely retarded children. AJOT 32(2):100-104, 1978.

Chapter 5

Overview of the Cognitive Process

Throughout the history of psychology, cognitive studies have been influential in the research and development of the field. Prominent studies include those of Bartlett, Piaget, Jung, Koffka, Kohler, Wertheimer, Lewin, Luria, Binet, Tolman, and Rotter. After World War II the elements of computer technology, the work in information and processing theory, and studies in linguistics led to the further development of cognitive psychology. Beginning in 1960 and into the 1980s, cognitive psychology was not only influential but it was a focal point in theoretical and applied psychology. Simultaneously the influence of cognitive psychology and neurology has been increasingly felt in occupational therapy theory and practice. Because of this influence, the growing interest in cognitive approaches to treatment, and the subsequent need to have a broad understanding of cognition in contemporary practice, the authors provide a summary of the cognitive process which will give basic information for understanding the cognitive approaches discussed in this text.

The applied and theoretical literature in medicine, psychology, and education which addresses the structure, organization, and functions of the brain is extensive and could not be adequately summarized in the space of this chapter. We have, however, summarized key aspects of cognitive theory in order to provide a basis for the application of three theoretical approaches in occupational therapy: (1) a *holistic neurological* approach based upon the work of Alekander Luria and elaborated in Chapter 9, Organic Mental Disorder, (2) a *cognitive-behavioral* approach influenced by the work of Piaget, Bandura, and cognitive-behavioral psychologists and exemplified in occupational therapy through psychoeducational treatment programs, as discussed in Chapter 6, Cognitive-Behavioral Frame of Reference, and (3) the cognitive arm of the *developmental* framework presented in Chapter 7, Developmental Frame of Reference.

The occupational therapy literature does not indicate that the profession has adopted a specific cognitive frame of reference. In physical medicine Luria's work is the more frequent reference, and it is this neurologic-holistic approach that serves as a basis for the discussion of the treatment of organic or physically based cognitive dysfunction. In psychosocial arenas, the psychoeducational programs (including that by Lillie and Armstrong, 1982) reflect early cognitive-behavioral theory, and the work of Claudia Allen (1982, 1985) suggests an emerging cognitive-developmental theory. The theoretical approaches discussed in this text are not the only possible cognitive routes.

In this chapter we draw from several sources to provide a foundation that will serve the neurological, cognitive-behavioral, and cognitive-developmental treatment frameworks. They are the information processing, structural-organismic, and social learning theories. The reader will find that cognition is approached more broadly than as conceived by Piagetian theory. When including some social learning tenets, we have taken the liberty of estimating when given social learning skills are most likely to emerge. While there exist diverse discussions regarding cognition, we have chosen Flavell, Bandura, and Perry and Bussey as primary references from the theoretical literature and Kaplan and Sadock and Lezak from the applied literature.

Theoretical Conception of Cognition

Since mental processes intrude into all aspects of human life, it is difficult to establish limits in defining cognition. Flavell suggests an encompassing conceptualization of cognition that combines the traditional view of cognition with the information-processing and structural-organismic perspectives.

The traditional view of cognition is that it is composed of "higher mental" processes which include "knowledge, consciousness, intelligence, thinking, imagining, creating, generating plans and strategies, reasoning, inferring, problem solving, conceptualizing, classifying, relating, symbolizing, and perhaps fantasizing and dreaming" (Flavell, 1977 p. 2).

In addition to the "higher mental" processes, the contemporary therapist will broaden her understanding if she includes other components such as "organized motor movements (especially in infant cognition), perception, imagery, memory, attention and learning . . . and social cognition" (Flavell, 1977, p. 2).

Information Processing View of Cognition

Man as Machine. The information processing view of cognition comes from the work of Herbert Simon, Allen Newell, Walter Reitman, and others. "The information-processing theorist thinks of man as a complex machine or device, in some ways analogous to a modern electronic computer, that possesses elaborate *programs* (sequences of instruction) for dealing with information in intelligent and adaptive ways. The programs consist of intricately interrelated and sequenced cognitive operations or *processes* that construct or create, receive, transform (recode, reduce, elaborate), store, retrieve, and otherwise manipulate units of information or knowledge" (Flavell, 1977, p. 5). In this view the individual receives information or *input* from the environment through his sensory systems (visual, auditory, tactile, olfactory). This sensory information is processed by short term and long term memory components as well as other sensory buffers. It is then analyzed and transformed according to rules of the cognitive system to produce thoughts, feelings, and behaviors. The rules provide the guides for constructing, monitoring, and executing information. They give meaning to stimuli and produce goal directed or planned behavior, called *output*. Although different from the structural-organismic perspective, the information processing view can complement the more traditional Piagetian perspective. Information processing theory provides an analogy for explaining the coding and organization of environmental stimuli and the role played by the person's beliefs and expectations during the process. In a sense it provides the "rules" for thinking and behaving. In recent years information processing vocabulary has become popular in everyday language, and it is being used increasingly in cognitive literature.

The Structural-Organismic Perspective

The writings of Jean Piaget (1952, 1957, 1962, 1963, 1973) and Heinz Werner (1948, 1957, 1963) represent the structural-organismic perspective, which sees cognition as a complex internal system of organization that influences how the person relates in his environment. It is an *assimilation-accomodation* model of cognitive functioning.

Assimilation and Accommodation. As man interacts every day with people and objects in his environment, he takes in new information. This information fits into existing cognitive structures (schemes) which will give meaning to the new event. This process gives a subjective view of the world and is called *assimilation*. During *accommodation* the person will notice the specific properties of objects, people, and events as well as the relationships that exist among them. He will take in this new information and alter the existing cognitive structures (ways of interpreting information) to meet the demands of the new experience and thus develop a more objective view (Flavell, 1977, p. 7). Both assimilation and accommodation occur simultaneously throughout the process of development, and if the two processes are in balance, adaptive intelligence exists (Flavell, 1977, p. 56).

Equilibration. The method of maintaining this balance is called equilibration. *Equilibration* is an internal self-regulatory process through which the individual controls the process of development and maturation as well as the experiences and social interactions that occur throughout life. (It is not the same as motivation.) For optimal cognitive growth there needs to be moderate disequilibrium (Flavell, 1977). That is, the individual must be exposed to experiences that blend both the familiar and the novel. Too much sameness is "boring" and fails to stimulate his interest; totally novel events or experiences have nothing in them that he can understand or relate to. Given a moderate amount of new information, the individual will change his thinking as needed to achieve harmony or balance and thus achieve a more sophisticated level of adaptability (Perry and Bussey, 1984).

During the assimilation and accomodation processes, schemes are developed. *Schemes* are the cognitive units or individual structures which house or give meaning to all experiences. Stated another way, schemes are the mental representation of experience. As the person grows and changes, more and more schemes are accumulated. They organize the person's perceptions and the events that are perceived by the person into information groups according to common characteristics (Flavell, 1977).

Motivation for Cognitive Development. Throughout development the basis for motivation expands and changes, and several motivators can exist simultaneously. Initially the system functions as a result of *intrinsic motivation*. The infant is believed to respond to its environment from birth because of an inborn mechanism which causes the child to respond to stimuli and explore his environment. As the child interacts in its environment and encounters novel experiences, he is also intrinsically motivated to achieve equilibration. Eventually, as the child interacts in and learns from its surroundings, he gains a sense of personal satisfaction and competence which become additional motivating forces for interaction (Flavell, 1977).

Development of Knowledge. Structural-organismic theory, commonly referred to as *cognitive developmental* theory, proposes that as children and adults develop, they come to think about their worlds in new ways (see note 1). That is, not only do they increase the quantity of their knowledge, but the nature or quality of their thinking changes also. As part of the developmental process, different kinds of knowledge come into existence. For the sake of discussion we can group this knowledge into three kinds of information (although the reader will quickly recognize that these categories are overlapping and interdependent): physical knowledge, symbolic-representational thought, and social cognition.

Physical knowledge encompasses the physical properties of objects and events (e.g., their size, shape, and color) and organizes this information according to principles of logic. These principles determine how the individual perceives the changes in and relationship of objects and actions over time and through space. It was the acquisition of physical knowledge that was a primary focus of Piaget's work. Physical knowledge both provides the basis for and is dependent on symbolic-representational intelligence and social cognition.

Symbolic-representational intelligence encompasses language development, the use of language (including reading and writing), and the formation of mathematical constructs. This knowledge allows the individual to correctly name objects, communicate his needs, and form logical sequences of thought and action.

Flavell describes *social cognitive development* as a "gradual process of differentiating self from nonself, persons from nonpersons, and one person from another" (Flavell, 1977, p. 59). These conceptions will be developed and elaborated to form rules, laws, morals, values, and ethics that assist a person as he interacts in his social world and uses verbal and nonverbal communication (Flavell, 1977). (While social learning theory has not been primarily concerned with establishing age parameters for social cognition, it has contributed to the understanding of the roles that imitation, modeling, and observation learning play in cognitive development. Therefore we will include this information in the discussion that ensues. Moral development will be discussed further in Chapter 7, Developmental Frame of Reference.)

The "rules" of cognitive development (especially Piagetian) are probably quite familiar to the reader. Briefly summarized, they are as follows:

1. Knowledge development (of all types) occurs in a invariant, sequential pattern of developmental stages, characterized by the use of given cognitive structures.
2. An individual operates primarily at one stage and then (incorporating the cognitive structures identified with this stage) proceeds to the next stage, at which he will utilize new structures.
3. Process through these stages is not automatic and is related to four broad conditions: (a) the physical maturation of the individual, especially the central nervous system; (b) physical experience with objects and sensory stimuli; (c) social "transmission" through interaction in which people exchange increasingly complex ideas; (d) the existence of a self-regulating, internal mechanism that operates within the individual to reconcile or "equilibrate" maturation and experience.
4. A person may not skip a stage and "jump" to a higher one.
5. Persons prefer to utilize the highest or most complex cognitive structures of which they are capable (Piaget, 1973, pp. 27-28).

While no one seems to challenge the general utility of cognitive-developmental principles in giving a typical picture of the progression of cognitive changes, recent literature has emphasized the following:

1. The child or adult may use cognitive structures representative of more than one "stage," depending on the situation.
2. Adults (and children) may "regress" and use cognitive structures typical of lower stages than what they have proven capable of using, as, for instance, when they are under stress or have unmet emotional needs. Therefore, a stage theory of cognitive development should not connote to the reader an all or nothing, acquisitional model. Further, and this cannot be overemphasized, an adult's behavior and thoughts can be characteristic of any of the stages to be discussed.

To illustrate this, as we proceed in our review of cognitive development we will pause often to exemplify given cognitive structures as represented in adult behavior. When lower levels of cognitive reasoning predominate, however, the individual tends to be limited in his ability to deal effectively with a variety of adult expectations. This should be kept in mind by the reader as she prepares to use the information from this chapter as a foundation for treatment.

The stages most frequently identified in discussions of cognitive development are chronologically organized as follows: infancy (birth to 2 years), early childhood (2 to 6 years), later childhood (7 to 11 years), and adolescence to adulthood (12 years and older). As we highlight briefly how the three threads of knowledge intertwine to create the fabric of cognition, we emphasize that what follows represents only the "tip of the iceberg" in regard to the infinite, complex, and unique knowledge structure developed by each of us.

Infancy (Birth to Two Years)

Physical Knowledge

The foundation of all three kinds of cognition are laid during the period Piaget called the *sensorimotor* period of logic development. At birth the child has a biological identity and an amorphous personal-psychological identity. As he develops during these first two years of life, the child is aware of and interprets bodily sensations; and he actively processes the information gained from his exploration, his body rhythms, and his feelings. An important part of this process in cognitive development is for him to distinguish the sensations that come from inside from those that originate outside himself. In other words, he establishes his boundaries and takes a big step in the process that will continue throughout life: establishing a sense of self.

The infant's beginning movements begin as random movements and initially lack goal direction. However, as he develops in this period, movement becomes more purposeful, and there is much practice play or experimentation with objects. From this he makes the important discovery that objects have permanence (they exist even when temporarily out of sight) and that motor acts have predictable results (e.g., release a toy and it will fall). A key developmental accomplishment in this stage is the infant's eventual ability to retain an internal image (symbol of an object).

As he develops, he will become capable of simple imitation: that is, simple gestures and sounds can be imitated but not coordinated sequences of events (Perry and Bussey, 1984, p. 126).

During infancy the child is egocentric, at the center of his reality. All his perceptions are generated from his center. Therefore, all things are as they appear to the child, and he can conceive of no alternatives. Because he can entertain only one alternative at a time, his problem solving is rigid and limited. To problem solve, the child uses trial and error manipulations that are tied to the obvious cues in any given dilemma. There is no sound reality testing as we think of it.

The present is the time frame that exists for the child. He cannot conceive of "tomorrow" or "later" in the way the adult can. One result is his need to have demands met immediately, also called the need for immediate gratification.

Some adult behaviors that are suggestive of this cognitive stage of development include those often described as "primitive" or regressed. For example, a confused individual may put objects in his mouth or may need to touch all objects in his environment in order to ascertain their physical properties, or he may become agitated when an important other is out of his sight, because of a disturbance in object permanence. These behaviors should not be confused with the continued enjoyment we all have in experiencing the sensory or sensual aspects of our world.

Symbolic Representational Knowledge

The ability to represent persons, objects, and events symbolically in images becomes the ability to use language. There are two broad aspects of language that we consider here — learning language and learning how to use it (Flavell, 1985; see note 2).

How is language learned? Researchers believe that the child has both innate and acquired mechanisms which promote language development and communication. There is believed to be an innate ability to discriminate and produce speech sounds. The acquired mechanisms which promote language development and communication are dependent upon the environment and the experiences that the person has with people and objects. For instance, the availability of models is believed to be important in speech development. The child imitates the speech he hears first as sounds and then words and later generalizes to learn the rules of grammar and syntax. Cognitive and motor development also influence language (e.g., the ability to speak depends on the ability to coordinate the mouth, tongue, and facial muscles in given patterns).

The child talks about the things he knows and experiences and uses language initially to communicate with significant others in his world. Language in infancy begins with nonverbal gestures (the child points to and reaches for objects) and the babbling or "gurgling" sounds we often refer to as baby talk. These babbling sounds can be regarded as the child's experimentation with and development of all the sounds he will need for later controlled, semantic speech. Near the end of this stage many children use one and two word structures as they learn the names of important objects and become increasingly capable of communicating their needs.

The infant not only is learning to "talk," he is learning to use language for its private purpose and for broader purposes of social communication. The private use of language refers to its function as "any sort of aid to one's own thinking, remembering, emotional control or other nonsocial endeavors." The social use "refers to the use of language to send and receive messages in interpersonal situations" (Flavell, 1977, p. 173).

Social Cognition

Social cognition is knowledge about oneself and people, the relationships between people, groups, and institutions, and the rules and customs governing these relationships (Flavell, 1977). Like physical knowledge, social cognition proceeds from an invariant formation to a more abstract, hypothetical form.

Attachment. The initial form of cognition is *attachment,* which is evident in the close bond that exists between the child and primary care-givers. While Freud emphasized the significance of attachment to the mother, cognitive developmentalists and social learning theorists stress that attachment occurs between the infant and other consistent persons in his life, e.g., father, siblings, grandparents, and baby-sitters. However, not all these figures may be of equal importance to the child. That attachment exists can be seen in the infant's signs of pleasure at being with the care-giver, the distress he displays when separated from the care-giver, and the efforts he makes to rejoin the care-giver (Perry and Bussey, 1984, pp. 45-57).

133

While contact (e.g., physical, visual) is believed to be necessary for attachment to occur, it is not yet clear what minimum amount of contact is necessary. Certainly physical contact, play, eye contact between the care-giver and the child, feeding, and other aspects of what we think of as sensitive and affectionate care-giving do affect the attachment process (Perry and Bussey, 1984, p. 55).

Through the attachment process, the child learns about himself and his effect on others. For example, when he cries, mother responds; when he is scared, the closeness of another is comforting. From successful attachment, the child gains essential cognitions related to the dependability (or undependability) of others, and he establishes a foundation of thoughts regarding his own effectiveness and acceptability.

The adult who makes frequent suicide gestures for the purpose of mobilizing a spouse or therapist may not have integrated cognitions enabling him to evaluate and count on the trustworthiness of others.

Once the child is able to represent himself, objects, and events internally (e.g., he knows that his mother exists even when she is not in sight), he has the confidence and sense of safety that allow him to go further in exploring his environment. It is through this exploration that separation or *detachment* begins.

Summary

We can summarize the infancy period as one in which essential cognitions or awarenesses are internalized. This knowledge gives the child a sense of himself as separate and as powerful within his world. While this is by no means a conclusive list of all the information he gains, we can suggest the following as basic cognitions established by the child in the infancy period (these should be read as beliefs internalized by the child and not as literal verbalizations made by him):

1. I am myself: I am no one else.
2. There are people who will keep me safe, fed, and comfortable.
3. There are people who want to be with me.
4. I am acceptable.
5. I am powerful: I make things happen.
6. People/objects continue to exist even if I don't see them (only partially established).
7. Some objects bring pain; some bring pleasure.
8. Given motor acts have predictable consequences (only partially established).

Early Childhood (Two to Six or Seven Years)

Physical Knowledge

During early childhood, which Piaget referred to as the *preoperational* period of development, verbal and nonverbal means of communication continue to develop, as well as behaviors which contribute to self-control. The child can communicate his desires, gains in muscle strength, and gains control in relation to the execution of purposeful action (including control over urination and defecation and control over selected aspects of his environment).

Establishing Simple Relationships

A childhood type of logic (or what Flavell calls *semilogic*) is evident in the child's knowlege of identities and functions. An *identity* "reflects an understanding that something has remained invariant while other things have changed" (Flavell, 1977, p. 98). The classic example of an identity is seen in Piaget's experiment in which the child can recognize that two identical beakers hold the same amount of water. *Functions* refer to "the child's increasing recognition of simple functional relationships and regular co-occurrences or covariations among everyday objects and events" (Flavell, 1977, p. 99).

For example, when Dad picks up his briefcase, the child knows that he is going to work; or when the baby-sitter comes, Mom and Dad are leaving. The limited usefulness of these functions results from the child's postulates regarding *causality.* Frequently the child at this period will conclude that if events occur together, one must have caused the other. Or he inaccurately concludes that two events that often occur together must occur together.

Preoperational causal thinking is evident in the conclusions of the following young adult: Joan was brought into the hospital by her family, who verbalized concern over her behavior in the preceding two months. They stated that she was increasingly argumentative and irritable, that she was buying an unusual amount at local stores and spending beyond her means. When the therapist asked Joan why she thought she needed hospitalization, Joan paused and recalled the most recent event preceding her admission, saying, "I think they're mad at me because I slept late this morning."

The child continues to be egocentric and is unable to consistently entertain the views of others. For instance, the child who desires sweets for lunch may not be able to consider the stance of the parent whose primary concern is that the child should have nutritious meals. (Piaget's contention that children at this stage are unable to consider the views of others has not been borne out by much experience and research. However, there are many limits on his ability to consider the views of others.)

There is a "magical" quality in the logic of the egocentric child, for in his egocentricity, he believes that he can control events with his thoughts. An example of "magical thinking" is evident in the following adolescent's conclusions:

After talking with his primary therapist, John was furious. Back on the hospital unit, he told everyone that his therapist was a "jackass" and that he did not want to see him any more, but he said nothing of his anger to the therapist. The following day John's therapist announced that he would be going on a two-week vacation. While the therapist was gone, John was extremely depressed and noncommunicative. He finally told one of the other patients that he felt "really awful" because he had (by his anger) "made" his therapist leave.

135

Symbolic Representational Knowledge

The increasingly sophisticated use of language is a key development during early childhood. The child learns to use all the parts of speech (nouns, verbs, pronouns, etc.) according to grammatical rules and builds a vast vocabulary.

In addition to adequate vocabulary and sentence structure, there are cognitive processes which will increase the effectiveness of communication: the ability to be specific in the identification of objects and people (referent-nonreferent array), the ability to be sensitive to the listener, and the ability to be sensitive to feedback (Flavell, 1977).

Referent-Nonreferent Array

First the child, as speaker, must adequately identify and describe the similarities and differences in his environment in order to help the listener distinguish the correct object, person, or event under discussion. For example, if there is a group of children and the child wishes to tell the listener about his brother, who is in the group, he might state, "See that boy in the red shirt on the blue bicycle, with the boy in the blue shirt on a yellow bicycle; the boy on the blue bike is my brother." The child speaker has distinguished his brother (*referent*) within the group of children (*nonreferent*) and can now further develop his conversation.

Distinguishing Among Listeners

The second process is the child's ability (as speaker) to be sensitive to his listener and the communication setting. This will allow the child to adapt his vocabulary as well as his method of communication. Thus, communication can be adapted to meet the need of the child versus the adult, the stranger versus a friend, the use of the telephone versus personal contact. The adult who has not mastered this level of skill, for instance, may seem to be overly familiar with casual acquaintances or strangers.

Using Feedback

The third process is the child's ability (as speaker) to receive and make use of feedback when he speaks. Feedback allows him to understand verbal and nonverbal messages conveyed by the listener and to respond to the feedback to improve the quality of his message. That is, he will amplify or clarify his communication if the listener seems confused, or he will modulate his tone and delivery if the listener appears to be angry (Flavell, 1977, p. 174).

Finally, as a listener, the child becomes increasingly able to attend to one and then more than one speaker, to ask questions when needed in order to increase his understanding, and to respond verbally and nonverbally to the communication he receives (Flavell, 1977).

As a result of improved communication, the child's self-control increases, his behavior becomes more purposeful, and he can profit from training and teaching experiences.

Social Cognition

During this early childhood period, the individual becomes increasingly able to separate or detach from parents. Now able to take an "image" of the parents when he leaves them, and trusting that they will be there when he returns, the child can leave parents for longer periods of time. (Emotionally, attachment remains strong.) At the same time he becomes capable of more *complex imitation*, *differentiation*, and *identification*.

Differentiation occurs when the child knows his own preferences for persons and objects and can identify his own feelings and the feelings of others. He will progress from a superficial awareness of another person's appearance and behavior to an in-depth understanding of the other's thoughts and feelings. During social cognitive development the child broadens his percepts: He not only recognizes his mother but also can see changes in facial expression and knows that different expressions have different meanings. He can identify feelings in a global manner, e.g., good versus bad and happy versus sad. He may break a dish, for instance, and then say "bad boy." He next learns to identify and represent his own thoughts and the thoughts of others. For example, he may come home from school and say, "The kids think I'm stupid."

The child begins to understand the concept of merit and blame and can consider the significance of individual intentions or motives. Even the four or five year old child who has done something wrong will, upon seeing a disapproving glance from his mother, respond with "I didn't mean to, Mommy," and then he may follow this statement with "I'm sorry; I won't do it again." Eventually he will be able to identify the motives and system of defenses he and others use. For example, you may hear a young child or adult say to another, "Oh, you're just doing that to be my friend."

As a part of cognitive development, the child expands upon his infantile ability to imitate the behavior of others and begins to imitate complex sets of behaviors of both parents and playmates. At first he will tend to look at superficial qualities (e.g., those related to size and strength) and imitate his parents (and peers he admires) in order to feel important. Soon he will select behaviors to imitate what he sees as most likely to bring him desired results. Thus, he becomes capable of selective imitation based on the *anticipation of consequences*. He also is believed to be learning about others through his observation of them, even when no direct imitation follows. That is, he becomes able to cognitively retain behaviors he sees modeled, and to extrapolate (and generalize) rules of social behavior that can be called upon later for use by him. (See Bandura, 1977, for a further discussion.)

Identification is a kind of complex imitation in which the child actively selects and retains the attitudes and beliefs of the parent or role model (Rosenthal and Bandura, 1978). In identifying with significant role models, the child may adopt their behaviors, their emotional responses, and the cognitions (he discerns) that occur during his observation of them.

During this period the child conceives of and describes himself in terms of observable or tangible characteristics. He may, for example, describe himself as "a boy" and describe his physical attributes (blue eyes, brown hair), and usually relates having the preferences and values of his parents. He adopts the framework of others in his self-conception, because it is their framework with which he is most familiar and because he depends on parents and significant others for his self-esteem.

Summary

Some of the key cognitions internalized during early childhood include the following:

1. What I want is most important, but other people have wants too.
2. I have (specific) skills. Things I can do include (the person can name his capabilities).
3. I can make things happen by wishing.
4. Some behaviors are rewarded; some are punished.
5. Things that look alike are alike.
6. People are not all the same.
7. Primary differences in people are in their size, strength, or possessions.
8. A mistake is not as bad if it is an accident.
9. Mom (or Dad or someone else) has predictable behaviors. These are (the person can name them).
10. Different people are treated differently.
11. My mother's (father's) face, voice, and manner can tell me if she is happy, sad, angry.
12. Yesterday is over; tomorrow has not yet come.

Later Childhood (Seven to Eleven Years)

Physical Knowledge

The cognitive accomplishments of the previous period are being expanded upon during the next period, which Piaget referred to as one of *concrete operational thinking*. The person becomes increasingly able to perceive the whole picture and have a "balanced view." That is, he is able to analyze the parts in relation to the whole object or event (*decentration*) rather than focus his attention on one particular stimulus (*centration*). Now the person is able to grasp the concepts needed for *transformations, reversibility, inversions, compensation,* and *reciprocity*. His thinking becomes quantitative and oriented toward measurement. This facilitates the use of number skills and knowledge that serve as the foundation for the logical thinking that occurs in conjunction with their use (Flavell, 1977).

Transformations can be physical or temporal. For example, the person can see that amounts may remain the same even if the shape differs (*physical transformation*); i.e., when a large rock is cut into pieces, the shape changes, but the weight of all the pieces is the same as that of the original large rock. *Temporal transformations* allow the person to have a firm grasp of the concept of past, present, and future time. Prior to this development the person could focus only on that one aspect of time which he perceived in the present moment (Flavell, 1977).

When a person's thoughts become reversible, he is able to "sense how one action can literally annul or negate its opposite (*inversion*)" and "also how one action or factor can more directly undo or make up for the effects of another which is not its opposite (*compensation*)" (Flavell, 1977, p. 99). For example, a person is shown two parallel lines of equal length, each containing 10 pennies, and is asked whether the lines are equal. Then the length of one line is changed by expanding the distance between each coin. If the person identifies the change in length of lines and attributes this change to the broader spacing of coins, he is demonstrating compensation.

Number knowledge and skills are evident in the person's ability to perceive sets of similar objects, to count the objects, to read and write numbers, to identify the cardinal and ordinal aspects of a number (i.e., to count objects using the correct sequence and identify the last number in a series as well as particular numbers prior to the last [e.g., of 16 items, the "fifth" item]), to identify similar sets of objects and compare the number and size of the objects in each set, to add and subtract objects, and to be able to see the reversible quality of the process (Flavell, 1977).

The individual functioning at this stage has a form of thinking which Flavell calls *logical*. That is, he is able to make propositions about specific aspects of reality and then test each proposition separately, in order to confirm the logical relationships that can exist. Flavell calls this process *interpropositional thinking*.

Interpropositional thinking uses inductive reasoning and is represented in psychology literature by the following experimental task: The child is shown two rows of beads, equally spaced and placed parallel to each other. He is asked to state whether there are equal numbers of beads in each row. Then the spacing of the beads in one line is changed, although the same number of beads still exists in each line and the lines remains parallel. The child is asked to state whether the numbers of beads in each row are still equal. The child who confirms his response by counting the beads in each line is using interpropositional thinking.

In occupational therapy there is an analogous example. The patient who is working on a tile trivet that is modeled after a sample trivet may seek to confirm his choices as he works by accurately counting the tiles in each row of both trivets (the sample and the one he is making).

Discovering the logical relationship between objects and events is a major aim of thinking in this period. However, logical relationships can be deduced about only perceptible tangible matters, not about hypothetical constructs. Whatever knowledge is discovered, information is viewed as "correct" or "incorrect." This is a stage of *absolutes*, and there is little ability for flexibility. In children the stage of absolutes is readily seen in their interpretation of rules or laws.

This stage of absolute thinking by an adult is illustrated in the following example: An older adult was evaluating the benefits of a travel club and deciding whether to become a member. He based his decision to join upon his desire to take a trip in the immediate future and the reimbursement on this first trip he would receive for joining the club. He could not determine whether there were long term intangible benefits for joining the club. That is, in the future would the club travel to sites of interest to him? Did the majority of club benefits meet his social needs?

Symbolic-Representational Knowledge

The ability to use language privately as well as socially increases during this period. Vocabulary and syntax become more complex. The individual can appreciate, for example, that the same word can have several meanings, that two words that sound alike are in actuality very different, and that several different words can connote an identical meaning.

The child or adult is able to use feedback in a way that was limited previously. Because he can now *decenter* (or imagine the views of someone else), he can *empathize* with a person with whom he engages. Thus, feedback is not restricted to taking in information to modify his own performance (although it can still be used for this). Feedback, both verbal and nonverbal, can now be used by the child to better understand the needs and concerns of another.

Social Cognition

The child has come far in the process of separation from parents and needs only occasionally to "touch base" with them through the day as he goes about his many activities. (The continuity of the emotional caring continues to exist.) Although still identifying with his parents, he has begun the process of distinguishing how his likes and preferences are at times different from theirs, in preparation for adolescence to follow.

The child's peer friendships have become very important to him, and increasingly he identifies with and imitates peers, as he had done previously with parents. Being like and being accepted by peers are important and can place the child in conflict with his parents' ideals.

In this stage of cognitive development the child will learn to grasp the concept of "personality" and will identify and discuss his own as well as the personality of others. Whereas initial descriptions of a friend used to be, "He is nice, he has toys that I like, and we ride bikes together," descriptions now become more precise than "nice," "good," or "bad" and are less tied to another's appearance and possessions. Thus, the child becomes able to say, "She is my friend because she is thoughtful and considerate and listens to my problems."

The child's sense of self, which comes from both the reflections and reactions of others to him and from his increased ability to think about his own experiences, has become much more firm. It not only includes a sense of himself as a physical and psychological being as he exists, but also has come to include an *ideal self* or thoughts about the person he would like to be. This ideal self develops from his observations of the results of given behaviors in others and from his incorporation of values. It may begin with the wish to change physical attributes ("I wish I looked like Jane; everyone likes her") and progress to more concern about psychological traits ("I like myself best when I'm kind and patient").

Summary

We can summarize some of the key cognitions established during later childhood with the following global statements:

1. Not everyone thinks and feels as I do.
2. Events have history; I have a history and a future.
3. Events have their opposites.
4. Objects and events can be organized logically.
5. I believe what I can see or prove.

6. I am mostly like my parents, but I'm different in the following ways (person can name).

7. Friends are important; being like my friends is important.

8. My friend's personality is more important than the possessions he has.

9. I have my own personality.

10. It is important that I consider the feelings of others.

Adolescence and Adulthood (Twelve Years and Older)

Physical Knowledge

As a result of cognitive, social, and motor skill development, the adolescent will begin to question how he has defined himself, the rules and beliefs that he has adopted unchallenged from parents and role models, and he will search for an identity that is self-defined (sometimes referred to as "autonomous" identity).

He continues to use trial and error problem solving but begins to experiment with a more scientific approach. He begins to focus on the future, raising such issues as, "Who do I want to be? What do I want to do? Whom do I wish to be with? What do I value? How will I accomplish my goals? How will I contribute to life?"

The Scientific Period

Prior to adolescence, one's knowledge is considered prescientific. That is, the person uses trial and error learning and primarily seeks experiences which provide consistency and regularity. At about age 15 to 20 years the individual sees the limitations of this knowledge and seeks to find variety in experiences and variables in his knowledge. As a result he begins to logically restructure his knowledge. When this occurs, the *scientific period of knowledge development* occurs.

During this period the person forms new hypotheses about himself and his world. He then sees experiences designed to systematically collect data in order to validate or reconstruct his knowledge and to amplify his information. This ability to carry out hypothetic-deductive reasoning has also been called *formal operational thinking*. Now the person can see possibilities and not just the "real situation." He can anticipate future outcomes when he is problem solving, is able to conceptualize an outcome after generating multiple combinations of given data, and can show planned, strategic problem solving (Flavell, 1977).

For example, the individual wishing to attend college will be able to identify his interests, the schools which can best satisfy his interests, as well as other resources which will help him to satisfy his needs and fulfill his goals. During this scientific process there is a cycle by which one's personal identity is continuously remodeled and problem solving promoted. Knowledge structures maintain a basic identity of oneself and the "real" world and at the same time incorporate information from life's experiences to allow for growth and changes in self-perception and increasingly sophisticated problem solving.

Symbolic-Representational Knowledge

The increased sophistication in language communication is that needed for and representative of the hypothetical thinking just discussed. The individual is able to use language privately to generate and "keep track of" many alternatives while weighing both the obvious and the more subtle differences in courses of action. He is able to think through a plan and imagine its consequences without actually needing to carry out actions in the physical sense. He can use language to both imagine himself and others in the future and reflect upon himself or others in the past in order to select the most suitable course of action.

While the very young child can enjoy fantasy because he can enter into it and lose his boundaries within it, an adult capable of this mature level of cognition can enjoy the freedom and symbolic play in fantasy yet not lose a sense of himself as real.

The language of the adult often includes a rich use of simile, metaphor, and allegory. Thus, words come to represent much more than the obvious (or literal), and they become capable of carrying a depth of private and publically shared symbolism. As a result, the adult thinking at this level can appreciate the puns and plays on words that make up sophisticated adult humor, such as satire.

Social Cognition

The most characteristic changes in social cognition occur as a part of the transition into adulthood as the individual goes about establishing an identity autonomous from his family. To achieve autonomy the person will work to further develop and formalize his self concepts. The mature self concept includes several dimensions which relate to the following:

1. Being able to recognize and relate comfortably in a variety of different roles (which may have very different role expectations) while retaining an overall sense of wholeness.
2. Having a sense of competency to meet challenges while being able to realistically acknowledge limitations.
3. Accepting the responsibility for one's own actions and feeling that the self has power over the outcome of personal events.
4. Being able to separate one's own ideas or ideals from those of others and to actively select those which will guide one's belief and value system (Perry and Bussey, 1984).

As he prepares to take his place as a mature individual, the person will philosophize about the world, how it should be, and how to make it better. From these philosophical ideals and from a long history of taking in and accommodating to information about his world will come an identity constructed from his own beliefs, not defined by others. He will take a stance and identify thoughts, values, and attitudes, many of which may differ from those of his parents, and he will behave more independently. This new self definition will allow him to separate from his parents and begin a search for a partner with whom he can have an emotional and/or sexual relationship.

Summary

Mature cognitions internalized as guiding structures by many (but certainly not all) young adults include the following:

1. Not everything is as it seems.
2. There are concerns (needs, causes, issues) more important than my own desires.
3. There are many courses of action I could take in my life; I must consider their consequences.
4. The greater welfare of mankind is my concern.
5. Most social issues are not "black and white."
6. I am separate from my parents: I am responsible for my own decisions.
7. There is a world of experience beyond the verifiable.
8. I do not have to control or organize everything in my environment.

Summary of Structural-Organismic Position. Reaching adulthood does not mean that cognitive development ends. Even when no new cognitive schemes develop, throughout his adult life the individual will continue to take in information, accomodate to changing role expectations, and learn new skills.

Not every adult achieves the so-called higher levels of cognitive function. Nor does the individual always use the most sophisticated cognitive schemes that he has shown himself capable of. In times of stress, for example, when motivation is diminished, when physical causes interfere with cognitive processes, or when emotional-affective needs are unmet, the person may revert to lower levels of cognitive function.

Perception, Metacognition, and Memory as Cognitive Processes

In addition to sensory-motor, symbolic-representational, and social knowledge, the broad definition of cognition includes perception, metacognition, and memory. These are discussed next.

Perception

In the literature, the development of perception is described as moving from a singular system during infancy and expanding to a perceptual-attentional system throughout life. The descriptions of the five senses and their development broaden to include the perception-attentional characteristics of development and descriptions of how these characteristics aid goal attainment.

Perception involves the ability to perceive space and objects, to integrate information from the multiple sensory systems (auditory, visual, tactile), to coordinate the sensory and motor systems, to remember visual images, to interpret perceptual illusions, and to grasp the concept of picture perception (Flavell, 1977, pp. 171-172).

Selective Attention

In the area of perception Flavell recommends the work of Eleanor Gibson (1969), which describes the theory of perceptual learning and development. Her theory emphasizes the selective nature of perceptual processing and attentional deployment. She describes the processes through which the person comes to differentiate perceptual data and identify similarities and differences between objects and events. This perceptual sensitivity occurs as a result of abstraction, filtering, and peripheral mechanisms of attention. The infant perceives, attends to, and responds to stimuli in the environment. As the person grows, his perceptions and attention become increasingly selective, focused, and under the control of his mind (Flavell, 1977, p. 167). This increased control over one's perception and attention influences learning and facilitates adaptation. The person comes to be able to decide when to attend, what to attend to, and the benefits of attending and thus develops an attending strategy (Flavell, 1977, p. 169).

Attention Span

With development we see that attention becomes increasingly planned and strategic. As attention becomes more strategic, it also occurs over longer periods of time. Attention does not occur in isolation, but over time. Thus the individual screens, selects, and retains the necessary data to respond and benefit from the feedback which comes from the environment and from within himself to determine whether he missed or overlooked something. He then sets about maintaining general contact with reality as well as selectively attending to and adapting to one or more situations simultaneously (Flavell, 1977).

Through experience the individual becomes increasingly aware of his ability to attend and of how to use his attention, to direct his behavior, and to accomplish a goal. This ability to monitor his attention, use planned attention, and develop strategies is part of metacognition.

Metacognition

Metacognition is a recently coined term used, with increasing frequency, in the fields of psychology and education. It has been defined, categorized, and exemplified in multiple ways. Briefly, metacognition is "cognition about cognition" (Flavell, 1985, p. 104). That is, a person is aware of what he does and does not know, what helps him to learn and to use his knowledge, and how and when to use his knowledge.

Metacognitive skills influence "oral communication of information, oral persuasion, oral comprehension, reading comprehension, writing, language acquisition, perception, attention, memory, problem solving, social cognition, and various forms of self-instruction and self-control" (Flavell, 1985, p. 104). Since the recognition of metacognitive skills, teachers and therapists have begun to teach these skills through strategies such as those used in cognitive behavioral therapy, social learning programs, and competency education.

Examples of metacognition include the person's recognition of universal qualities such as "people make mistakes" and "man is fallible." This information increases his tolerance of errors, his own and others'. Metacognition is also the information in man's memory which tells him whether he has a good or a poor memory, whether he learns best from visual or auditory stimuli, and his learning strengths (e.g., he learns social sciences more easily than biological sciences). Metacognition encompasses the strategies that a person uses to achieve a goal. For example, he knows when to make written lists to assist him to remember information when studying for an examination, or he knows how to read and learn material in a textbook versus leisurely reading a novel. Further, metacognition helps a person keep track of his progress toward the goals he sets. Overall, metacognition assists a person in learning from his own experiences, whether an increased awareness of the techniques that improved his golf score or racquet ball game or his favorite recipe.

Memory

The next component to be discussed that contributes to an expanded definition of cognition is memory. To understand memory and its development we will look at the basic memory processes — knowledge, strategies, and metamemory. The reader will recognize the use of information processing vocabulary in the contemporary conceptualization of memory.

The basic processes of memory are called the *hardware* of the human memory system, the fundamental operations and capabilities of the system (Flavell, 1977, p. 216). Storage, recognition, and recall are examples of basic processes. Basic memory operations influence the person's capacity to learn and know. In discussions of memory the reader may have noticed that it is difficult to separate the meanings of memory from knowledge. Flavell describes this interrelationship when he states, "What a person knows influences what he learns and remembers" (Flavell, 1977, p. 216).

In Flavell's discussion two types of knowledge are referred to: episodic memory and semantic memory. *Episodic memory* is the knowledge that a person has from specific, personal experiences. *Semantic memory* is acquired knowledge that comes from multiple sources. It is the knowledge that allows us to name objects, people, places, and colors. For example, when a child hears the word "bike," he will visualize the object which he has learned is his bike (semantic memory) as well as remember how he learned to ride his bike, or the times he has fallen off the bike, or the friends with whom he rides his bike (episodic memory).

The process by which this knowledge is stored is called *construction*, and the method by which it is retrieved is called *reconstruction*. When a person remembers something, he does not make an exact copy of the information that is stored. He cannot make copies that replicate information as a tape recording or as a photograph does. Rather he may add or omit information and emphasize points that are meaningful to him. Thus he conceptually organizes and reorganizes data until he has a meaningful representation of the information (Flavell, 1977). For instance, when the child described previously tells someone about his bike and the experiences that he has had with his bike, he reconstructs the information (constructions) about his bike that has been stored. With each reconstruction one will probably find some variation in the stories shared about his bike because of the difficulty in exact reproduction.

In order to remember information, a person may use specific conscious activities to help him remember. These memory activities are called *memory strategies*. Strategies are used for the storage and retrieval of information. Some examples of storage strategies include:

1. *Rehearsal:* the process in which a person repeats stimuli or an experience until it is remembered; e.g., a child counts from 1 to 10 until he knows the sequence perfectly.

2. *Organization:* the process in which a person organizes or categorizes information into knowledge groups with similarities. For example, the child learns that there are dogs, cats, birds, and horses and then learns that they all are part of the category, "animal." The student organizes information into categories to be remembered for his examination.

3. *Elaboration:* the process in which the person uses visual images to create a picture or a story to remember two nonrelated items (Flavell, 1977, p. 217). (Note: more will be said about using these strategies in the discussion of organic brain syndrome later in the text.)

Metamemory means "knowledge about anything concerning memory." It has two distinguishing categories — sensitivity to and knowledge of person, task, and strategy variables (Flavell, 1977, p. 218). That is, the person knows when to store or retrieve knowledge as well as what will improve or decrease his memory performance. Metamemory exists when the person is able to describe his ability to remember and/or limitations in remembering, the tasks that help him to remember or that are more easily remembered, and the aids that he uses to store and retrieve information.

Problem Solving

The last aspect of cognition to be included in our overview is that referred to as problem solving. Problem solving is an active process that incorporates all the components of cognition that have been discussed that contribute to (1) recognizing that a dilemma (mental and/or physical) exists which requires attention, (2) identifying its salient features, and (3) creating a sequence of responses. The nature of the logic used in problem solving depends on the development of cognitive structures, as has been described.

When investigating the ability for problem solving, the occupational therapist (as well as other clinicians) has most frequently assessed the patient's ability to identify the problem, look for alternative solutions to the problem, choose one of the alternatives, make a plan of action, implement the plan, and evaluate the outcome.

In addition to this general problem solving format, Bara (1984) suggests that the therapist also consider categories of problem solving. Bara identified six types of problems: formal, mundane, physical, interactive, personal, and self problem solving. *Formal problem solving* has limited application to clinical settings and uses mathematical and logical procedures to solve problems. *Mundane problem solving* uses "common sense" knowledge to interact in everyday life and solve day to day problems (e.g., the person has learned not to touch fire, not to run in the street in front of a car, and not to pick things up from the ground and put them in his mouth).

Physical problem solving uses procedures that help us solve physical reality problems. For example, spatial and temporal orientation helps us to see interrelationships among physical events. We know enough to put on our boots and raincoat when it is raining, or we know that we need a certain amount of space in order to walk through a doorway without hitting our head, or to wear lightweight clothing when it is hot.

Interactive problem solving uses the social rules acquired from one's family and social network to understand and participate in social interaction; i.e., the rules for interacting with one's parents, "house rules" that must be observed when one lives at home (times to be home, calling to notify parents that you will be late), or knowing how to greet and make a new acquaintance (e.g., shaking hands).

Personal problem solving, like interactive problem solving, uses social rules, but a personal touch is added to these rules. Eventually the person learns to interpret rules using his own frame of reference rather than just doing what he is told or expected to do and perhaps has learned to manipulate social rules. Thus the person uses personal experience and social rules to interact and problem solve in social situations. For example, the street person, the blue collar worker, and the professional have each developed their own standards and style of interaction and method of problem solving. Each has learned from daily experiences or observing his social network how to solve problems and the codes for interaction.

As one learns from other problem solving experiences, one learns *self problem solving*. A person learns from his own experimentation. How often has a parent heard a child state, "Let me do it my way or try it myself." New innovations may come from self problem solving. Self problem solving may reflect one's attitude toward oneself. In the previous example the child is asserting himself and seeking independence and permission to be a problem solver. This image of independence may be an accurate one or may differ from what he thinks and feels about himself.

Cognition in the Context of Therapy

The cognitive system and its limits have been described within the context of therapy by the behaviorist who would "conceptualize the system as a structural network of external and internal stimulus-response connections" and by the psychodynamically oriented therapist who would talk about the "structure and functions of the ego" (Flavell, 1977, p. 4). Rather than repeat the descriptions of these conceptualizations, which are referenced in other chapters of this text, the authors present here the application of cognition in mental health from the perspective of the psychiatrist, psychologist, and occupational therapist with an emphasis on the assessment of cognition. Specific assessments and the occupational therapy interventions that incorporate cognitive theory are described in Chapters 6, 7, and 9.

The Psychiatrist's Assessment of Cognition

Through the assessment of cognitive processes, the psychiatrist seeks to identify or to increase her understanding of psychopathology. During the initial interview she seeks to identify the patient's motivation, needs, and family experiences as well as his social and occupational experiences and interests, and how they have influenced the patient's perceptions, his method of processing information, and his cognitive development. She then evaluates the relationship between the patient's signs and symptoms and his perceptual interpretation, his system of information processing, and his developmental picture (Kaplan and Sadock, 1981).

The psychiatrist carries out a general examination of cognitive function when she uses a *mental status examination*. The mental status examination is designed to establish the patient's general fund of knowledge, his orientation to time, place, and person, his recent and remote memory, his ability for behavioral control, his judgment, his insight, the accuracy of his perceptions, his thought processes, his expression of affect, his general behavior, his speech patterns, and his attitude toward himself and others (Kaplan and Sadock, 1981, pp. 199-200). This information is then documented in the patient's permanent record and used by the mental health staff as they plan and implement intervention strategies.

The Psychologist's Assessment of Cognition

Should the general examination of the patient by the psychiatrist or primary therapist not produce the data necessary for diagnosis, problem identification, and the treatment plan, a psychological assessment administered by a clinical psychologist or neuropsychologist may be requested. The clinical psychologist will use skilled observation and interview in conjunction with standardized tests (a test which has identified validity and reliability criteria) to augument previously acquired data elicited by the psychiatrist.

The test batteries most frequently used with psychiatric populations include an individual intelligence test, an association technique (e.g., person drawing or Rorschach), a story telling test (e.g., Thematic Apperception Test), completion methods (e.g., Minnesota Multiphasic Personality Inventory), and graphomotor tests (e.g., Bender-Gestalt Test) (Kaplan and Sadock, 1981, pp. 208-215).

The results of the previously mentioned tests are then documented by the psychologist, who summarizes the patient's test behavior, his intellectual ability and present functioning, his capabilities and limitations, his reality testing, his ability for self-control, his personal and interpersonal conflicts, his self concept, his system of defenses, his symptoms, his motivation, and the possible diagnosis and prognosis. The reader will note that tests are used to assess cognitive function as well as other areas influenced by cognition (Kaplan and Sadock, 1981, p. 216).

Psychological Testing for Brain Damage

During the general examination the psychiatrist may suspect that the patient has brain impairment and thus may request psychological testing to validate her impressions and to provide additional information regarding the patient's intellectual performance and personality (Kaplan and Sadock, 1981). The data from the test will be used to describe, predict, modify, or control behavior (Lezak, 1976).

When assessing brain damage, tests are used to analyze three functional systems. The three functional systems identified by Lezak (1976) are intellectual functions, personality-emotional variables, and control functions. Each of these systems is briefly described. The reader is referred to the original source (Lezak, 1976) for a detailed neuropsychological assessment approach.

Intellectual Function. Intelligence has four major classes of function: receptive, memory and learning, cognition-thinking, and expressive functions. *Receptive functions* include the intact sensory systems (e.g., visual, auditory, tactile) and the active process of perception, which is aware of, registers, recognizes, discriminates, organizes, and processes sensory information. The *memory functions* facilitate learning and depend upon registration of information, short term storage, and long term storage (see note 3). *Thinking* is a function of the entire brain. It is evident in the patient's ability to make computations, reason and make judgments, form concepts, abstract information and generalize behavior, and organize and plan. The *expressive functions* are the means by which the patient communicates and include his ability to speak, draw, write, use physical gestures and movements, and express affect (Lezak, 1976).

The efficiency of these intellectual functions is influenced by the patient's ability to attend, attend over time, his level of consciousness (e.g., alert, drowsy), and his activity rate (i.e., the patient's speed of motor response and the speed of the activity performed; Lezak, 1976).

Personality and Emotional Variables. The patient's personality can change and behavior problems can result when the patient with a neurological disability cannot meet the demands of society. Therefore the psychologist seeks to determine whether the patient is dull, inhibited, euphoric, anxious, depressed, or hypersensitive and whether he has a social sense which allows him to recognize and respond to the standards and expectations of daily life.

Control Functions. Control functions are inferred from the patient's activity response. Can he initiate and complete activities? Can he adapt his work pace as needed, i.e., more slowly or quickly? Can he shift his attention? Are his solutions to problems rigid and inflexible?

Should the mental status examination and psychological testing fail to provide the depth of understanding necessary for diagnosis, problem identification, and patient treatment, modern technology can provide assessment alternatives, such as computed cranial tomography (CT scan).

The Occupational Therapist and the Concept of Cognition

Given the previous applications of cognition and the data resources available from the mental status examination, psychological testing, and modern technology, what can the occupational therapist contribute to cognitive assessment and treatment? Before answering this question, the conceptualization of cognition in occupation therapy as described by Mosey (1970), Smith (1983), and Spencer (1983) will be presented.

Mosey (1970) refers to conceptualizations of cognition in *Three Frames of Reference for*

149

Mental Health. Definitions in the text are based upon the work of Piaget, Arieti, Bruner, Flavell, Sullivan, and others. Detailed descriptions are given of "the process of perceiving, representing and organizing stimuli" (p. 49). The processes of representation and organization are emphasized in the object relations frame of reference. The acquisitional (behavioral) frame discusses cognition as a "learned adaptive skill" (p. 140). The developmental frame sees cognition as a skill which is "stage specific and . . . appropriate to one's cultural group" (p. 171) and expounds upon the subskills and their components that exemplify cognition.

In *Willard and Spackman's Occupational Therapy,* cognition is defined and evaluated as follows:

"Cognition. The conscious process of awareness and knowledge of objects through perception, memory, and reasoning; mental process of knowing and understanding; an ego function — thinking, judgment" (p. 918).

"Cognition is the mental process by which knowledge is acquired; it is the ability to think and reason. Following disease or injury in which impairment of cognitive functioning is suspected, the following should be evaluated:

1. Ability to follow simple or complex instructions.
2. Ability to carry over learned skills from one day to the next.
3. Ability to attend to a task (attention span).
4. Ability to follow numerous steps in a process.
5. Ability to understand cause and effect.
6. Ability to problem solve.
7. Ability to concentrate.
8. Ability to perform in a logical sequence.
9. Ability to organize parts into a meaningful whole.
10. Ability to interpret signs and symbols.
11. Ability to read.
12. Ability to compute" (Smith, 1983, p. 153).

Cognition is also defined and applied in assessment and intervention strategies in the discussions of brain injury and other disabilities which affect the patient's memory, communication, sensory, perceptual, and other cognitive processes. Within this context and using an information processing analogy, Spencer describes cognition as follows:

"Cognition is knowledge and understanding of the environment gained through the information processing capability of the brain. It involves the mechanisms of perception, memory storage and retrieval of information, organization, and language expression. Cognitive behavior is related to the character and effect of interpersonal relationships. Difficulty in handling input of stimuli (reception, interpretation, organization, order of importance) can hinder ability to store necessary information in the brain for retrieval, resulting in poor concentration for intellectual processing or a deficit in long-term memory. Language deficits may be evident due to lowered comprehension and thought organization. Personality changes, loss of inhibitions, distortions of judgment, and lack of abstract reasoning combine with memory loss to hinder cognitive function, problem-solving, and learning ability" (Spencer, 1983, p. 400).

The discussions of head injury by Spencer (1983) and others such as Abreu (publication in press) reflect a broader conceptualization of cognition than has been previously applied in occupational therapy. In mental health the authors wish to broaden the application of cognition, to incorporate recent conceptualizations, in order to augment the assessment and treatment strategies utilized by occupational therapists. These are discussed in Chapters 6, 7, and 9.

In response to the initial question posed, "What does the occupational therapist contribute to cognitive assessment and treatment?" the following general response is provided. Contributions are influenced by the varied role of the occupational therapist, which may be defined by the setting in which she works. Being sensitive to the needs of the setting prevents duplication of services. Therefore the therapist may or may not have a formalized assessment responsibility. When doing a more formal assessment, the occupational therapist may use the guides provided by Smith (1983) or may use tests such as those described in Chapter 9.

However, regardless of the setting, the therapist is responsible for a continuing assessment of patient functioning during activities and personal interactions in the occupational therapy environment. This includes noting cognition as it is reflected in daily living, work, and leisure performance. Stated another way, cognition is evaluated as the ability to formulate a coherent, well integrated response(s) we call *problem solving*. Of all the helping professionals, the occupational therapist often has the most information about the patient's ability for daily problem solving. This is discerned not merely through "testing" but through the varying treatment experiences available in the treatment setting. The occupational therapist's observations are shared with other treatment team members to increase staff understanding of patient behavior, to change and update intervention strategies, and to increase consistency in treatment approach. These observations can also be shared with the patient to enhance his understanding of the gains made during the treatment process.

The occupational therapist also makes referrals for testing based upon her observations or the results of her initial occupational therapy screening. She may recommend that a patient be tested by a psychologist or by a "high tech" method.

Regardless of the therapist's role in assessing cognition, there are multiple benefits to patient care that result when the clinician has a broad understanding of cognition and its potential application in assessment and treatment, benefits evident to the reader in the discussions of cognitive-behavioral, developmental, and organic brain syndrome frameworks.

End Notes

1. Guidano and Liotti (1983) integrate stage specific and information processing models and have identified two kinds of knowledge: *tacit* knowledge and *explicit* knowledge. *Tacit* knowledge is the original kind of knowledge and consists of the information that cannot be

verbalized. This information is prelogical, helps the individual focus his attention and pursue a goal, communicates to the person his perceptions of himself and the world, and eventually will serve as coordinator between experience and "higher" cognitive function. *Explicit* knowledge is information that exists after language develops. This information can be verbalized, is in or "has a conscious component" that allows the person to explore and control the environment, and gives him the ability to reflect upon experiences to form concepts that endure over time and that can be manipulated. The person manipulates these concepts to form reality, to consciously control himself and his environment (Guidano and Liotti, 1983).

2. In his discussion of communication and language, Flavell acknowledges the work of Noam Chomsky, George Miller, Roger Brown, and other scientists who have made significant contributions to the study of language acquisition and development. The reader is referred to these sources. Social learning theory also provides detailed discussions of language development and related research. In Chapter 9 we discuss the ability to read and write as part of language development.

3. Atkinson and Shiffrin (1968) have classified memory into three categories based upon the length of time that the information is stored: sensory memory, short term working memory, and long term memory. *Sensory memory* is information housed very briefly in one of the sensory systems. Examples of sensory memory are short term visual memory or *iconic memory* and short term auditory memory or *echoic memory.* Sensory memory is complex owing to the complex nature of the sensory systems, particularly the visual and auditory systems. Problems in these areas are usually described as perceptual problems rather than memory problems. *Short term working memory* is the "system responsible for temporarily holding information while learning, reading, reasoning, or thinking." *Long term memory* is the "system that preserves information for anything ranging from minutes to years" (Atkinson and Shiffrin, in Wilson and Moffat, 1984, pp. 9-10).

References

Allen C: Independence through activity: The practice of occupational therapy (psychiatry). AJOT 36(11):731-739, 1982.

Allen C: Occupational Therapy for Psychiatric Diseases: Measurement and Management of Cognitive Disabilities. Boston, Little, Brown, and Co., 1985.

Atkinson R, Shiffrin R: Human memory: A proposed system and its control processes. In Spence K, Spence J (Eds): The Psychology of Learning and Motivation. Vol. 2. New York, Academic Press, 1968.

Bandura A: Social Learning Theory. Englewood Cliffs, NJ, Prentice-Hall, 1972.

Bandura A: Social Learning Theory. Ed. 2. Englewood Cliffs, NJ, Prentice-Hall, 1977.

Bara B: Modifications of knowledge by memory processes. In Reda M, Mahoney M: Cognitive Psychotherapies. Cambridge, MA, Ballinger Publishing Co., 1984.

Flavell J: Cognitive Development. Englewood Cliffs, NJ, Prentice-Hall, 1977.

Flavell J: Cognitive Development. Ed 2. Englewood Cliffs, NJ, Prentice-Hall, 1985.

Gibson EJ: Principles of Perceptual Learning and Development. New York, Appleton-Century-Crofts, 1969.

Guidano V, Liotti G: Cognitive Processes and Emotional Disorders. New York, The Guilford Press, 1983.

Hopkins H, Smith H (Eds): Willard and Spackman's Occupational Therapy. Ed 6. Philadelphia, Lippincott, 1983.

Kaplan H, Sadock B: Comprehensive Textbook — Modern Synopsis of Psychiatry III. Ed 3. Baltimore, Williams & Wilkins, 1981.

Lezak M: Neuropsychological Assessment. New York, Oxford University Press, 1976.

Lillie M, Armstrong H: Contributions to the development of psychoeducation approaches to mental health service. AJOT 36(7):438-443, 1982.

Newel A, Simon H: Human Problem-Solving. Englewood Cliffs, NJ, Prentice-Hall, 1972.

Perry D, Bussey K: Social Development. Englewood Cliffs, NJ, Prentice-Hall, 1984.

Piaget J: The Origins of Intelligence in Children. New York, International Universities Press, 1952.

Piaget J: Logic and Psychology. New York, Basic Books, 1957.

Piaget J: Plays, Dreams and Imitation in Childhood. (Translated by Gattegno C, Hodgsen F). New York, W. W. Norton and Co., 1962.

Piaget J: The Psychology of Intelligence. Patterson, NJ, Littlefield, Adams, 1963.

Piaget J: The Child and Reality. (Translated by Rosin A). New York, Grossman Publishers, 1973.

Rosenthal TL, Bandura A: Psychological modeling: Theory and practice. In Garfield SL, Bergin AE (Eds): Handbook of Psychotherapy and Behavior Change. New York, John Wiley, 1978.

Smith H: Assessment and evaluation — Specific evaluation procedures. In Hopkins H, Smith H (Eds): Willard and Spackman's Occupational Therapy. Ed. 6. Philadelphia, J.B. Lippincott Co., 1983, pp 149-174.

Spencer E: Functional restoration — Specific diagnosis. In Hopkins H, Smith H (Eds): Willard and Spackman's Occupational Therapy. Ed. 6. Philadelphia, J.B. Lippincott Cp., 1983, pp 381-445.

Werner H: Comparative Psychology of Mental Development. Chicago, Follett, 1948.

Werner H: The conception of development from a comparative and organismic point of view. In Harris D (Ed): The Concept of Development. Minneapolis, University of Minnesota Press, 1957.

Werner H, Kaplan B: Symbol Formation: An Organismic Developmental Approach to Language and the Expression of Thought. New York, John Wiley, 1963.

Wilson B, Moffat N (Eds): Clinical Management of Memory Problems. Rockville, MD, Aspen Systems Corporation, 1984.

Chapter 6

The Cognitive-Behavioral Frame of Reference

Some readers may ask whether there a difference between behavioral therapy and cognitive-behavioral therapy. The answer is "yes." Cognitive-behavioral approaches seek primarily to change the thoughts believed to result in or cause specific behaviors and to develop a knowledge base for problem solving. Behavioral approaches give primary attention to the behaviors that need to be changed through the use of reinforcement strategies. Secondarily the behaviorist gives consideration to the thoughts that may influence behavior.

During the 1970s, from within behavioral and social psychology there was a growing interest in cognitive processes and self-control. *Self-control* refers to the person's ability to influence his own growth and development rather than being controlled by outside reinforcers. This interest in cognitive processes and self-control conflicted with basic tenets of behavioral theory and therapy and led to a polarization between cognitive-behavior therapists and noncognitive behaviorists. This polarization caused many disputes among behavior psychologists. However, during the 1970s a special interest group for cognitive-behavioral research was formed within the Association for the Advancement of Behavioral Therapy and the Association for Behavioral Analysis. This special interest group supported cognitive research and the study of the "inner person" in behavioral psychology. Out of the differing opinions, the conflictual discussions, and the research and literature came *cognitive-behavioral psychology.*

The occupational therapy literature has not made a firm distinction between behavioral approaches and cognitive-behavioral approaches. There is a clear distinction, as noted earlier,

155

and the authors have chosen to discuss it and identify it with psychoeducational occupational therapy programs which exemplify cognitive-behavioral theory. The psychoeducational approach in occupational therapy seeks to strengthen or establish a knowledge base and to change the patient's thoughts about himself from "incapable" to those of "capable" and "competent" and prepared to respond to life's daily challenges.

Definition

The cognitive-behavioral frame of reference in psychosocial settings is an emerging frame of reference in which man's *cognitive function* is believed to mediate or influence his affect and behavior. It provides an assessment guide for determining cognitive function, affective states, and generalized behaviors which are apparent as the patient participates in his environment. It suggests that treatment include verbal and behavioral techniques to change the patient's thoughts, to bring about behavioral change, and to improve function. When applying the framework, the occupational therapist uses graded activities to provide progressive challenges and success experiences in order to develop cognitive abilities; to expand the knowledge and strategies that the patient can use to act upon, interact in, and gain control of his environment; to increase his self knowledge; to problem solve; and to cope with life's challenges.

Theoretical Development

Occupational Therapy Literature

In 1982 Lillie and Armstrong described a psychoeducational program for psychiatric problems. Although they did not identify it with a cognitive frame of reference, they acknowledged social learning, cognitive, and behavioral theories as influential in the program development. Because of the influence of these theories, the authors feel that the program's description exemplifies cognitive-behavioral theory. More will be discussed about psychoeducational programming in this chapter.

Cognitive-Behavioral Literature

In the 1970s the theories of rational emotive therapists, cognitive therapists, social psychologists, and some behavioral theorists merged to form cognitive-behavioral theory. The work of Ellis, Beck, and Bandura and the studies and writings of Davidson, Kanfer, Phillips, Lang, Lazarus, Mischel, Peterson, Mahoney, Meichenbaum, Goldfried, Kazdin, Wilson, and other cognitive behavioral theorists are represented in cognitive-behavioral theory. The merger emphasizes the role of cognitive processes in understanding behavior, developing self-control, planning assessment and treatment strategies, and furthering the efficacy of behavioral treatment strategies (Stone, 1980). The psychologists who contributed to the cognitive framework of therapy have emphasized the importance of cognition in the mediation of behavior and interpreted classical conditioning and reinforcement in cognitive terms.

In the literature the terms cognitive therapy and cognitive-behavior therapy have been used interchangeably. Sources representative of those in which both terms were favored have been used by the authors in the discussion of cognitive-behavioral theory and its application in this text.

Mahoney and Arnkoff (1978) have identified three major forms of cognitive-behavior therapy: rational psychotherapies, coping skills therapies, and problem solving therapies.

The *rational psychotherapies* include Ellis' rational emotive therapy (RET), Michenbaum's self-instructional training (SIT), and Beck's cognitive therapy. *Coping skills therapies* use existing methods to facilitate coping with stressful events. Methods include covert modeling (Kazdin, 1974), modified systematic desensitization (Goldfried, 1971), anxiety management (Suinn and Richardson, 1971), and stress inoculation (Meichenbaum, 1973).

The *problem solving therapies* exist in behavior therapy and are exemplified by Fairweather's treatment program for institutionalized adults (Fairweather, 1964) and by the work of D'Zurilla and Goldfried (1971), Mahoney (1977), and Spivack, Platt, and Shure (1976). The therapist teaches skills which are used to find specific solutions for a presenting problem as well as strategies which can be used to solve similar problems that may be encountered in the future. This is in contrast to the problem solving of the behavioral approach in which the therapist uses reinforcement methods to modify the patient's behavior to solve the immediate problems but does not prepare the patient for coping with future difficulties. Problem solving therapy has the least representation in the clinically applied cognitive-behavior literature.

Since the cognitive frame of reference is in the process of development in psychosocial occupational therapy and little has been published by occupational therapists in this area, we have chosen to summarize three major contributions to cognitive-behavior theory, in order that the reader might become more aware of cognitive-behavioral principles and their potential application in occupational therapy. These contributions are: Bandura's social learning theory, Ellis' rational emotive therapy, and Beck's cognitive therapy (see note 1).

Cognitive-Behavioral Theory

Bandura's Social Learning Theory. Albert Bandura's social learning theory has had a significant impact on contemporary psychology and particularly on cognitive-behavior therapy. While Bandura's work has been noted in our discussion of behavioral therapy, we emphasize in this chapter how it is applied in cognitive therapy and discuss its utility in the practice of cognitive-behavioral occupational therapy. Social learning theory is comprehensive and has multiple applications in occupational therapy practice; therefore the authors suggest that Bandura's work (Bandura, 1977; Rosenthal and Bandura, 1978) be given serious consideration even if the reader chooses not to apply a cognitive-behavior frame of reference.

Through an increased understanding of social learning theory one broadens one's knowledge in multiple areas: the role of internal and external reinforcers, the role of cognition in mediating environment and person interactions, the role of cognition in modeling and

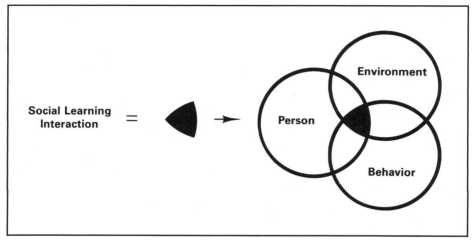

Figure 6-1. Social Learning

observation learning, the role of self-control and self-regulation in learning social responses and principles of corrective learning and treatment, and the alternative sources of motivation for behavior and treatment.

Social Learning Paradigm. When applied by the cognitive-behavior therapist, it is an *interactive-interdependent* paradigm of social learning that is conceived. Learning is viewed as an outcome of the interaction of behavior, person, and environment. Behavior is not just the outcome of the interaction between the person and his environment, nor is it determined solely by the environment. Rather behavior is seen as an *interacting determinant* of the outcome or response (Fig. 6-1). How the person reacts and his unique perceptions of the environment act on the environment as much as the environment acts on him.

For example, the occupational therapist in rehabilitation frequently encounters spinal cord injured patients who may have a lesion at the same spinal cord level and have similar physical abilities and limitations of function, but each patient's response to rehabilitation and what he accomplishes in treatment and in life will vary. This variation in performance and accomplishment comes in part from the patient's unique view of his disability and what he hopes to accomplish as well as his actions in his environment. His behavior can elicit empathy, sympathy, anger, acceptance, or assistance from those with whom he interacts. The reaction of others will affect his self image and the kinds of opportunities that become available to him as well as his ability to progress and cope in the future.

In the mental health setting, this interactive-interdependent paradigm can be seen in an adolescent treatment setting where several adolescents with similar problems may participate in the same therapeutic milieu but each will vary in his response to treatment as well as his own progress. The patient's view of peers and adults, his beliefs about treatment, and his values and expectations all influence his behavior and his ability to profit from treatment. His behavior influences what parents, staff, and peers expect and think of him, the goals they hold for him, the support they offer him, and the reactions that they have based upon judgments of previous behavior. Ultimately the adolescent influences and can control many of the current and future reactions of others with his behavior, and he can create an environment which will influence his quality of life.

From these examples we see that both the environment and the person may regulate behavior and influence the outcome of interactions. It is the correlation of events rather than the pairing of events that determines behavior (Bandura, 1977, p. 204).

The Importance of Cognition in Modeling. Traditional behaviorists acknowledge that learning may occur when the individual *models* his actions after those of someone he observes. Social learning theorists emphasize that cognition plays a significant *intervening role* in modeling. They remind us that people do not imitate or model every behavior that they observe. Rather individuals actively think about and select those behaviors which they will try to reproduce. The behaviors they choose to imitate will depend largely on what Bandura calls *anticipated consequences* (Perry and Bussey, 1984, p. 123). Therefore individuals are more likely to model behavior that they believe will lead to a positive consequence. They learn this in part by noticing the consequences that result when another engages in a particular behavior. For instance, if an adult sees another patient being praised for the care given to a craft project, the adult (our observer) may choose to imitate this behavior.

Modeling and imitation can play a part not only in skill building but also in "rule" and attitude formation. The patient who observes another patient or staff member consistently displaying certain attitudes (sharing, concern for others feelings) may discern the common thread that runs through diverse actions and situations and repeat, in his own interactions, a similar attitude.

As noted previously, a person is more likely to imitate someone he perceives as being like himself (i.e., a male will more likely imitate a male; a member of one group will more likely imitate another group member) or someone whom he regards highly. However, an individual is not likely to model behaviors which he feels incapable of (i.e., a patient who believes that he is incapable of mastering weaving is unlikely to model a weaver, no matter what regard he may have for the model). Work by Bandura in this area is pertinent to occupational therapists. His studies suggest that if the observer (here, the patient) can see the model performing individual motor steps while the patient imitates and practices each of these steps, the patient increases his own perception of self-efficacy. This is referred to as modeling of gradual mastery (see Bandura, 1977, and Rosenthal and Bandura, 1978).

Cognition in Reinforcement. There exist internal and external sources of reinforcement, and both may stimulate and maintain behaviors and thoughts. It is not just the tangible outcome or "measurable" reinforcement that must be considered. It is equally the individual's interpretation of and expectation regarding the reinforcement. This interpretation will be modulated by his cognitive abilities, as discussed. In the social learning view, reinforcement may be an *external,* a *vicarious,* or a *self-produced* consequence (Bandura, 1977, p. 97).

External reinforcers may be money, food, or material goods or social approval, privileges, or penalties. *Vicarious reinforcers* are symbolic (images a person has as a result of observing and learning from others) and include the individual's values and his images of success or failure (Bandura, 1977). For example, the student who is studying for a profession is reinforced or rewarded for his efforts and the sacrifices that studies demand by the images he has of mentors, the prestige of the profession, and the values and salary associated with the position and which will be his when he completes the professional studies.

Successful performance during tasks leads to a sense of efficacy and competence. *Competence* means that the patient has internalized behaviors which are maintained even when external reinforcers are withdrawn. From a patient's success and sense of competence he gains a sense of self-control. *Self-control* indicates that the patient is capable of setting standards, judging his own behavior against these standards, comparing his performance with previous performance, and maintaining an internal reward.

Self-produced consequences come from the individual's sense of accomplishment, his sense of self-control, and his sense of competence that come from success (Bandura, 1977). Stated simply, feeling competent and in control is a "good" feeling and is rewarding.

Hierarchy of Reinforcement. Social learning theory conceptualizes a hierarchy of reinforcement which is based upon the view that reinforcers acquire meaning and change as a result of developmental experiences. *Initial reinforcers* are more often external, such as smiles of approval, attention from significant others, and food. As cognition develops, symbolic reinforcers play an important part in influencing behavior. *Symbolic reinforcers* are memories, verbalizations, and internalized pictures (Bandura, 1977).

For example, a person learns social control in part from his parent's verbal discussion or reprimands which identify the laws of God, nature, and society. His knowledge of these laws becomes reinforcement for social conduct. He can control his behavior because he knows the consequences of speeding, trespassing, or stealing. Or a child can remember his mother's warnings, or perhaps recreate an image of a tragic newscast which describes a child's abduction, and he will refuse a stranger's overtures or offer of a ride.

Next in the hierarchy is social contracting. A *social contract* is the system that identifies the rewards and privileges and the punishments and censure that accompany specific behaviors (Bandura, 1977). When an individual assumes the roles and responsibilities of a job, through contractual agreement his employer provides benefits and a salary. Or when a parent neglects or abuses a child, he violates his "social contract" for parenting and is reprimanded by society.

Personal satisfaction, the last reinforcer in the hierarchy, is an intrinsic, self-produced reward, and it is regarded as the "best" reinforcement of behavior. Because, as a reward, personal satisfaction is probably the least dependent on changing (sometimes "fickle") external circumstances, behavior based upon personal satisfaction is difficult to extinguish (Bandura, 1977). Self-satisfaction comes from self-evaluation and self-produced consequences. The person who perfects intellectual, creative, or physical skills and pleases himself rather than the public and is comfortable with this pleasure has personal satisfaction.

Whatever the reinforcement, cognitive theorists emphasize that the ability to think about or anticipate reinforcement frees the individual from needing an immediate reinforcement for behavior. The reader will recall that traditional behaviorists state that positive reinforcement should follow immediately a desired response. Cognitive behaviorists disagree with this as a general requirement, but do acknowledge that given cognitive structures must exist for the individual to recognize and wait for a nonimmediate reward.

Further Influence of Cognition in Social Learning Theory. Cognition influences motivation, goal setting and attainment, the achievement of insight, and the acquisition, retention, and expression of behavior. Once a person has the ability to represent events symbolically (that is, once he can have a visual picture in his head of people, objects, and events), he is able to identify similar experiences of his own and others, remember previous outcomes, and evaluate these events to anticipate possible consequences of behavior. It is this symbolic process that allows a person to learn from vicarious experiences (i.e., those he hears or reads about) and to problem solve in thought without needing trial and error learning experiences. In other words, he can imagine "what would happen if . . ."

The ability to anticipate consequences of behavior influences the person's motivation and regulates the goals he tries to achieve. *Goals* are statements of the *general standards of conduct* which regulate behavior; thus, they serve as guides for self-regulation of behavior. People use goals to evaluate their performance and their accomplishments. In the application of social learning theory, behavior is evaluated by contrasting the patient's behavior with his goals and by comparing his present behavior with previous behavior. (Note: The patient's behavior is not contrasted with that of other people or the "norm.")

As with traditional behavior therapy goals should be specific enough to make identification of accomplishment possible; this includes stating the conditions for behavior and the type and amount of behavior required. Consistent with the principle of creating "moderate disequilibrium," the goals should be moderately difficult in order to maintain the person's interest and effort. If they are too easy, the patient loses interest, and if they are too difficult, he is unable to perceive himself as attaining them. Social learning theory emphasizes that the individual's perception of himself as being capable of goal attainment actually increases his ability to accomplish goals (Perry and Bussey, 1984).

Goals are accomplished through the satisfaction of subgoals. *Subgoals* are the immediate goals which can mobilize effort and indicate what the patient is to do in the "here and now." When successfully accomplished, they increase the image of the self as capable and reinforce the effort needed to attain remote goals. *Remote goals* identify behaviors desired or required in the distant future to produce self-satisfaction and control. They do not serve as incentives for the present, because they are usually too far removed from the "here and now," which makes competing demands for the person's attention.

Cognition also allows the person to accurately interpret reality and develop insight. As in traditional behavioral practice, social learning theory states that when a person has *insight,* he is aware of the relationship between contingencies, events, and what is reinforced (Bandura, 1977). This knowledge is believed to enhance learning, and increasing insight is a key aim of many social learning strategies. When a person knows the reason for and benefits of treatment, he is more inclined to try new experiences or is more motivated to learn, provided the benefits are compatible with his needs and interests. Insight also increases his ability in self-control.

Learning is also affected by the person's use of cognitive structures to interpret reality. A patient can misread reality, overgeneralize, have false or rigid beliefs, or use faulty cognitive processing and thus misinterpret reality. Since behavior is governed by a person's beliefs and by his anticipation of the outcome of his behavior (Bandura, 1977), such misinterpretations must be corrected if adaptive learning is to take place.

Relevance of Bandura's Work to Occupational Therapy. In his discussion of modeling and observation learning, Bandura proposes that the efficacy of treatment is increased by actual performance or cognitive-behavioral learning rather than by relying solely on cognitive-verbal methods (see note 2). This is, of course, consistent with the underlying premise of occupational therapy.

Bandura's study provides a circular, interactive model of treatment: (1) Change a patient's thoughts from "incapable" to "capable" (in order that he will engage in activity). (2) Use activities in which he can experience himself as capable. Grade these, use physical guidance, or use a model engaged in gradual mastery in order to ensure success while at the same time increasing the patient's perceptions of himself as capable. (3) Use verbal techniques to help the patient identify his own success, generalize his learning, and increase his sense of self-control and competence. Success will lead to feelings of satisfaction, competence, and control, which in turn help the patient to cope with other day to day (and future) demands (see note 3; Bandura, 1977).

Bandura's work on modeling raises a question about the typical grouping of patients in occupational therapy. One often finds, for example, that patients with similar needs and abilities are grouped together by the therapist. One can consider the potential merit of pairing more functional, interactive patients with those who are perhaps less involved or less functional. If the less functional patient can identify with the more functional patient, he may profit in that he may imitate the adaptive behaviors he observes. (Therapeutic experiences of this nature have proven successful in remedying social learning problems with children. See Perry and Bussey, 1984.)

Bandura's conclusions are consistent with the behavioral practice of incorporating both external and internal reinforcements. Bandura and social learning theorists go further, however, in proposing that the treatment staff actively help the patient to identify properties of anticipated reinforcements and that they assist the patient to achieve a sense of control in order that he can moderate his need for immediate gratification.

Bandura's work also supports active intervention by the therapist to assist the patient in identifying his own strengths, limitations, and the cognitions he uses to solve problems in order that he can feel that he has control of and responsibility for his own action.

Individuals within the occupational therapy profession who have supported the application of social learning theory in occupational therapy practice include Koestler (1970), Mosey

162

(1974), and Conte and Conte (1977). The reader is referred to articles by these authors for their comments.

Ellis' Rational Emotive Therapy. Of the identified cognitive therapies, rational emotive therapy may be the one best known to the reader. Rational emotive therapy was originated by Albert Ellis in 1955. He disagreed with the Freudian view that instincts determine behavior and the existential view that the authenticity of and acceptance by a therapist could change a patient's beliefs and habits.

Ellis was also dissatisfied with the results of his psychoanalytic practice and decided to take a cognitive approach. This approach assumes that thoughts, feelings, and behaviors interact and have a reciprocal cause and effect relationship. The approach has been summarized in what is called the ABC theory: (A) There is a fact, event, behavior, or attitude, which causes or influences the patient's belief (B), which determines the consequence (C). It is the belief, not the activating event, that determines the consequence. Thus the therapist uses interventions that dispute the patient's beliefs.

Rational emotive therapy as a form of psychotherapy strives to help the patient develop a rational basis for living through disputing those irrational views that produce neurosis or problems in living, or "self-defeat." These irrational views are summarized by Ellis in three statements called *musturbatory thinking:*

1. I must perform well and be approved by significant others. If I don't, it is awful, I cannot stand it, and I am a rotten person.
2. You must treat me fairly. When you don't, it is horrible and I cannot bear it.
3. Conditions must be the way I want them to be. It is terrible when they are not, and I cannot stand living in such an awful world (Corey, 1982, p. 173).

In order to counteract these irrational views and promote rational living, the rational emotive therapist does the following:

1. Gets the patient to acknowledge his irrational ideas that motivate his disturbed behavior and challenges him to validate the ideas.
2. Uses logical analysis to demonstrate the illogical nature of the patient's thinking and to minimize his beliefs.
3. Shows how the beliefs are ineffective and how they will lead to future emotional and behavioral disturbances.
4. Uses absurdity and humor to confront the irrationality of the patient's thinking.
5. Explains how these ideas can be replaced with more rational ideas that are empirically grounded.
6. Teaches the patient how to apply the scientific approach to thinking so that he can observe and minimize present or future irrational ideas and illogical deductions that foster self-destructive ways of feeling and behaving (Corey, 1982, p. 176).

During individual and group treatment sessions, and depending upon the need of the patient, the rational emotive therapist utilizes cognitive, emotive, and behavioral techniques. The cognitive methods used include disputing irrational beliefs, cognitive homework, bibliotherapy, and employing new "self statements."

When *disputing irrational beliefs,* the therapist helps the patient to see that it is his view of an event or belief about himself that is causing the patient's problem, his symptoms, or sense of defeat. The therapist then tries to get the patient to give evidence that supports his beliefs or interpretations of reality. Later during treatment the patient will be asked to do the disputing himself and to work systematically to diminish his distorted views. Ellis' homework assignments are given to the patient to demonstrate the rational or irrational nature of his thoughts and behaviors.

For example, during a public demonstration of rational emotive therapy for marriage and family problems, Ellis gave an assignment to a woman whom he had interviewed during a 15 minute period in which they discussed her marital stress. He asked her do do the following: During the next week prior to jogging each day (jogging was the woman's chosen reward), sit quietly, ask yourself these questions, and then answer them. (1) Why must I have a perfect marriage? (2) State the reasons for the belief that "If I don't have a perfect marriage, I'm an awful person." (3) What would I change to make the marriage more perfect?

With this assignment Ellis tried to help the woman see that she had unrealistic expectations, that no marriage was perfect, and that while she may have had feelings about herself and her contributions to the relationship, they did not make her an "awful" person. He also asserted that she must begin to identify what she could change in the relationship or what she would like her spouse to change.

Task and reading assignments may also be used to diminish distorted thoughts and change behavior. *Cognitive homework assignments* are tasks given to the patient by the therapist. These tasks are usually completed between sessions and/or during the treatment sessions. The tasks are used to help the patient deal with anxiety and to help him dispute irrational beliefs. For example, a person who is afraid of heights may be asked to take an elevator to the top of a building, or a person who is afraid of crowds may be asked to go to a place where a crowd of people is present. (This strategy is similar to implosive therapy, a classic behavioral approach in which the therapist accompanies a patient as he experiences a threatening situation.)

Bibliotherapy is the method of cognitive treatment in which the therapist "assigns" the reading of literature that relates to the patient's problem. Rational emotive therapists would be inclined to have the patient read *The Rational Emotive Approach* (Ellis, 1973) or *A New Guide to Rational Living* (Ellis and Harper, 1975) or other similar literature.

Emotive techniques utilized in rational emotive therapy include unconditional acceptance, rational emotive role playing, modeling, self statements (which may be voiced out loud or said to oneself), rational emotive imagery, and shame taking. The therapist teaches the patient to accept himself. The ideas that "we all make mistakes," that "nobody is perfect," that "it's OK to be yourself," and that "one needs to learn to live with oneself" are emphasized to develop *unconditional acceptance.*

The therapist is a model for the patient. Therefore, she actively participates in therapy sessions to verbalize rational thoughts and model effective task behavior, to model courage when she tries new experiences and takes risks, and to model unconditional acceptance of herself and the patient.

Imagery and role playing allow the patient to try out the expression of new thoughts, feelings, and behaviors in thought or fantasy or in contrived (but safe) settings prior to risking expression of rational thoughts and feelings or new behaviors in the "real world."

Operant conditioning, self-management principles, systematic desensitization, instrumental conditioning, biofeedback, relaxation techniques, and modeling are behavioral techniques used by rational emotive therapists (Dryden, 1984). Incorporation of these techniques into therapy reflects a broadened view of rational emotive therapy. Ellis has called this a "second type" of rational emotive therapy, and he sees it as being the same as other cognitive-behavioral therapies (Dryden, 1984). However, not all cognitive-behavioral therapists would agree with Ellis. Therefore, a different presentation of cognitive-behavioral therapy as conceived by Beck will be outlined, and then the similarities and differences between Beck's cognitive-behavioral therapy and rational emotive therapy will be summarized and their application to occupational therapy discussed.

Beck's Cognitive Therapy. Beck (1976; Beck et al., 1976 and 1979) has been very influential in his contributions to cognitive-behavioral therapy. Beck refers to his model as cognitive therapy and defines cognitive therapy as "an active, directive, time-limited, structured approach used to treat a variety of psychiatric disorders (depression, anxiety, phobias, pain, somatic problems). It is based on an underlying theoretical rationale that an individual's affect and behavior are largely determined by the way in which he structures the world (Beck et al., 1979, p. 3).

Beck assumes that an individual's cognition influences how he perceives and experiences everyday events, that his cognitions are based upon internal and external stimuli as well as past and present experiences, that his cognitions influence his feelings and behavior, and that therapy can heighten the individual's awareness of his cognitions and how they influence his feelings and behaviors (Beck et al., 1979).

To heighten the patient's awareness of cognition and its influence, cognitive therapy techniques and a "scientific" approach are used to help the patient to identify and test reality, to correct distorted thoughts and concepts, and to master problems and situations by reevaluating and correcting the thoughts which contribute to dysfunction. The scientific approach helps the patient to monitor his thoughts, recognize the relationship between thoughts, feeling, and behavior, identify data that support or negate his cognitions, or reinterpret his thoughts.

The techniques incorporate a collaborative "here and now" relationship in which the therapist uses behavioral techniques to elicit cognitions (help the patient to identify his beliefs or thoughts) to change behavior and discusses with the patient alternate, more healthy responses and the benefits and liabilities of changing or maintaining present beliefs and behaviors. The techniques and discussion help the patient to develop a scientific attitude through which he learns to recognize and monitor his thoughts and behavior and systematically test his assumptions.

Some of the cognitive techniques that facilitate effective performance include graded task assignments, modeling, coaching, behavioral rehearsal, homework, stress inoculation, cognitive modeling, and scripting. Patients are taught to identify irrational thoughts and cognitive distortions through rational and emotive imagery and discrimination training. Techniques develop assertive beliefs, identify personal rights, use thought-stopping, role reversal, and symbolic modeling, and incorporate educational methods (Rathjen, Rathjen, and Hiniker, 1978).

Contrast Between Rational Emotive Therapy and Beck's Cognitive Therapy. Both theories hold that behavior change comes from cognitive change. Differences arise in the terminology for the belief system, the therapeutic approach, the methodology used to rethink, and the homework assignments given (Table 6-1).

Beck suggests that the therapist work with the patient's rules for living (the patient's philosophy of life), not just the "musts" in life or irrational thoughts which are the focus of the rational emotive therapist. The rational emotive therapist has a more forceful approach. She is directive in identifying the patient's beliefs, confronting irrational beliefs, and providing methods of dispute for irrational beliefs. Beck envisions the therapist engaged in a collaborative effort in which the patient and therapist mutually explore the patient's beliefs to identify those that lead to cognitive distortions and overgeneralizations and then mutually to negotiate behavioral assignments.

During treatment, the process for rethinking varies with the two therapies. The rational emotive therapist quickly identifies the "musts" in the patient's life, evaluates these thoughts, and then goes about disputing these "musts." The therapist's philosophy of life is very influential in this process. In contrast, Beck supports the use of inductive questioning and a Socratic dialogue method. In this method of questioning the therapist helps the patient to identify thoughts and find the evidence to support his beliefs and then works cooperatively to find the means to correct his thoughts. Later the therapist will propose to the patient that he evaluate his beliefs and consider changing his philosophy of life (Dryden, 1984).

Another major contrast is the difference in approach to behavioral assignments. While both therapies use behavior assignments, Beck proposes that these assignments be negotiated by the patient and the therapist, and he would consider the patient's present ability and place increasing demands for performance. Tasks are graded in difficulty and work periods are increased. The rational emotive therapist does not use graded tasks and feels that they limit the patient's capabilities. The rational emotive therapist usually determines the homework assignment and demands high performance or behavior contrary to that which a patient exhibits (Dryden, 1984). This poses an interesting question for the occupational therapist. Does the use of graded activities promote success? Or does this approach convey to the patient that he has limitations and cannot manage a greater challenge? Is it acceptable to convey to the patient that he has limitations?

The patient in rational emotive therapy undergoes a logical analysis of his belief system based upon the ABC theory; there is an activating event (A), which influences what a person believes (B), which influences subsequent behavior or the consequence (C). Beck's cognitive-behavioral therapy uses a scientific method to identify and test the patient's beliefs. The patient will make a hypothesis about the reason behind his behavior and then will sys-

Table 6-1
Contrasting Rational Emotive Therapy
and Cognitive Therapy

	Rational Emotive Therapy	Cognitive Therapy
Treatment Focus	Focus on "musts" and individual's irrational thoughts.	Look at individual's philosophy of life.
Nature of Therapist Interaction	Therapist is directive; challenging.	Therapist collaborates with patient in mutual exploration.
Role of the Therapist	Therapist disputes irrational beliefs; models rational behavior.	Therapist uses inductive methods; asks patient to support or dispute beliefs.
How Activities Are Determined	Therapist determines treatment activities.	Therapist and patient collaborate to select treatment activities
Nature of Therapeutic Activities	Does not typically use graded tasks; patient confronts the task which he had been incapable of performing.	Uses tasks graded in difficulty.

tematically test his hypothesis and participate in corrective experiences. These experiences will promote cognitive functioning and thereby enhance coping and problem solving.

The discussion in this section may make it appear that the occupational therapist is more likely to incorporate social learning and cognitive-behavioral approaches similar to those of Beck rather than rational emotive therapy techniques. However, all have been influential in formulating cognitive psychoeducational interventions.

Current Practice in Occupational Therapy

The Person and Behavior

The therapist who utilizes cognitive-behavior theory sees the patient as a cognitive psychosocial being whose knowledge develops and changes throughout life. Knowledge is housed in schemes which are stored, retrieved, and reorganized to produce a self concept, a view of others, the rules for interacting with others in the environment, and behaviors and skills which are used to respond to and control one's environment. The way in which this occurs has been described in Chapter 5.

Cognitive-Behavioral View of Cognitive Dysfunction. In the previous chapter we highlighted the "normal" or "ideal" progression of knowledge development. However, with the patients who are seen in psychosocial treatment settings, knowledge development may be delayed or interrupted or may have resulted in maladaptive behavior. In the cognitive-behavioral frame of reference, cognition or "thinking" is seen as the basis for a psychiatric syndrome.

Dysfunction occurs because of insufficient, inflexible, or distorted knowledge. Cognitive dysfunction is identified by behaviors that reflect a rigid attitude, limited exploration of one's environment, a failure to establish an autonomous identity, misinterpretation of reality, and limited problem solving skills.

A person explores and learns from his environment when he senses that it is safe and permissible to do so. Ideally this sense of safety is conveyed to the child by adult role models who provide a safe and consistent environment and who communicate that they believe he is capable of controlling his environment and that he can learn from exploration. In this safe, consistent, as well as appropriately stimulating environment and from exploration, the person gains a knowledge base (tacit and explicit knowledge) which will shape his view of reality, future learning and knowledge acquisition, and his unique approach to problem solving. Negative experiences or limited exploration can lead to fear of the environment, distorted or limited knowledge, a rigid and defensive attitude, and poor problem solving skills.

As the person grows and interacts in his environment, he gathers information not only about the environment but also about himself. This self-knowldege is influential in his emotional development. Emotional development can be seen by the individual's position on continuums representing "dependence and independence," "self-interest and interest in others," "personal views of reality and the ability to be empathetic," "identity with others and an autonomous identity," and "ability to express and control feelings." Optimum function reflects a balance of the two extremes for each of these continuums and is associated with a feeling of *competence*. Dysfunction is usually seen when the predominant behaviors are at the extremes of the continuum or when cognitive function does not meet developmental expectations and is associated with feelings of *incompetence*.

The patient with distorted self-knowledge will often use a reasoning process that tends to be dogmatic or unrealistic. This method of reasoning may be illogical, not coinciding with reality, or involve inferences that do not have a basis (Guidano and Liotti, 1983). For instance, when the patient reasons, he makes inferences which may be incorrect. He may personalize information unnecessarily and may view events from "extremes" (i.e., issues are seen as black versus white, good versus bad, possible versus impossible). He may selectively abstract information and thus gets a distorted view; he may make global generalizations (e.g., all women are bad, blonds have more fun). His thoughts are unidimensional rather than holistic with multiple perspectives, and his thoughts cannot be easily reversed or varied (Beck, 1976; Beck, Rush, Shaw, and Emery, 1979, in Guidano and Liotti, 1983).

Cognitive distortions and deficiencies that occur have also been identified within the context of specific diagnostic categories (e.g., agoraphobia, depression, eating disorders, and obsessive-compulsive disorder; Bowlby, 1977). However, psychiatric labels are not necessary for understanding and describing cognitive dysfunction.

The Role of the Occupational Therapist

The role of therapist is not that of the "expert" and may vary from teacher (original role) to that of "personal scientist." The occupational therapy literature indicates that thus far, the occupational therapist has chosen the role of a *teacher*. This role is identified in the early theoretical development of cognitive-behavior theory. In the role of a teacher the therapist is a facilitator and participant-observer who designs and implements corrective learning experiences.

Educator-Facilitator. As an *educator-facilitator*, the therapist provides a structure. The educational structure in treatment is not like that in a traditional school setting. Rather it is a structure in which patients help develop the course, identify their learning needs, and participate in determining the course content and homework assigned. The therapist designs learning experiences which occur in a classroom atmosphere and during academic and skill development groups. During the learning experiences the therapist-educator carefully explains the rationale behind treatment approaches and assignments, and gives specific and frequent feedback regarding the patient's thoughts, behavior, and his accomplishments in relation to short and long term goals. She facilitates a learning process which helps the patient to gain new information and skills, knowledge which will increase his self-understanding, expand his resources for problem solving, and increase his ability to control himself and his environment.

The reader should also consider the benefits that come from modeling a "personal scientist" attitude. The *scientist attitude* requires the patient and therapist to recognize the relationship between thoughts and behaviors, to create ways to prove or disprove relationship theories, to explore life and its multiple possibilities and probabilities, and to question "absolute certainties."

Model of Scientific Attitude. In modeling the "scientist," the occupational therapist provides a secure base for exploration and encourages the patient to explore life in a systematic manner. This systematic manner is one in which he will hypothesize about and recognize cause and effect relationships in life, and in which he will plan and carry through with experiments or learning activities to confirm or disprove hypotheses. As a "personal scientist," the therapist helps the patient to "step back" from his beliefs, to postpone judgment of himself and the world, and to logically challenge the self theories that he constructs. This "scientific" process can be pursued through cognitive-behavior techniques.

The scientist attitude is illustrated in a response to a comment frequently heard in occupational therapy: "I am all thumbs" or "I'm not good with my hands." The occupational therapist replies, "What has happened to cause you to state that 'I'm not good with my hands'?" Or she might ask, "Does this comment refer just to occupational therapy activities or have you had difficulties at work or home?" With these responses the occupational therapist does not accept the patient's statement as fact and asks the patient to either validate or question his generalization. Next the therapist might ask the patient to perform specific tasks that did not relate to previous task failure, and that gave him the opportunity to re-evaluate his capabilities.

Participant-Observer. In the *participant-observer* role the therapist strives to be flexible, to individualize learning experiences, and to adjust her approach to the patient. The therapist strives to find a style that fits the patient's needs. As a participant, the occupational therapist provides support and gives feedback to the patient in response to the thoughts and feelings that he shares as well as his behavior. She also shares her views of the problems that the patient confronts. When observing the patient, the therapist views the whole cognitive system and tries to increase the patient's awareness of the interrelationship of his thoughts, feelings, and behaviors, both past and present. When appropriate, she tries to help him come to new conclusions about himself and others. This can be seen in the following example: An 18 year old head injured patient had multiple physical and behavioral problems as a result of her injury. She shifted from childlike attention seeking, dependent behavior to "acting out," adolescent behavior, to expression of concern regarding such young adult interests as living independently, finding an intimate relationship, and being employed. (These interests were realistic provided she could gain control of her behavior impulses.)

One day during one of her "acting out" adolescent periods, she ran away from the rehabilitation center. It was not easy for this young woman to run away when she was wheelchair bound and had many physical limitations. The therapist decided to share with the patient her view of the experience. Instead of again reminding the patient of the dangers of her behavior (many other staff had done this), the occupational therapist decided to focus on the tremendous amount of energy required to run away and to challenge the patient to learn to use this energy in a positive manner rather than in the negative self-destructive manner that

170

running away represented. This strategy helped avoid the usual authority struggle that the patient evoked during most interactions and turned the patient's attention to reconsider how she could use some of her energy.

Another example of an individualized approach that took into account the interaction between thoughts, feelings, and behaviors is recalled in the following exchange between a patient and therapist:

The patient saw himself as "superior" and was very intolerant of other patients' "ignorance." One day the therapist chose to confront a statement the patient made to another patient, "You mean you don't know that? Everybody knows that!" The therapist suggested to the patient that although he might know things that others do not, rather than "put another down because of his lack of knowledge," he might see an opportunity to teach this person and share his knowledge with others. She helped him to recognize that he could gain respect for his knowledge from others rather than the contempt that he seemed to elicit for being "bright."

In summary, in the teacher-student relationship the occupational therapist works collaboratively with the patient to identify problems and to plan and implement learning activities. The therapist provides a nonjudgmental attitude and a secure base from which the patient can re-evaluate his assumptions. She communicates to the patient that she respects him and his ability to learn and solve his problems.

The Function of Activities

The occupational therapist applying a cognitive-behavior frame of reference uses activities to determine the patient's cognitive function (see note 4), to facilitate cognitive development, to increase the patient's knowledge of himself, of others, and of his environment, and to prove or disprove the assumptions that the patient holds about himself, his life, others, and his environment.

Assessing Knowledge and Skill Level. The patient's present level of cognitive function is identified through activities in which he expresses thoughts, feelings, and behaviors. Activities also require the patient to demonstrate his general fund of knowledge (e.g., the information he has, his ability to read and write and to use tools), as well as the strategies (skills) he uses to apply this knowledge. During assessment of cognitive function, the therapist uses activities to identify the strengths and limitations in the patient's knowledge and skills.

Increasing Knowledge and Increasing Competence. Cognitive development is facilitated through engagement in activities which provide an opportunity to develop sensory, perceptual, motor, social, and academic knowledge, facilitate logical thinking, and learn skills and strategies for applying this knowledge in multiple contexts. Specific experiences which require the patient to "do" something are used to develop a broad knowledge base, to provide opportunities for self-assessment, to provide a successful outcome, to build self-confidence, and to develop a sense of self-control.

Educational Modules. Activities may be presented within the context of an educational format which may be identified as the program curriculum or class schedule. The occupational therapist develops course syllabi for the activities or educational modules presented. Syllabi have been developed in multiple arenas: Getting Credit, Consumer Awareness, Social Networks and Social Support Systems, How to Ask for a Dinner Date, Housing Rights and Responsibilities, Job Search, and Nutrition on a Budget, to name a few (Talbot, unpublished paper). In general, courses could be grouped according to basic living skills, community awareness, and personal growth and development.

Utilizing Homework. Courses may include homework activities. Rathjen et al. (1978) give guidelines for increasing the effectiveness of homework and increasing the likelihood of its completion. These may be utilized by occupational therapists. Assignments should be written and should identify the specific tasks to be completed by the patient or, at times, by the patient and the therapist. Specifics should identify the purpose of the assignment, instructions for the task, and other data which will help the patient determine whether he has met his responsibilities and completed the assignment. The assignment should be individualized to meet the patient's needs and should allow for patient input when the required tasks are assigned. (See also Maultsby, 1971.)

At the beginning of each treatment session the therapist checks to see whether assignments are complete and asks what the patient thinks and feels about the assignment. Was the task too easy? Too difficult? Was it meaningful? If the patient has not completed his tasks, the therapist seeks to identify the reason for noncompletion. Were directions and expectations clear? What interfered with completion? To support the completion of assignments, the therapist may use follow-up reminders or calls or contingency contracts.

Theoretical Assumptions

When applying cognitive-behavior theory in occupational therapy, the occupational therapist who utilizes the cognitive frame of reference makes the following assumptions to formulate the basis for evaluation and treatment:

1. The patient's emotions and behavior reflect his cognitive function.
2. Treatment does not eliminate the disorder but provides cognitive, affective, and behavioral learning experiences to teach skills, strategies, and methods of coping.
3. The person develops as a result of the interaction of the cognitive system, behaviors learned, and the social and physical environment.
4. Treatment is more effective when specific techniques and skills are learned (i.e., tasks and psychoeducational experiences) than when only verbal methods are utilized.
5. The patient benefits from psychoeducational programs which integrate educational procedures and psychological techniques.
6. The patient learns skills and strategies which he can use independently to face problems and find solutions.
7. When the patient masters the use of his body and objects, he has a resource for problem solving.

8. When a patient learns new cognitive strategies to respond to the present, he is preparing to confront and solve future problems.
9. When the patient changes his present knowledge and skill level, he changes his past knowledge and self-image.
10. The principles of change can be understood by the patient as a result of cognitive experiences and the therapist's feedback that describes the rationale for treatment.
11. Treatment activities can help the patient to act upon his environment as well as help him to monitor his thoughts, feelings, and behavior.
12. The self-monitoring process can be learned during treatment.
13. During treatment activities a patient can change negative self-thoughts and feelings into a positive self-image.
14. The arrangement of the learning environment influences cognitive function and can facilitate cognitive development and stimulate problem solving.
15. The patient can benefit from a structured treatment setting which controls distractions and provides repeated opportunities for skill practice and problem solving.
16. Cognitive developmental theory can be applied when designing tasks to modify the complexity of the experience and to promote successful learning.
17. The therapeutic tasks used during educational experiences consider the patient's cognitive knowledge, his level of cognitive function, and his interests.
18. Tasks with a high probability of success can stimulate cognitive development.
19. Self-regulation is the tendency toward equilibration. That is, the person can maintain a balance in which present knowledge and cognitive functioning and new learning and challenges complement each other to facilitate growth, optimum function, and the quality of life.
20. Therapy should stress the highest degree of equilibration, not the highest cognitive developmental level.
21. A person has acquired self-regulation when he can monitor relevant data that come from himself and his environment, use these data to choose and implement new behaviors, and practice these behaviors until they become automatic.

Evaluation

Environment, Attitude, Knowledge, and Skills. As with other therapeutic approaches in occupational therapy, the therapist applying the cognitive-behavioral framework believes that assessment is an ongoing process; "assessment and change are interdependent" (Meichenbaum, 1977, p. 259, in Guidano and Liotti, 1983, p. 131). Thus the information that follows could be applied within the context of the initial or the ongoing evaluation process.

We can take the premise that has been repeated throughout this text: patients are individuals who have not been able to cope to their own satisfaction and need help in changing. The questions that the therapist and patient ask are, What needs to change, and how can this change be accomplished? The cognitive-behavioral framework suggests that change

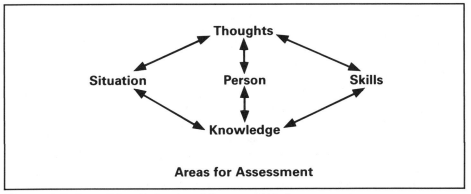

Figure 6-2. Cognitive-Behavioral Frame of Reference

be targeted in terms of four factors: What environmental situation(s) would the patient like to feel more competent in? What thoughts (or attitudes) does he need to reassess? What does he need to know more about? What skills does he need to learn? (See Figure 6-2.)

The patient may not always be aware of the information or skills he needs, the thoughts he needs to change, or even the situations in which he wishes to achieve competence. He may only know that he is uncomfortable at present. One reason for this is that many of the thoughts we have and behaviors we all engage in daily are automatic; we do not think about our own problem solving or recognize our own internalized cognitions.

For example, when we drive a car and encounter problems suddenly presented by heavy traffic or poor road conditions or a child running in the street, we respond without thinking about how we should react and the problem solving process that occurs. Nor may we be aware of how stimulation influences our behavior, what determines how we formulate cause and effect relationships, or the process of remembering.

This lack of awareness can also be seen in examples of other automatic reactions — overeating, for example. If you speak to an overeater, he may tell you that he will eat if food is present without thinking about whether he feels hungry or whether his body needs nourishment. Another example is the person who automatically withdraws from social interaction without considering the pleasure from, need for, or benefits of responding to family, friends, or new acquaintances. Finally, there is the person who expects to fail even before he hears instructions or initiates an activity.

An individual does not typically have immediate access to the rules of the cognitive process which influence his behavior, feelings, memory, and problem solving. Since the cognitive process is not in our immediate awareness in most instances, the therapist and the patient make assumptions regarding the impact of cognition upon behaviors and affect, and depend upon keen observation of verbal and nonverbal interactions that occur during evaluation and treatment activities to gain an understanding of how thoughts are processed and to identify situations in which change would be desirable.

Assessing Cognitive Structures. A key aim of the assessment is to *assess cognitive structures*. To do this the occupational therapist uses observation, testing, and the interview to assess the patient's cognitive functioning. When observing the patient, the therapist tries to determine the following:

1. The patient's ability to remember, his perception, and his attention.
2. The patient's ability to observe and accurately interpret his own behavior (the logic he employs in learning from events), including his ability to identify the historical data that relate to current problems and successes, his ability to identify stimuli (events, rewards) which support given behaviors, and his ability to identify his problems.
3. The adequacy of the patient's knowledge base — his knowledge of information related to the activities of daily living, vocational endeavors, and leisure pursuits (e.g., his awareness of community resources and of learning strategies.
4. The strategies the patient uses to problem solve and their effectiveness.
5. The existence and effectiveness of specific skills needed for daily function.

Listening for a Life Theme. In addition to assessing specific cognitive structures and skills during the assessment, the therapist tries to listen for the patient's "life theme" and "rules for living." Internalized rules for living emerge from the patient's behaviors and statements during the evaluation. Examples might be: I can take care of myself; I don't need my parents to run my life; people can't be trusted; I have to do as my spouse wants or he'll get angry.

Usually a theme emerges (Mahoney and Kelly, in Guidano and Liotti 1983). The theme is the message that underlies the rules for living and comes through consistently as the patient speaks and interacts in the interview and completes tasks. Typical life themes include: I am a victim of circumstance; people and life have always been against me; I am unworthy; I have never been able to use my hands; my father thinks I'm stupid; I can't be independent. Just as a patient's thoughts convey a "life theme," his problem solving may reflect a life style (e.g., a tendency toward patterns of behavior that are outgoing, withdrawn, intellectual, dependent, haphazard, cautious). The therapist will be looking for indications of such a life style, especially when this style is one that tends to limit rather than enhance coping skills.

Evaluating the Person-Environment Match. The therapist will want also to assess the extent of the "match" between the patient and his environment. In relation to this she may assess:

1. The patient's self-image: What are his interests? His goals? Does he appear to accept himself? Can he tolerate mistakes? Take risks? Can he exert self-control? In what areas does he feel capable, or incapable? Do others perceive him as he perceives himself? Are his self-expectations reasonable? Is he flexible, or does he respond in a rigid manner?
2. The patient's view of the environment: Is he aware of or interested in the environment? Does he see the environment as demanding, hostile, accepting, ignoring, rejecting?

What aspects of the environment does he especially attend to? What kinds of situations and settings does he prefer? What does he expect of others? Is he tolerant of others? Is his view of the environment and others realistic?

3. The patient's learning style: Does he initiate tasks? Does he sit back and observe? Whom does he admire? With whom does he identify? Can he postpone gratification? Maintain diligence? What reinforcements maintain current behavior? What reinforcements might be used to build new behaviors? What strategies help him learn — verbal instruction, use of diagrams, hands-on guidance, memory strategies? In what settings does he learn most easily — large group, small group, quiet, stimulating environment? Can he generalize his learning?

4. What are the current (and expected) environmental demands the patient is preparing to meet? What knowledge and specific skills are required? What stimuli, cues, models, and reinforcements are available? What demands will there be for patience, tolerance, self-control? To what degree will the patient's "rules for living" enhance his success or diminish the likelihood of success?

In summary, the occupational therapist uses her assessment to learn more about the patient's cognitive structures and the extent of the information and skills he possesses, the "rules for living" that underlie (and either support or undermine) his effectiveness, his learning and problem solving strategies, and the effectiveness of these in meeting his current and expected needs. With this information, she and the patient will emphasize in each area what he will work to change (*thoughts, skills, knowledge, situation*) and identify cognitive learning strategies that best match his learning needs.

Assessment Instruments

Task Check List. The task check list designed by therapists at the Life Skills Program adapted Hewett's hierarchy of educational tasks (see note 5) to assess the learning needs of the adult psychiatric population. The check list itemizes key behaviors for each of the seven learning levels identified by Hewett: entry, acceptance, order, relationship, exploratory, mastery, and achievement levels. The check list is used to develop an education plan for the patient (Lillie and Armstrong, 1982). (See Appendix K.)

Allen Cognitive Level Test. (Allen has designed two instruments for assessing cognitive performance. They are included here because the assessments are designed specifically for occupational therapy assessment and this text seeks to acknowledge the existing resources in the profession. However, Allen's theory is a developmental one, and her approach is based on developmental and not cognitive-behavioral principles. Also the definition of cognition used by Allen refers only to "voluntary motor acts" and is not the one used in this chapter. [In this chapter, cognition includes thoughts, affect, and behavior and their interaction]. Allen's approach to cognitive dysfunction is discussed in Chapter 7.) The purpose of the first interview is to establish rapport. Then, in a "here and now" atmosphere, the patient is asked to do a leather lacing task. The task tests the patient's ability to do simple and complex leather lacing stitches: running stitch, whip stitch, and single cordovan stitch. Allen states that it is a "competence measure . . . inference about the individual's capabilities from observation of performance" (Allen, 1985, p. 105). The patient's performance is identified with a particular level of cognitive function. Six levels are identified. Test details and the discussion of the strengths of the test are available in Allen's book, *Occupational Therapy for Psychiatric Diseases: Measurement and Management of Cognitive Disabilities* (1985).

Lower Cognitive Level. In a test originated by Allen to test the patient who is unable to do the leather lacing task, the patient is asked to imitate motor actions. The therapist claps her hands in specific rhythms and asks the patient to repeat the sequence that she performs. Test details are available in the previously mentioned text (Allen, 1985).

Treatment

Since the mid-1970s, multiple definitions of the therapeutic process for cognitive change have evolved. Guidano and Liotti list six definitions. Of the six, two seem most applicable to occupational therapy: The therapeutic process is (1) a teaching relationship in which the therapist facilitates the development of coping strategies and self-control (Goldfried 1980) and (2) a "scientific" process which helps the patient to question his beliefs and judgments and then systematically confirm or disprove his thoughts, a definition first used by Kelly (1955) and later by Mahoney (1976, 1980), Mahoney and Demonbreun (1977), Meichenbaum (1977), and Guidano and Liotti (1983).

Re-establishing the Cognitive System as Self-regulating. In general, the cognitive-behavioral change process in occupational therapy encourages shared authority and responsibility in treatment by the patient and the therapist. The goal of treatment is to facilitate cognitive growth and improve cognitive function in order to re-establish the cognitive system as a self-regulating system. To be a *self-regulating system* the person needs a broad knowledge base, skills to function competently in his environment; knowledge of himself, others, and the environment; and the ability to use his knowledge for problem solving. The therapist will frequently try to improve the ability to problem solve in a variety of daily situations, such as those proposed by Bara (1984). (Refer to the discussion of problem solving in Chapter 5.)

When the individual possesses adequate knowledge and skills and perceives himself as able to cope with a range of daily problems, he experiences himself as competent. The more competent he feels, the more able he is to act flexibly and respond to a broad range of available options. Thus, the more competent he becomes.

Treatment Goals

As with the establishment of treatment goals described previously for other frames of reference, the cognitive-behavioral frame of reference sets behavioral goals to bring about behavior change and uses them to evaluate the treatment outcome.

Changing Behavior and Changing Thoughts. Although behavioral goals are utilized, it is not sufficient for the patient to change just his behavior. He must also change the way he thinks about himself and his experiences. For example, the patient may learn the skills for interpersonal interaction, such as how to initiate a conversation, communicate with his peers at work, and effectively assert himself with authority figures. However, in addition to the skills described, he must also change his thoughts about his interpersonal capabilities, his competence in social situations, and his awareness of when and how to use the communication skills that he has learned. Changes in the patient's thoughts, attitudes, and values may also be written as goal statements. For example, the patient can verbally identify his interpersonal skills (his abilities and limitations) and then verbalize what he has gained from occupational therapy.

The cognitive-behavioral framework emphasizes the release of "power" (see note 6) by the occupational therapist to the patient in order that he might determine his own goals and assume increased responsibility for intervention strategies and the evaluation of the efficacy of the treatment outcome. Therefore, authority tends to be more readily shared between patient and therapist.

A unique approach to goal setting is described by Lillie and Armstrong (1982) and could be replicated, if desired. They describe a process of "group goal setting." The goal attainment through education (GATE) group is one in which each participant selects his psychoeducational experiences based upon his needs and interests. The group is analogous to the high school "homeroom group" in which the students meet, learn about the available courses, and then set their goals for participation in the program.

Occupational Therapy and Cognitive-Behavioral Strategies

The occupational therapist who chooses the cognitive-behavioral approach chooses a framework that has an interactive focus rather than the traditional behavioral cause and effect relationships; that is, thoughts, feelings, and behaviors interact. The strategies she selects will utilize this interaction.

Listening for Musts

Occupational therapy does not focus extensively on "musts," nor does the therapist typically dispute the patient's beliefs in the forceful manner described by Ellis. However, the occupational therapist listens for the "must" messages in the patient's dialogue, such as might be communicated by the patient who "must" make a perfect bowl the first time that he uses the potter's wheel and then gives up trying because he failed the first time. Or the therapist may ask the patient to identify the things he "must" do on an activity configuration, an activity discussed by Mosey (1970) in which the patient completes a schedule that identifies the week's activities and then categorizes them (e.g., "want to," "have to"). She will then help the patient to see how these "musts" are controlling his life and how he can cope with the constraints and givens in life and increase his sense of success and control rather than feel defeated and apathetic.

For example, the husband who shuns responsibilities and "runs away" from home because he feels overwhelmed by his job, his family roles, and his need to be perfect in all these roles can be helped to modify his standards, and learn to express his feelings, and learn to ask for help from his family. (This example also applies to the woman and her role in the family.) Through behavioral and activity experiences the therapist will help the patient to gain control of his life through understanding the relationship between his thoughts, problems, and behavior.

Homework

In occupational therapy, the occupational therapist more frequently gives tasks rather than mental or verbal exercises like those of Ellis. These homework tasks typically can be accomplished in a brief period of time. For example, the patient is asked to make a draft of his resume prior to the next employment readiness class or to make a list of the geographical areas where he will look for an apartment, and the benefits of each area, prior to the next community transition group meeting. It should be noted that "homework" need not be done at "home." The inpatient may be asked to do things on the ward or in his room before the next occupational therapy session.

Building Knowledge Through Reading

When using bibliotherapy, the occupational therapist is not likely to assign an entire book, as may be done by the rational emotive therapist. Rather the therapist in psychoeducational programs more frequently uses mimeographed materials, short articles, or brochures that could describe a budget process, nutrition and meal planning, or first aid and what to do in an emergency, for example. Literature can be provided by the occupational therapist, guest lecturers, community agencies, or service providers that affect the patient's life. Professionals from social service and community agencies invited to occupational therapy groups have provided literature regarding Medicare benefits, unemployment benefits, veterans benefits, the effects of alcohol, and weight control, to name a few.

Patients Learn Their Rights

Like the cognitive-behavioral therapist, the occupational therapist may use intervention strategies for developing assertive beliefs and identifying personal rights, may utilize symbolic modeling and role reversal, and may incorporate instructional models.

The occupational therapist may be responsible for running assertiveness training or social skills training groups. (Note: The assertive group process is described in Chapter 4.) To develop an assertive belief system, the therapist uses lectures, therapist modeling, and role playing. The patient learns that he has specific rights and that he can learn assertive behavior for effective interpersonal communication.

To identify rights, the therapist may use bibliotherapy and group discussion and role playing to help the patient identify and accept his rights and to challenge such socialized messages as "think of others first." The occupational therapist helps the patient learn to ask for what he needs. For example, the patient who sits "waiting" for someone to notice that he needs the paint or other necessary material for him to continue his project will learn to express his needs. Or following a cooking group, the occupational therapist may discuss the experience with the patients and ask them to share their thoughts about working together and how they helped each other, or their concerns regarding the work process and how it affected individuals as well as the outcome of the activity.

Films and Visual Media

A form of *symbolic modeling* describes the use of films and tapes to demonstrate effective interactions. During a film, a narrator explains the "rules" for the competent social interactions which are exhibited in the film (Goldstein, 1973). In addition to the narrator's comments, when a film or video is used in occupational therapy, a discussion follows in order to heighten the patients' understanding of the film's content. Further, the patient group may be given an opportunity to role-play similar social encounters.

Modeling and Role Playing

Three aspects of role playing are *rehearsal, modeling,* and *coaching*. When using role playing, the therapist actively participates to portray effective methods for responding to problematic situations. The patient then rehearses the verbal and behavioral techniques demonstrated, and the therapist and patients give verbal and nonverbal feedback. Role playing is used in multiple contexts in occupational therapy. Through role playing the patient may practice job interviewing, asking for a date, introducing himself when meeting a new person, registering to vote, or applying for a library card, for example.

Modeling and Physical Guidance

Modeling may be used to build task skills, such as those involved in learning an unfamiliar craft, self-care task, or sport. The therapist may act as a model or have another patient model the sequence of steps in a task, giving the patient the opportunity to practice and achieve competence in each step before attempting the next (modeling of gradual mastery). The therapist may also use physical guidance, placing her hands on the patient's hands as he attempts a motor act and guiding him through the process to ensure success. (The therapist will gradually remove her physical support.) As an important adjunct to such skill building, the therapist will help the individual acknowledge his accomplishment and, when appropriate, help him identify the skills and reasoning he employed in order that these might become generalized.

Identifying Cognitive Distortions

The occupational therapist may also help the patient identify cognitive distortions and learn to test his cognition. Beck et al. (1976) suggest that the patient write down his thoughts, look for underlying themes, and then identify distorted thinking. To identify cognitions the occupational therapist may use a log in which the patient writes his thoughts, feelings, and behaviors that occur during tasks throughout the day. For example, the patient taking a city bus for the first time might note his concern that he would miss his stop, or his belief that other passengers were "looking at me strangely." Log notes are then discussed with the patient to help him understand his thoughts and their effects. The notes and discussions will also influence the choice of task and treatment strategy that is used subsequently.

Testing Cognitions

Testing cognitions means that the patient learns to distinguish thoughts from reality. In the previous example, the therapist may ask the patient to identify what happened or what people did that indicated that they saw him as strange. Thus, the therapist helps him to confirm or negate his thoughts. She will treat his thoughts as hypotheses to be tested by inductive analysis, not as statements of fact. If indeed the patient acted strangely, she will identify acceptable behavior for riding the bus. Through these verbal interactions that occur within the context of activity and the teaching relationship, the occupational therapist helps the client develop a scientific attitude and plan strategies for behavioral change.

Educational Experiences

Knowledge builds competence, and the therapist may use a classlike format to increase knowledge. Sample education experiences include money management (the patient learns to make a budget, open bank accounts, and manage his check book), body movement and relaxation (the patient may participate in exercise or aerobic sessions, or learn body mechanics and energy conservation and relaxation techniques), and home management (the patient may learn meal planning and cooking [Neistadt, 1984] and basic home repair or time management). Other examples include memory training (the patient may learn rehearsal strategies and how to use external aids or cueing methods), effective communication (the patient may learn to use the telephone, practice oral and written communication, and express himself in dyadic and group situations), and understanding sexuality (the patient can learn about his own sexual needs as well as how to ask for a date, courting protocol, and expression of sexuality). Still other education experiences might include anger management (the patient can learn how to identify his angry feelings, sources of anger, and alternative methods of expressing anger), leisure interests and skills (after identifying his interests the patient can learn to use community resources to develop the necessary skills [Lillie and Armstrong, 1982]), and vocational readiness (the patient can learn resume writing and job interviewing skills [Kramer, 1984]). These experiences may be planned and implemented by the occupational therapist or in cooperation with other health professionals.

Because of the educational and didactic nature of the therapeutic experience, groups are frequently used in treatment. Depending on the nature of the activity, class groups usually contain six to ten patients. Groups provide an opportunity for patients to help each other and to discuss methods of problem solving. During the discussions the patients functioning at high levels can help those functioning at lower levels; patients can give each other support and support risk taking; and patients can give each other feedback regarding their thought feelings, and behaviors. The groups also make possible the use of role playing and modeling which may be used for learning new interpersonal skills and problem solving strategies.

Sample Psychoeducational Group in Occupational Therapy

A comprehensive example of a psychoeducational group is represented by the SCOR program (Solving Community Obstacles and Restoring Employment) designed by Kramer (1984). The SCORE program identifies the patient as a student and the therapist as a teacher and uses an educational format to establish realistic career objectives, to teach job seeking and social and interpersonal skills, and to improve self-presentation (Kramer, 1984).

The program consists of 15 educational modules which help the student (patient) assess the advantages and disadvantages of employment, evaluate work and leisure skills, practice completion of employment forms, write resumes and job inquiry letters, role play and videotape employment interview questions and situations, and criticize his performance and that of his peers (Kramer, 1984).

The modules identify learning goals and provide the teachers (co-leaders) with guidelines for task presentation, implementation, and discussion. Teachers lecture on relevant topics, give instruction in employment seeking skills, and encourage discussion of tasks and feedback to peers. Modules may be presented in a flexible schedule, but Kramer recommends eight consecutive, three hour sessions. Each student must complete the 24 hours of class and may do so outside class time if necessary. Modules also allow for some flexibility in presentation, allowing the course to be individualized to meet the student's needs (Kramer, 1984).

The reader is referred to the original source for detailed module descriptions, sample forms, and a comprehensive discussion of the group format used to assist the physically and mentally disabled in the re-employment process.

When designing educational modules such as those described in the SCORE program, the occupational therapist uses her ability to analyze activities to provide graded learning experiences. (See Appendix G for a sample psychoeducational learning format.) The experiences are designed to develop knowledge and skills and to provide an opportunity to apply new information and skills in different situations and settings (an opportunity for generalization). They provide a vehicle for the patient to recognize error and to find a method to correct error as well as an opportunity for him to identify and use his strengths and abilities. It is through these graded learning experiences that the patient masters new information and skills. "*Mastery*" suggests that as a result of experience, the patient has acquired necessary knowledge and skills, can identify the action needed in a particular situation, will be able to apply this knowledge effectively, and will be able to use his knowledge and skills to meet future demands. Mastery also indicates that he has met the goals that he set for himself rather than those based upon the "norm" or those of other patients in the group.

Treatment for Peripheral or Deep Change

As the occupational therapist plans treatment strategies designed to bring about change in the patient's pattern of behavior, his cognitions, his skills, his "life theme," or his method of problem solving, there are some issues the therapist keeps in mind as treatment ensues.

The occupational therapist and patient may choose to bring about *peripheral* or *deep change*. A deep change requires a remodeling of personal identity. Remodeling requires continuous stimulation from experiences which allow the patient to gain knowledge and skills, form new self-statements, form new rules for interaction, try various methods of problem solving, and then process the experiences to give data that will enable him to change his attitude toward himself and incorporate this knowledge into a modified personal identity.

To change the patient's personal identity or change deep cognitive structures, the patient and therapist would have to work to bring about a change in the patient's tacit knowledge. To change tacit knowledge the therapist uses logical debate and logical challenge through the following techniques: (1) The therapist shows a patient how he has exaggerated an event (*decatastrophizing*). (2) The therapist challenges the patient's thoughts using logic and does not permit the patient to refuse responsibility for his thoughts and feelings (*reattribution*). (3) The therapist takes the patient's illogical reaction and substitutes a logical response (*rational restructuring*). (4) The therapist uses techniques which require the patient to confront his self-concept and the impact it has on his adjustment in life (*semantic techniques*) (Guidano and Liotti, 1983).

Prior to using these techniques in which the therapist challenges the patient's philosophies or beliefs and/or the personal identity that the patient holds, the therapist must assess the patient's strengths and stresses. She should try to answer the following questions: How much support does the patient need? Is it a good time to confront the patient? Can he benefit from a logical restructuring of his knowledge? Is he capable of developing more adaptive thoughts, attitudes, and behaviors? Not every patient should, needs, or can obtain a deep cognitive change (Guidano and Liotti, 1983).

In most instances the occupational therapist does not work in the realm of deep structural changes. In occupational therapy the patient and therapist usually work to bring about a "peripheral" change. A *peripheral change* occurs as a result of a reorganization of attitude toward reality. This reorganization need not include a change in personal identity but may lead to changes in behavior and thoughts, increased adaptation to the environment, decreased emotional stress, and improved problem solving. The cognitive-behavioral literature identifies a variety of superficial change techniques: success experiences, role playing, assertiveness training, coping skills training, social skills training, cognitive modeling, self-instructional training, stress inoculation training, problem solving, brainstorming, and thought stopping (Guidano and Liotti, 1983, p. 150). In this list the reader will recognize familiar activities used in occupational therapy settings already discussed in this chapter.

In summary, whether the therapist seeks a superficial or a deep change, throughout the therapy experience the therapist gives a secure base for exploration and models the "scientist attitude."

During the scientific change process of treatment there are three issues that the therapist and patient should keep in mind:

1. Cognitive change is a gradual process; to change one's knowledge base and one's attitude toward oneself takes time.
2. The therapist respects the patient's personal thoughts, feelings, and views. She encourages the patient to openly express these. This does not mean that she has to agree with them.
3. The therapist is aware of the patient's history (thoughts, feelings, behaviors) because it will influence treatment experiences and their outcome and also the quantity, rate, and manner in which new knowledge is absorbed.

Chapter Summary

The cognitive approaches in occupational therapy are derived from emerging theoretical frameworks. Thus, in most instances, the new approaches are not adequately supported by research which can specifically identify the benefits and limitations of cognitive interventions. However, the authors will share their initial reactions to cognitive theory and its application and make some conjectures about the possible contributions and limitations of cognitive-behavioral theory as it is applied in occupational therapy practice as well as pose questions that have arisen as we pursued our cognitive studies.

In all the other chapters that discuss specific frames of reference, we addressed "contributions" and then "limitations." Because it is an emerging theoretical approach, the nature of the information is speculative and therefore the limitations are discussed first.

Limitations

In recent years, study in the fields of psychology, education, and medicine have expanded the definition of cognition and have increased our understanding of the growth, development, and function of cognition. There remains, however, much that we do not know about cognition and many questions we cannot answer.

In regard to theory, we lack the depth of knowledge needed to clearly delineate the extent to which physiology, biology, heredity, environment, and experience contribute to cognitive growth, development, and performance. While we know that cognition is a complex interactive process, we do not adequately understand the interaction of the physical and psychosocial factors previously mentioned. Therefore, one can only hypothesize about the relationship between the biopsychosocial nature of an individual and the underlying organization and function of the cognitive processes that he uses as he grows, changes, and adapts throughout life.

It is not only the complexity of the cognitive process that makes it difficult to unravel, it is also the ever-changing nature of the cognitive process that makes any adequate definition elusive. We do know that changes in cognition occur slowly and in a manner similar enough to be conceived as "stage specific." However, most research has been in the area of child development. Researchers now must ask, "What are the factors that influence cognitive development and performance during the adult years?" More attention must be given to the adult years and how theory can be used to develop cognitive intervention strategies for young, middle-aged, and older adult populations in occupational therapy as well as for other treatment disciplines.

Given the status of theoretical development and research, occupational therapists must acknowledge these limitations and the speculative aspect of their own practices. Questions that arise include: How can therapists easily and accurately assess and identify problems of cognition? How can they determine what procedures and assessment tasks should be used? To date, few cognitive assessment tools have been developed in occupational therapy. Of those available in the field of psychology, most are more appropriately given by a psychologist. Future assessment tools must be able to help determine whether a particular cognitive skill has or has not been acquired. Because skills can develop simultaneously, how can we accurately identify the cognitive developmental level? Cognitive performance may be identified with a particular developmental level, but there are many degrees of function within that level. Therefore, the therapist must determine: Does the patient lack a skill? Does he have a skill and refuse to use it? Or, does he have a skill and use it infrequently?

When treating a patient, the therapist continues to ask: What really influences the nature and the growth rate of cognition? What strategies can enhance cognitive ability and performance? Because science does not know exactly what happens between the presentation of a problem and the patient's response, it is difficult to accurately assess the impact of cognitive treatment strategies utilized.

In addition to the previous issues that arise from the relationship between theory and practice, the occupational therapist must consider this question: What is the cognitive demand made by a particular cognitive treatment approach? Does the patient need to function at a "high" level in order to benefit from a cognitive approach? If, as many suggest, the answer is "no," it is imperative that the therapist match the particular cognitive demands made by a given treatment approach with the cognitive capabilities of her patient. Although Allen (1982, 1985) makes it clear that her cognitive therapy is designed for the patient operating at a low cognitive level, it becomes the job of the therapist utilizing many of the cognitive models to determine their appropriateness for given individuals, and the guidelines for doing so tend not to be explicit.

Contributions

In spite of the limitations and questions that exist, there is research to support the effectiveness of cognitive treatment. The information in this chapter is based upon cognitive-behavioral theory and therapy and represents the hypothesized relationship that exists between cognition and adaptive behavior. This marriage between cognitive and behavioral theories seems to be a good one for describing the relationship between thoughts, affect, and behavior and the interactive process that occurs between the three elements. While emphasizing the validity of subjective experience, as does the object-relations framework, the cognitive-behavioral therapist objectifies behavior change and uses such change to measure the effectiveness of intervention. To this extent, cognitive-behavioral treatment is verifiable through research.

The psychology literature summarizes research that supports the use of cognitive-behavioral strategies with multiple age groups and diagnostic problems. These have been referred to in this chapter. In addition to these citations, there is literature to support cognitive-behavioral approaches with children who are experiencing psychosocial and learning problems (Kendal, 1984; Meyers and Craighead, 1984; Kneedles and Hallahan, 1984). There is also information in the literature to support giving the patient information which would increase his awareness and understanding of the intervention strategies used by the therapist (Murray, 1984). Information regarding treatment strategies may be presented to the child or adult and takes into consideration the patient's ability to understand and use the information to enhance therapeutic outcome.

The hierarchy of reinforcement which is proposed by Bandura and has been influential in cognitive-behavioral therapy has multiple applications in occupational therapy. These applications note the many levels of reinforcement that come into play in occupational therapy treatment and have been discussed previously in this chapter.

The application of cognitive-behavioral theory as represented by psychoeducational programs promotes an education-learning focus rather than an illness-treatment focus and is compatible with the environment of many health and community settings. In addition, an education-learning model is well suited to the area of prevention, a speciality that continues to be of interest to the occupational therapist.

The occupational therapist has adopted or adapted some of the more useful components of behaviorism and has combined them with cognitive developmental theory to form strategies for developing the patient's basic knowledge and skills for personal self-care, interpersonal interaction, and work-leisure performance.

The psychoeducational strategies used in occupational therapy facilitate "doing" or action through activities that provide graded challenges. This is in accordance with the basic tenets of the profession. The classes, tasks, and homework facilitate educational experiences that promote mastery of skills and competent function through individualized learning experiences, and reflect the humanistic philosophy that has permeated the occupational therapy profession since its inception.

The educational model promotes treatment in groups. The group model has been recognized as both cost- and time-effective as well as a useful vehicle for enhancing patients' ability to give to and support one another.

The cognitive-behavioral frame of reference has the goal of promoting generalization, a goal clearly necessary if independence and/or reduced treatment demands are sought.

However, whether or not generalization is necessarily an outcome of education and treatment experiences is debatable and one that needs to be pursued in research.

End Notes

1. There are many other theorists who have contributed to cognitive-behavioral theory. Among them are Frank, Kelly, Rotter, and Meichenbaum. The reader is referred to the original sources for discussion of their theories.

2. The emphasis of actual performance during learning is similar to Bruner's concept of *enactive learning,* which is noted in the developmental frame of reference chapter.

3. The sense of efficacy and control that comes from success is also supported in the theory of life development intervention (LDI), which is discussed in Chapter 7.

4. Cognitive function includes the patient's thoughts, feelings, and behaviors. This conceptualization of cognition is broader than the definition used by Allen (1985), who defines it in terms of a "voluntary motor act."

5. Frank Hewett is an educator who has numerous publications regarding educational approaches for the exceptional learner. He identified six levels of competence that are necessary for effective learning to occur: attention — "the level of competence associated with receiving and perceiving sensory stimulation, coming to and sustaining attention and retention"; response — "the level of competence associated with motor responding, verbal language skills, and active participation"; order — "the level of competence associated with following directions and routines"; exploratory — "the level of competence associated with gaining an accurate and thorough knowledge of the environment through sensory-motor experiences"; social — "the level of competence associated with gaining the approval and avoiding the disapproval of others"; mastery — "the level of competence associated with self-help skills, academic skills, and vocational and career development" (Hewett and Forness, 1984, p. 86).

6. Therapists at the West Haven Veterans Administration Hospital, West Haven, Connecticut describe the patient as being "empowered" (Talbot, unpublished paper).

Ms. Judith Talbot is an occupational therapist at the West Haven Veterans Administration Hospital. At the time that she shared some of the examples that appear in this chapter she was designated the Educational Director for the Veterans Resource Program on G9W of the hospital.

References

Allen C: Independence through activity: The practice of occupational therapy (psychiatry). AJOT 36(11):731-739, 1982.

Allen C: Occupational Therapy for Psychiatric Diseases: Measurement and Management of Cognitive Disabilities. Boston, Little, Brown and Company, 1985.

Bara B: Modifications of knowledge by memory processes. In Reda M, Mahoney M: Cognitive Psychotherapies. Cambridge, MA, Ballinger Publishing Company, 1984.

Bandura A: Social Learning Theory. Englewood Cliffs, NJ, Prentice-Hall, Inc., 1977.

Beck A: Cognitive Therapy and the Emotional Disorders. New York, International Universities Press, 1976.

Beck A, Rush A, Kovacs M: Individual Treatment Manual for Cognitive/Behavioral Psychotherapy of Depression. Philadelphia, University of Pennsylvania Press, 1976.

Beck A, Rush A, Shaw B, Emery G. Cognitive Therapy of Depression. New York, The Guilford Press, 1979.

Bowlby J: The making and breaking of affectional bonds. I. Etiology and psychopathology in the light of attachment theory. Br J Psychiatry 130:201-210, 1977.

Bowlby J: The making and breaking of affectional bonds. II. Some principles of psychotherapy. Br J Psychiatry 130:421-431, 1977.

Conte J, Conte W: The use of conceptual models in occupational therapy. AJOT 31:262-265, 1977.

Corey G: Theory and Practice of Counseling and Psychotherapy. Monterey, CA, Brooks/Cole Publishing Co., 1982.

Davidson G: Behavior modification techniques in institutional settings. In Franks C (Ed): Behavior Therapy: Appraisal and Status. New York, McGraw-Hill Book Company, 1969, pp. 220-278.

Dryden W: Rational-emotive therapy and cognitive therapy: A critical comparison. In Reda M, Mahoney M: Cognitive Psychotherapies. Cambridge, MA, Ballinger Publishing Company, 1984.

D'Zurilla R, Goldfried M: Problem solving and behavior modification. J Abnorm Psychol 78:107-126, 1971.

Ellis A: Humanistic Psychology: The Rational Emotive Approach. New York, McGraw-Hill Book Co., 1973.

Ellis A: A New Guide to Rational Living. New York, Harper & Row, Publishers, 1975.

Ellis A, Whiteley J: Theoretical and Empirical Foundations of Rational-Emotive Therapy. Monterey, CA, Brooks/Cole, 1979.

Fairweather B: Social Psychology in Treating Mental Illness: An Experimental Approach. New York, Wiley, 1964.

Foreyt J, Rathjen D (Eds): Cognitive Behavior Therapy. New York, Plenum Press, 1978.

Frank J: Persuasion and Healing. Baltimore, John Hopkins University Press, 1973.

Frank J: Therapeutic components of psychotherapy. J Nerv Ment Dis 159:325-342, 1974.

Frank J: Psychotherapy and the sense of mastery. In Spitzer RL, Klein DF (Eds): Evaluation of Psychological Therapies. Baltimore, John Hopkins University Press, 1976.

Goldfried M: Psychotherapy as coping skills training. In Mahoney M (Ed): Psychotherapy Process. New York, Plenum Press, 1980.

Goldfried M: Systematic desensitization as training in self-control. J Consult Clin Psychol 37:228-234, 1971.

Goldstein A: Structured Learning Therapy: Toward a Psychotherapy for the Poor. New

York, Academic Press, 1973.

Guidano V, Liotti G: Cognitive Processes and Emotional Disorders. New York: The Guilford Press, 1983.

Hewett F, Taylor F: The Emotionally Disturbed Child in the Classroom. Ed 2. Boston, Allyn & Bacon, 1980.

Hewett F, Forness S: Education of Exceptional Learners. Boston, Allyn & Bacon, 1984.

Kanfer F, Phillips J: Learning Foundations of Behavior Therapy. New York, Wiley, 1970.

Kazdin A: Effects of covert modeling and modeling reinforcement on assertive behavior. J Abnorm Psychol 83:240-252, 1974.

Kelly G: The Psychotherapy of Personal Constructs. New York, Norton, 1955.

Kendal P: Social cognition and problem solving: A developmental and child-clinical interface. In Gholson B, Rosenthal R (Eds): Applications of Cognitive-Developmental Theory. New York, Academic Press, 1984.

Kneedles R, Hallahan D: Self-monitoring as an attentional strategy for academic tasks with learning disabled children. In Gholson B, Rosenthal R (Ed): Applications of Cognitive-Developmental Theory. New York, Academic Press, 1984.

Koestler F (Ed): Reference Handbook for Continuing Education in Occupational Therapy. Dubuque, Iowa, Kendall/Hunt Publishing Company, 1970.

Kramer L: SCORE: Solving community obstacles and restoring employment. Occup Ther Ment Health 4(1):1-135, 1984.

Lang P: The mechanics of desensitization and the laboratory study of human fear. In Franks C (Ed): Assessment and Status of the Behavior Therapies. New York, McGraw-Hill Book Company, 1969.

Lazarus A: Behavior Therapy and Beyond. New York, McGraw-Hill Book Company, 1971.

Lillie M, Armstrong H: Contributions to the development of psychoeducation approaches to mental health service. AJOT 36(7)438-443, 1982.

Mahoney M: Scientist as Subject: The Psychological Imperative. Cambridge, MA, Ballinger Publishing Company, (1976).

Mahoney M: Personal science: A cognitive learning therapy. In Ellis A, Greiger R (Eds): Handbook of Rational Psychotherapy. New York, Springer Verlag, 1977.

Mahoney M, DeMonbreun B: Psychology of the scientist: An analysis of problem-solving biases. Cog Ther Res 1:229-238, 1977.

Mahoney M, Arnkoff D: Cognitive and self-control therapies. In Garfield S, Bergin A (Eds): Handbook of Psychotherapy and Behavior Change. Ed 2. New York, Wiley, 1978.

Mahoney M: Cognition and Behavior Modification. Cambridge, MA, Ballinger Publishing Company, 1974.

Mahoney M: Behaviorism, cognitivism and human change processes. In Reda M, Mahoney M: Cognitive Psychotherapies, Cambridge, MA, Ballinger Publishing

Company, 1984.

Maultsby M: Systematic written homework in psychotherapy. Rational Living 6:17-23, 1971.

Meichenbaum D: Cognitive Behavior Modification. New York, Plenum Press, 1977.

Meichenbaum D: Cognitive factors in behavior modification: Modifying what clients say to themselves. In Franks C, Wilson G (Eds): Annual Review of Behavior Therapy: Theory and Practice. Vol 1. New York, Brunner/Mazel, 1973, pp 416-431.

Meyers A, Craighead W: Cognitive Behavior Therapy with Children. New York, Plenum Press, 1984.

Mischel W: Personality and Assessment. New York, Wiley, 1968.

Mosey A: An alternative: The biopsychosocial model. AJOT 28:137-140, 1974.

Murray F: The application of theories of cognitive development. In Gholson B, Rosenthal R (Eds): Applications of Cognitive-Developmental Theory. New York, Academic Press, 1984.

Neistadt M, Marques K: An Independent Living Skills Training Program. AJOT 38(10):671-676, 1984.

Newel A, Simon H: Human Problem Solving. Englewood Cliffs, NJ, Prentice-Hall, 1972.

Perry D, Bussey K: Social Development. Englewood Cliffs, NJ, Prentice-Hall, 1984.

Peterson D: The Clinical Study of Social Behavior. New York, Appleton-Century-Crofts, 1968.

Rathjen D, Rathjen E, Hiniker A: A cognitive analysis of social performance: Implications for assessment and treatment. In Foreyt J, Rathjen D: Cognitive Behavior Therapy. New York, Plenum Press, 1978.

Reda M, Mahoney M: Cognitive Psychotherapies. Cambridge, MA, Ballinger Publishing Company, 1984.

Rosenthal R, Bandura A: Psychological modeling: Theory and practice. In Garfield S, Bergin A (Eds): Handbook of Psychotherapy and Behavior Change. New York, Wiley, 1978.

Rotter J: Social Learning and Clinical Psychology. Englewood Cliffs, NJ, Prentice-Hall, 1954.

Spivack G, Platt J, Shure M: The Problem-Solving Approach to Adjustment. San Francisco, Jossey-Bass, 1976.

Stone G: A Cognitive-Behavioral Approach to Counseling Psychology. New York, Praeger Publishers, 1980.

Suinn R, Richardson F: Anxiety management training: A nonspecific behavior therapy program for anxiety control. Behavior Therapy 2:498-510, 1971.

Talbot J: Methods of psychosocial education. In Ryan E, Anderson J, Weiner H, Feidelson S, Talbot J, Bell M: Preventive Psychosocial Rehabilitation Psychology for Schizophrenics: Ideology, Practice and Outcome. Paper presented at the annual convention of the American Psychological Association, Toronto, 1984.

Additional Readings

Cotler S, Guerra J: Assertion Training. Champaign, IL, Research Press, 1976.

Kendall P, Hollon S, (Eds): Assessment Strategies for Cognitive-Behavioral Interventions. New York, Academic Press, 1981.

Kendall P, Hollon S (Eds): Cognitive-Behavioral Interventions. New York, Academic Press, 1979.

Liberman R, King L, DeRisi W, McCann M: Personal Effectiveness: Guiding People to Assert Themselves and Improve Their Social Skills. Champaign, IL, Research Press, 1975.

Mahoney M: Cognition and Behavior Modification. Cambridge, MA, Ballinger Publishing Company, 1974.

Mahoney M: Cognitive and Non-cognitive Views in Behavior Modification. In Sjoden PO, Bates S, Dockens WS (Eds): Trends in Behavior Therapy. New York, Plenum Press, 1979.

Mahoney M: Psychotherapy and the Structure of Personal Revolutions. In Mahoney M (Ed): Psychotherapy Process: Current Issues and Future Directions. New York, Plenum Press, 1980.

Meyers A, Craighead W: Cognitive Behavior Therapy with Children. New York, Plenum Press, 1984.

Sank L, Shaffer C: A Therapist's Manual for Cognitive Behavior Therapy in Groups. New York, Plenum Press, 1984.

Chapter 7

Developmental Frame of Reference

Occupational therapists have as their primary concern the ability of the individual to achieve meaning, mastery, and optimal well-being through engagement in purposeful activity. As such, occupational therapists have been concerned with defining the skills that lead to mastery of given activities and that are consonant with the physical and emotional maturation of the individual, as well as with societal expectations of given life periods. Historically, in occupational therapy literature, particular emphasis has been given to the maturational changes of childhood, and to the older years.

In looking at the entire life span developmentally, one is given an excellent basis not only for conceptualizing the changing role that activities serve as the individual grows and matures, but also for appreciating the ever-changing strengths and limitations that need to be considered in relation to skill building.

Such a life span developmental approach suggests, beyond the everyday events that may seem fragmented, an underlying order or natural progression in the development of purpose. Working within a life span developmental understanding allows the patient and therapist to cope with the patient's presenting or immediate demands for change, as well as to anticipate and prepare for expected changes.

Consistent with this text's focus on the adult, we will in this chapter summarize pertinent work in the area of adult development, relate this to treatment, and propose avenues for further study.

Definition

The developmental frame of reference is a biopsychosocial framework for occupational therapy assessment and intervention. Adult development is conceived as following a predictable, sequential pattern of age-related stages or phases: phases that are shaped by and respond to physical maturation, cognitive maturation, and psychosocial intrapersonal need as well as environmental expectation. Within the context of biological, psychosocial, and cognitive developmental theories, age-appropriate life tasks and enabling adaptive skills and behaviors are identified. These behaviors, skills, and tasks are stage-specific and interdependent, and occur sequentially during the life cycle. During assessment, the occupational therapist identifies behaviors, skills, and task accomplishments that permit normal development and promote well-being, as well as identifies skills that are lacking or behaviors that serve as barriers to the developmental process. Through the use of purposeful activities, occupational therapy promotes integrated learning and personal competence in sensorimotor-integrated functioning, academic skills, self-care and daily living activities, social interaction, leisure activities, and work performance. Through skill development, the patient gains personal competence and competence to meet life's challenges and master life's tasks.

Theoretical Development

The occupational therapy literature in development weighs heavily at each end of the life span continuum in pediatric and gerontology specialty areas. There are discussions of theory and practice specific to occupational therapy evaluation, treatment, and research with some infant, child, adolescent, and elderly populations and fewer discussions that emphasize middle adult development or the entire life span. Some of the contributors to occupational therapy developmental theory include Gilfoyle and Grady, Llorens, Lewis, Ayres, Mosey, Moore, Fiorentino, and Rogers. In general, the literature proposes physical or holistic approaches in which multimodalities are used as purposeful activities to facilitate normal development, treat or prevent disease and disability, respond to developmental delay, minimize chronic disability, improve physical-psychosocial function, promote adaptation, and maintain quality of life.

In mental health, Mosey's presentation of an adult developmental framework (Mosey, 1970 and 1968) and the adaptation of A. Jean Ayres' sensory integrative theory for the adult population has predominated. Sensory integrative theory proposes a neurodevelopmental sequence in the acquisition of skills.

The first published approach of sensorimotor-integrative therapy for an adult population was in 1974 by Lorna Jean King. Since then numerous articles have appeared that incorporate sensorimotor-integrative techniques for adult and child populations with a chronic disability (Rider, 1978; Endler and Eimon, 1978; Huddleston, 1978; Baily, 1978; Beck, 1980; Eimon, Eimon, and Cermak, 1983; Blakeney, Strickland, and Wilkinson, 1983). King's articles and subsequent literature support a neurophysiological approach for chronic but nonparanoid schizophrenic populations. These patients show perceptual deficits, poor sensory integration, inadequate motor planning, specific posturing patterns, and poor body image. The occupational therapy programs proposed in the literature support the use of gross motor activities and noncompetitive games. These programs will be summarized later in the chapter.

The principles of Ayres and the neurophysiological approach have also been used with the geriatric-psychiatric population by Ross and Burdick and others. In *Sensory Integration,* Ross and Burdick (1981) provide an activity analysis, a sensorimotor assessment, and a format for sensory integrative groups that may be used with the geriatric or psychiatric patient.

The work of A. Jean Ayres also influences Mosey's conceptualization of a developmental framework. Reed identifies Mosey's developmental frame of reference as being based upon the "integration of the ideas of Ayres, Azima, Fidler, and Sechehaye" (Reed, 1984, p. 406). The authors have identified Azima and Fidler as well as others with the object-relations frame of reference and note that Mosey's developmental model is one that, in its discussion of developmental skills and skill building, is strongly influenced by traditional object-relations theory as well as behavioral principles. Mosey's work (1970) lists seven adaptive skills and their subskill components. The theoretical presentation includes a discussion of assessment and intervention, some of which needs further clarification. These skills are summarized later in this chapter and are elaborated in Appendix H.

In order to put theory into a meaningful framework, this chapter organizes theory according to the following format. First, development will be discussed in terms of the adult's life stages. *Life stages* are consecutive time spans in the individual's life that provide an overarching structure for understanding development. Each life stage has a unique flavor or character, as fashioned by both the internal priorities of the individual as well as societal expectation. Integral to life stages are developmental tasks and marker events. *Developmental tasks* are the "physiological, psychological and social demands a person must satisfy in order to be judged by others and judge himself or herself to be a reasonably happy and successful person" (Chickering and Havighurst, 1981, p. 25; cited in Rodgers, 1984, p. 488). These include such major accomplishments as establishing a marriage relationship, beginning a career, and formulating guiding religious or political philosophies. Developmental tasks have an open-ended quality in that they often evolve to other tasks, or need to be reworked in subsequent life stages.

Marker events are more circumscribed in time and are pivotal events within life stages. Such events include marriage; the death of a parent, spouse, child, or close friend or graduation from college.

Finally, we will address what we refer to as *enabling skills.* These are the specific cognitive, psychosocial, and sensorimotor learned behaviors that enable everyday activity and serve as a basis for the accomplishment of the more encompassing developmental tasks. We have selected the term "enabling" to indicate that these skills make it possible for the individual to meet his developmental needs. These skills are also seen as "adaptive" in that they allow the individual to respond to change. Enabling skills include, for example, the ability to read and write, the ability to speak comfortably in front of peers, and the ability to drive a car or find one's way about town. Enabling skills also include the broader, more global skills, such as those identified by Mosey, i.e., "Drive object skill: the ability to control drives and select objects in such a manner as to ensure adequate need satisfaction" (Mosey, 1970, p. 135).

Some enabling skills and their components may be relatively easy to identify — as, for example, the ability to read and write. Other skills, such as those related to the integration of self-esteem, or the ability for appropriate human and nonhuman object cathexes may be much more open to interpretation and consist of a virtually endless number of component skills. Skill building has been the primary goal of occupational therapy in developmentally oriented practice models. In this chapter, we will discuss the enabling skills related to cognition, moral reasoning, social perspective, and sensorimotor-integrative function.

It is from the fields of psychology and social psychology that one is given a conceptual picture of the life span and the developmental tasks to which enabling skills contribute. Therefore, we now turn to these areas.

Theories of Life Span Development

Life Stages

The psychology literature has a wealth of contributions to life span developmental theory. Of these, the more frequently referenced in occupational therapy literature are Erikson, Freud, Jung, Gesell, Havighurst, Neugarten, Bruner, and Buhler.

Farrell and Rosenburg (1981; cited in Rodgers, 1984, p. 484) summarized the process by which adult developmental theories most often have been formulated. Typically the theory starts with a descriptive study of adults (the study may be cross-sectional or longitudinal). These adults are observed and interviewed extensively. They are asked to give a phenomenological account of themselves, their life history, and their goals. Spouses and significant others may also be interviewed, and pertinent data regarding occupation, health, social affiliation, and so on will be obtained. The researcher then compiles the data and looks for discernible "patterns" or clusters that can be verified through other similar studies. It should be noted that many of the theories to be discussed are based on the conclusions of a researcher or clinician who has studied rather limited populations. Levinson (1978) for example, studied 40 men; Jung (1933, 1963, 1964) based his conclusions on the observation of his clients, plus on his interviews with some individuals from other cultures. Buhler's work (1953) is based on the biographical case study of 200 elderly Viennese in 1930. Erikson's (1950, 1959, 1968) conclusions are based on the observation of his own patients, plus the retrospective study of several well-known, accomplished individuals. Other recent studies, including those of Gould (1972, 1975) and Vaillant (1971, 1977), involved less than 300 people. Despite this limitation, the reader will discern enough similarity across theories as to be convinced, we believe, of their essential viability. We will begin by looking at the seminal work by Jung on life stages, and then we will examine the more recent study by Levinson.

Jung. Jung made a significant departure from Freud in his conceptualization of adult life span development. Freud believed that primary development ended with adolescence, and he viewed adult behavior as a repetition of patterns established during childhood, and as a living-out of beliefs gained through early experiencing. Jung envisioned a life span structure in which adults continue to develop, reassess goals, give up old values and embrace new ones, make new commitments, and develop parts of the self that had been undeveloped.

Jung identified four primary stages of life: (1) Childhood, (2) Young Adulthood, (3) Middle Age, and (4) Old Age.

Jung was cognizant of the extrinsic or social parameters of each stage and was interested in social institutions such as religion as well as the internal or intrapsychic activity throughout development. Jung's stages are reviewed here because his work made a clear and significant impact on more recent, subsequent research in adult development.

Childhood (Birth — puberty). This stage goes from birth to sexual maturity. During this time, the individual is typically protected by and lives within his parents' world. His sense of "I-ness" is shaped by the beliefs, values, and psychic atmosphere created by his parents.

A transition to the next stage begins in adolescence. The adolescent has an increased sense of self as separate and independent from his parents. He must give up childish behaviors and fantasies; he must test out new decisions, and be able to envision himself as separate from parents. He does this partly by questioning the "givens" of their world, and by re-assessing these precepts from his own perspective.

Young Adulthood (Puberty — 35 to 40 years). As adolescence concludes and the individual embarks into the world, he must adapt to social demands. He will select and pursue a suitable career, marry, and oftentimes, establish a stable family. He will continue to redefine his relationship to his parents, though he will never be entirely separate from them.

Adaptation is primarily to outer or environmental demands, as the individual seeks to gain status, and be recognized as accomplished by his peers.

Young adulthood ends at midlife. The individual has adapted (more or less) to societal expectations, but he finds himself beginning to question his own accomplishments and values. He asks himself "What have I done with my life? Has it really been worthwhile?" Even where accomplishments and youthful strivings have been attained, mere revelling in success is not enough. The individual feels the need to "take stock" and consider where his life is going.

Middle Age. Middle age begins somewhere around the age of 40, and with it begins what Jung called the second half or "afternoon" of life. During this phase the individual begins to know himself more deeply, and to respond to inner callings rather than societal expectations. Jung had special interest in this stage. As discussed in the Object Relations Chapter, Jung conceived of the self as comprised of polarities. These included a tendency to relate to the world in a fashion either deemed as extroverted (interest in others or in the environment) or introverted (a tendency toward contemplation and introspection); the existence of both a masculine and a feminine side in all individuals; and a tendency to evaluate information either through rational (logical, discernible means) or nonrational (intuitive) means. Whatever polarity is favored in the individual's actual behavior and thinking, the opposite polar function is latent in the self. During the second half of life, these unexpressed parts of the self are believed to emerge and develop. For example, a man who tended to act quickly and relate superficially to others during the first half of his life might in the second half become more

197

thoughtful and introspective. Likewise, a man who was very "masculine" during the first half of life (masculine as used by Jung was in the traditional sense of "strong," or aggressive) might in the second half of life allow his more "feminine" (sensitive, intuitive, creative, vulnerable, nurturing) side to emerge. This man might develop a wish to be emotionally closer to his wife and children, or may develop a desire to garden, or to create through the arts. For women, the opposite will occur. The nurturing, vulnerable woman will allow herself to exert more direct control and authority, and will feel more comfortable with getting out of the home for longer periods.

While it was not believed that one preference or polarity would be totally replaced by its opposite in the second half of life, the task of midlife and beyond was to allow these latent potentialities to be given some expression. Two processes needed to occur. Each part of the self needed to be given expression through the process Jung called *individuation*; then all parts, all polarities, needed to be united into a unified whole through the process Jung called *integration*.

Another important aspect of the second half of life was to respond to what Jung called spiritual values. The individual becomes more concerned with philosophy and belief systems, and less concerned with materialistic comforts or accomplishments related to physical prowess. Along with individuation and integration, the response to spiritual values helps the individual more toward the ultimate development of selfhood Jung called *transcendence* (see end note 1). While the individual in the first half of life might be especially concerned with his own accomplishments and "climbing the ladder of success," he might in the second half of life use his knowledge to teach or enhance the accomplishments of those younger. This person has more leeway because he has established himself in his career, or because his children are older; however, the need to deal in a new way comes from an inner urge. A failure to deal with these issues and engage in reappraisal renders the individual increasingly narrow and ultimately unfulfilled as increasing age brings more demands for him to change.

Toward the end of this stage, as the person moves towards very old age, he must face his own bodily decline. He will leave the formal work setting, if he has not already done so, and generally move from positions of authority, both in the larger society and within his family. The individual must seriously confront the inevitability of his own death, which he sees reflected in the death of many associates.

Old Age. Old age for Jung was "extreme" old age (no exact years were given). The individual is typically infirm, and often taken care of by others. He actively contemplates his own death as well as the prospect of life after death. Jung saw the belief in a hereafter as *archetypical*, or innately present in all persons; and considered the continuation of life through the soul as a reasonable possibility.

The Jungian influence is seen in the work of Levinson (1978) and Sheehy (1976), and is compatible with the findings of Erikson, (1950, 1959, 1968), Neugarten (1964, 1969, 1979), Buhler (1953, 1961, 1962, 1968), Havighurst (1972), Gould (1972, 1975, 1978) and other well respected developmentalists.

Levinson. Daniel Levinson (1978) and his associates at Yale expanded upon Jung's thinking and further refined the stages that Jung conceived. Levinson gives special emphasis to the early and middle adult years or late teens to late forties, a period which Levinson believes has historically been handled vaguely by those in the human sciences.

Levinson states that in shaping his life the individual must constantly make choices in the area of occupation, family, friendships, leisure and belief systems. The individual must commit to his choices and ultimately exclude from his attention that which he has not chosen. These choices will mutually determine and be determined by the roles each individual assumes, his unique manner of relating within these roles, and activities specific to role fulfillment.

Stage Cycles. Starting with an in-depth study of 40 men, Levinson found that the life structure is an alternating sequence of stable and transitional stages. A *stable stage*, believed to last from five to seven years, is the time in which the individual commits himself to the developmental tasks of that stage. (Table 7-1). These developmental tasks include accomplishing externally oriented goals, i.e., building a career and establishing one's niche in society; as well as grappling with internal reappraisals and developing intrapsychic polarities, such as those conceived by Jung. As a part of task accomplishment, the individual assumes social and occupational roles specific to each stable stage. He may, for example take the role of novice or apprentice in early adulthood, and be the authority or "elder statesman" in middle adulthood. Having accomplished the developmental tasks of a given stable stage, or having reached an age where task expectations change regardless of what has been previously accomplished, the individual moves into a transitional stage (usually lasting 3 to 5 years) during which life is reviewed.

During a *transitional stage*, decisions are made to discard elements of the former stage no longer experienced as meaningful, to retain those elements still viable, and to move on to the tasks and roles of the next stable stage. During a transitional stage one is, according to Levinson, "suspended between past and future" (Levinson, 1978 p. 51).

Midlife. Levinson discusses at length the midlife transition (occurring around ages 40 to 45), seeing it, as Jung, as an especially significant time during which internal polarities need to be reworked. The inner forces that Levinson identifies as opposing within the individual are those pertaining to (1) *destruction-creation*, (2) *feminine-masculine*, (3) *attachment-separation*, and (4) *young-old*. Levinson describes the midlife as pivotal in terms of the individual's need to confront his own loss of youth and deal with the recognition that he is not going to live forever. In confronting his own mortality, the individual experiences more urgently the need to give all aspects or potentialities of his being expression.

Common to all transitional periods are feelings of inner conflict; often, grief ensues as sadness is felt at what must be given up, and anxiety is experienced regarding the uncertainty of the future. Some preoccupation with death is common in all transitional stages because the process of termination and re-engagement is evocative of death and rebirth (Levinson, 1978, p. 51). In order for the transition to end successfully, the individual must make new, critical choices. Once choices are made and commitment given them, the next stable stage ensues.

Table 7-1

Levinson's Life Stage and Developmental Tasks

Ages		Stage	Key Tasks
E **A** **R** **L** **Y** **A** **D** **U** **L** **T** **H** **O** **O** **D**	17	Early Adult Transition	Question pre-adult world, imagine self as member of adult world; Give up adolescent behaviors; make some preliminary choices for adult life; change nature of relationship to parents; gain more training; learn more about oneself.
	22	Entering The Adult World	Establish own home base; make and try out choices related to occupation, love-relationship, and peer friendships; find a balance between creating a stable life structure and keeping a sense of adventure. Begin to form a "dream"; begin to establish mentor relationship.
	28	Age Thirty Transition	Take steps to modify areas not satisfactory. Find out what is "missing" and either take new steps or strengthen commitments. Continue to develop one's dream; establish mentor relationship.
	33	Settling Down	Invest self in major components; work, family, community activities; settle for a few key choices; work at "making a niche" and climbing the ladder of success; develop a firm sense of authority; change mentor-relationship; feel more self-assured and independent while being tuned into the needs of others.
	40	Mid-Life Transition	Reappraise life structure; redefine goals, values; deal with polarities within self (midlife individuation); polarities related to (1) young/old, (2) destruction/creation, (3) masculine/feminine, and (4) attachment/separation; Accept own mortality. Become mentor to another.
M **I** **D** **D** **L** **E** **A** **D** **U** **L** **T** **H** **O** **O** **D**	45	Entering Middle Adulthood	Commit self to new choices.
	50	Age 50 Transition	Modify life structure; can continue to work further on tasks of midlife transition.
	55	Culmination of Middle Adulthood	Build a second middle adult structure. Prepare to face a new era where physical decline and loss of status must be squarely met.

Table 7-1

Levinson's Life Stage and Developmental Tasks

Ages	Stage	Key Tasks
L A T E A D U L T H O O D 60	Late Adult Transition	Deal with physical decline; give up (or prepare to give up) formal authority; firm up values that maintain integrity.
65	Late Adulthood	Give up formal authority and status; form a broader life perspective; be less concerned with external rewards; contribute wisdom as elder in a supporting role; rely on inner resources. Face prospect of death.

This information is summarized from Levinson, D. *Seasons of a Man's Life*, New York, Alfred A. Knopf, 1978.

However, Levinson emphasizes that certain issues (i.e., separation-attachment, or finding a place among peers) will continue to emerge and need to be readdressed throughout the life span.

The Mentor Relationship. A concept introduced by Levinson and now in popular use is that of the *mentor.* The mentor relationship is seen as an important, complex relationship for both men and women during young adulthood. Most often viewed in relationship to the work setting, the mentor is usually several years older than the younger individual (though not old enough to be a parent). He acts informally as a teacher or sponsor — helping the individual to enhance his skills and abilities and acquainting him with the customs and values of the occupational and social world. Frequently, through his own accomplishments, the mentor may inspire and serve as an example for the younger individual to emulate (Levinson, 1978, pp. 97-101). Although one tends to hear of the mentor in relation to higher status occupations, Levinson found this relationship evident across social and economic boundaries.

Levinson noted little variability in terms of the ages in which periods begin and end, and he found that the stages occurred in a fixed sequence. However, it is not that one stage is better or higher than those preceding (Levinson, 1978, p. 319). Levinson suggests the metaphor of the four seasons: spring, summer, fall, and winter. None is intrinsically better than another, but each is essential to the unfolding life cycle.

Transitional Stress. Although Levinson's work is not about therapy, it is evident in the histories of those he interviewed that transitional stages are especially likely to cause the individual to experience stress, and to prompt him to contact others for some assistance with transition. Further, failure to work through or accomplish the tasks of any stage may prevent successful task resolution during subsequent stages, and unresolved problems may continue to emerge and plague the person.

For example, the young man or woman who is in conflict regarding their sexuality during their late teens may behave in a manner that is especially inhibited or conversely, promiscuous. If this individual marries in their mid-twenties without having integrated a satisfying sexual self-image, they may experience difficulties with both the sexual and emotional intimacy necessary for a fulfilling marriage. As the family unit expands to include children, concerns about sexual adequacy or attractiveness may exacerbate, and commitment to the marriage relationship may dwindle. This same person, at the age of 45 to 50 years (if still unresolved regarding his sexual self), may display rigid or exaggerated same-sex behaviors (as in the "macho man" or "sweet defenseless woman") at a time when his or her peers are comfortable with expanding beyond sexually stereotypic behavior.

The therapist cognizant of a life stage conceptualization such as Jung's or Levinson's perceives an underlying order in the events of the patient's life, and she can assess his strengths, limitations, and needs from a perspective much broader than the immediate demands of a given stress. Restoring comfort and order are not necessarily regarded as a therapeutic goal, since the necessity of re-evaluation and new commitment bring inevitable turmoil. This perspective on treatment will be discussed later in the chapter.

Developmental Tasks. As defined, developmental tasks are the major social, vocational, avocational, philosophical, and psychological accomplishments necessary for a person to relate in his world satisfactorily. These tasks are understood within the framework of age-related life stages and include changes within social, occupational, and avocational roles, or adjustments in the style of relating within a role. If developmental tasks are achieved, the individual tends to feel pleased, and subsequent developmental tasks are more likely to be accomplished. If they are not accomplished, then he tends to feel like a failure, societal disapproval ensues, and there is more likelihood of difficulty with future tasks. As Levinson suggests, implicit in the idea of any task is the concept that it may be carried out well or poorly. Some tasks are easily evaluated; developmental tasks tend not to be as easily evaluated and often require the distance of time to be adequately assessed (Levinson, 1978, p. 53). For example, it is relatively easy to identify if one has gained the necessary formal training prerequisite to entering a profession. It is far more difficult to determine if one has gained in self-knowledge (both of these are generally seen as developmental tasks of early adulthood). Speaking very generally, one may assess a task as successful when it is "viable in society and acceptable for the self" (Levinson, 1978, p. 53).

We will look at the developmental life tasks posited by Erik Erikson and Robert Havighurst, in order that they may be compared to those of Levinson.

Erik Erikson. Erikson (1950, 1959, 1968) also presented a life span theory of development. He conceptualized eight stages, four of them specific to adulthood. He saw each stage as necessitating the resolution of a psychological issue or crisis. Thus, the developmental tasks he delineated might be termed psychological tasks. The resolution of the psychological issue at each stage is necessary if the individual is to achieve internal harmony and successfully respond to the emotional issues of subsequent stages. Each major task is seen in terms of a polarity. At each stage the task is mastered within a particular context which has been referred to by Newman and Newman (1979) as the "central process" and which frequently identifies the social network in which the person operates to resolve the crisis, i.e., within a peer group, in school, or within the family (Table 7-2).

Psychological Issues. Adulthood begins with the need to resolve "Identity versus Role Confusion." The adolescent must struggle to see himself as separate and meaningful, with some sense of direction, aims, and goals for his future. From ages 20 to 40, the issue is between "Intimacy versus Isolation." The individual must see himself as worthy of love and capable of loving, and develop the ability for close friendships as well as a love-relationship. Failure to do so leaves him feeling alone and isolated. From ages 40 to 65, in middle adulthood, the individual needs to develop concerns beyond his own family. He struggles with "Generativity versus Stagnation." He desires to be more creative — to create products of value, to contribute ideas, and to contribute to the general well-being of others. This psychological adjustment requires a reappraisal of work and relationship goals in order that new directions responsive to his inner values can be pursued. Failure to do so, or attempting to stick with old goals, results in the individual feeling that life is stagnated; accomplishments lose their meaning.

The psychological task of late adulthood (65 years of age and later) relates to the need to achieve a sense of "Integrity versus Despair." Integrity comes about when one can reflect on his life and see his own progression. It means looking realistically at success as well as failures, and accepting that failures can no longer be corrected. While there may be some realistic disappointment at what cannot be done and cannot be remediated, the person feels that he has done reasonably well and sees his good qualities as outweighing the bad. Failure to achieve integrity finds the individual desperately trying to make amends, making unreasonable demands on others to ease one's discomfort, or withdrawing from all involvement with others in a gesture of defeat.

In summary, Erikson's psychological tasks, if successfully accomplished, result in an autonomous person who is able to value himself while achieving closeness and relatedness to others, is able to look realistically at his successes and failures and to ultimately feel that his life has been worthwhile.

The reader will notice that while Erikson's tasks are compatible with those of Levinson and Havighurst (to be discussed), Erikson's tasks are essentially intrapsychic or internal. Havighurst's are external (oriented to society), while Levinson's are both intrapsychic and externally oriented.

Erikson's theory is implied or evident in occupational therapy literature and more recently applied by Zemke and Gratz. They use Erikson's eight stages and developmental tasks as a guide to assess the patient's adjustment to a psychosocial and/or physical disability. They

Table 7-2

Life Developmental Tasks

Life Stage Process	Developmental Tasks	Psychosocial Crisis	Central Process
Infancy (birth to 2 years)	1. Social attachment 2. Sensorimotor primitive intelligence causality 3. Object permanence 4. Maturation of motor functions.	Trust versus mistrust	Mutuality with the caregiver.
Toddlerhood (2-4 yrs.)	1. Self-control 2. Language development 3. Fantasy and play 4. Elaboration of locomotion	Autonomy versus shame and doubt	Imitation
Early school Identification age (5-7 yrs.)	1. Sex role identification 2. Early moral development 3. Concrete operations 4. Group play	Initiative versus guilt	
Middle school age (8-12 yrs.)	1. Social cooperation 2. Self-evaluation 3. Skill learning 4. Team play	Industry versus inferiority	Education
Early adolescence (13-17 yrs.)	1. Physical maturation 2. Formal operations 3. Membership in the peer group 4. Heterosexual relationships	Group identity versus alienation	Peer pressure
Later adolescence (18-22 yrs.) Experimentation	1. Autonomy from parents 2. Sex role identity 3. Internalized morality 4. Career choice	Individual identity versus role diffusion	Role
Early adulthood (23-30 yrs.)	1. Marriage 2. Childbearing 3. Work 4. Life style	Intimacy versus isolation	Mutuality among peers
Middle adulthood (31-50 yrs.)	1. Management of the household 2. Child rearing 3. Management of a career	Generativity versus stagnation	Person environment fit and creativity
Later adulthood (51 and older)	1. Redirection of energy to new roles 2. Acceptance of one's life 3. Developing a point of view about death	Integrity versus despair	Introspection

Material in this chart is reproduced with permission. Newman and Newman *Development Through Life: A Psychosocial Approach,* Homewood, Illinois: The Dorsey Press, 1979, pp. 30-31.

remind the reader to be sensitive to the impact of disability upon the time line that is identified for the resolution of psychosocial crises. (Zemke and Gratz, 1982).

Havighurst

Task Mastery. The theory of developmental tasks as described by Robert Havighurst (1972) identifies a life span consisting of six stages or periods: infancy and early childhood, middle childhood, adolescence, early adulthood, middle age, and later maturity. In each period, specific tasks are mastered in response to a combination of forces: physical maturation, the pressures of society, and the desires, aspirations, and values of the person and his personality which form from daily interactions throughout his life. The tasks may be universal (i.e., walking, or talking) or culturally defined such as those tasks required for role expectations and social skills. Some tasks are recurrent and others are not. *Recurrent tasks* are the ongoing challenges throughout life such as making friends and defining masculine and feminine roles. The developmental tasks which are not recurrent have learning periods with time limits. These are periods in which the person is physically prepared and psychologically motivated to meet the demands of society.

Newman and Newman have presented the developmental life span concept in ten stages of development which incorporate those periods identified by Erikson and Havighurst. These stages are presented with the specific developmental tasks of each period and the central process through which development occurs (Table 7-2).

The developmental tasks seen as integral to each stage are more specifically occupational, cognitive, values-related, and relationship oriented, or external than the internal orientation of either Jung or Erikson. The reader might wish to compare the major tasks described by Levinson with those of Havighurst to see their complementary relationship.

The occupational therapist is concerned about developmental tasks, for these represent the larger or longer term goals towards which therapy is directed. In selecting activities and building identifiable enabling skills, the therapist seeks to enhance the ability of the patient to meet the greater demands of these developmental tasks. While developmental tasks would not likely be written into a treatment plan, both the patient and therapist use their understanding of these to place treatment in a meaningful life context.

Marker Events. Within the context of life stage structure, and whether the life cycle is perceived as consisting of four to eight or 10 periods, the individual is seen as necessarily encountering specific life events, called marker events by Levinson. Certain predictable marker events are experienced within the context of a "mental clock" each individual carries internally telling him when the event should occur (Neugarten, 1979, p. 888). People can state, for example, when they feel it is the optimal time to leave home, marry, have a first child, or to retire. These life events necessitate changes in self-identity and reappraisals of values, and are regarded as stressful insofar as they require change. However, Neugarten postulates, most often these events can be reasonably well tolerated when they occur "on time." If on time, they can be anticipated and rehearsed, and peers may be observed and imitated. For example, having a child may be anticipated and relished by a 28 year old woman; having a child at age 44 could be very disruptive to a woman who has been enjoying her increased independence. Further, failure to meet a marker event at the time expected may itself be considered a problem. For example, when a young man or woman fails to leave their parent's home by age 30, people (including the parents) often frown on this and view it as immature or clinging behavior.

Not all marker events are viewed as positive, nor can they be necessarily controlled by the individual. The death of spouse and forced early retirement, for example, would be marker events that might be both negative and unexpected. Whatever the marker event, the event requires change and adaptation by the individual. The individual's ability to deal effectively is influenced by his successful adaptation in the past, his confidence and esteem, and his cognitive abilities, as well as by the support and expectations of others, as influenced by role expectations, socioeconomic status, and the nature of his peer and broader social network. To illustrate, if a woman with a high-paying job chooses to have a child "off time" at age 40, she may be given a great deal of support by her associates, who find her decision daring but positive. If a woman of low economic status, perhaps one receiving government welfare, chooses to have a child at age 40, she may not only be criticized but her very right to childbearing questioned.

It is generally agreed that when an event is "off schedule," or nonnormative, it is less likely to be anticipated and is therefore more likely to have lasting detrimental effects. The early death of a spouse, for example, is generally more difficult for the individual to deal with than when a spouse dies at a much older age. Even positive events, off time, can be problematic. For example, when a long awaited job promotion occurs at a late age, much of the potential satisfaction may have dissipated, and the individual experiences an almost bitter sense of "why couldn't this have happened sooner?"

Marker events are to the authors like the events in a photo album. One can look back and remember "the day we got married" or "moved to our first home" or "Susan went off to college." They may relate to such developmental tasks as establishing a family or succeeding at an occupation, but are more limited in duration. This should not lead the reader to lose sight of the fact that, even though an event is limited in time, its effects may be long awaited or long lasting. As noted by Danish et al., "Events do not occur in a vacuum; they occur in a rich life space of the individual, including competing demands from a variety of areas. . . and people significant to the individual" (cited in Danish, D'Augelli, and Ginsberg, 1984, p. 525).

Marker events may or may not contribute to the particular stress which results in a patient seeking occupational therapy. Where a patient appears to be having difficulty dealing with a marker event, the therapist will pay special attention to the internal and external resources the patient has to cope with the event. Whether or not the event is "on" or "off" time influences the individual's preparedness to respond to the event and the availability of support from friends, family, and community to meet the challenge of the marker event confronting the patient. As with developmental tasks, marker events provide a background for the selection of activities which are chosen according to their ability to enhance or build needed enabling skills.

Mediating Factors in Understanding Development

Before we proceed there are several factors we would like the reader to bear in mind as she considers the prospect of using a life span developmental approach in understanding adult behavior.

1. Developmental tasks are not like chapters in a book to be read and completed; they better approximate themes in a novel, weaving themselves throughout the story, to be constantly reconsidered. Therefore, while one may speak of the ability to engage in give-and-take peer relationships as emerging in middle childhood, the adult needs to consistently readdress the task of establishing meaningful peer relationships — redefining his roles with peers in each developmental stage. To cite another example, marriage is not simply an event to be accomplished; the marital-relationship is reworked in each developmental stage as each partner brings into the relationship his own unique, evolving needs and perceptions. Separation from one's parents is never fully (emotionally) achieved, but the nature of the parent-child relationship is renegotiated in each developmental stage, from birth of the child to death. Sexual identity is not simply established by a given age; it is periodically redefined in accordance with biological, emotional, and social changes. Development may be viewed as an ongoing, unfolding process that ultimately moves the individual toward greater wholeness. As a part of that ongoing process, the individual renegotiates the self's relationship to the world. A life span developmental approach assists one in keying in on the "nature of the renegotiation," and it provides some guidelines for affirming that this renegotiation is occurring. But the life span approach should not be used to create artificial boundaries or suggest unyielding closures.

2. The degree of flexibility within developmental hierarchies is not clear with many aspects of adult development. It may be apparent, for example, that a child who has not learned to walk is not going to be able to run; but can we state uncategorically that a person who has not been able to settle on and satisfactorily pursue an occupation or career by the age of 45 or 50, will therefore be unable to deal with the subsequent development tasks of being creative and passing his ideas on to mankind? Or, one might ask, what if a woman becomes divorced at age 38? Will she be able to address the issues usually predicated on stability? If one needs to start over and create a new stable structure, how might this be experienced at age 38 or 44 or 64?

3. It is uncertain if a life stage developmental framework that is based on experiences common to adults is as useful for understanding the needs of individuals whose life course has been atypical. From the standpoint of the mental health treatment community one might ask, how is the life span conceptualization applied when an individual has been marginally functional throughout his life, perhaps even requiring residential or parental care? Does any of the hierarchy apply? Life span theory addresses normative structures and events, and these

questions are not easily answered. It becomes the task of the therapist utilizing a life span framework to determine how disruptive events or an unusual life structure mesh with the expectations of a society to impact on the individual, influence his perceptions of himself, and determine the options available for meaningful activity.

4. Finally, one needs to consider that societal expectations for adults are not static, and may change as a society itself develops. The adult life span approach to understanding psycho-social development is in a somewhat ironic position. It has been relatively recently, especially in the 1970s and 1980s, that an adult life cycle has been vigorously postulated. But, just as clinicians and researchers are consolidating their information and offering viable, conceptual frameworks, our society is at a stage of re-evaluating many of its own age and gender related expectations. For example, women are becoming more career-oriented and at an earlier age; many relatively older women are bearing first children, and men are becoming more active in the parenting of young children. Older grandparents are more often starting second careers, and young men and women are moving into professions and positions of authority, i.e., as judges, lawyers, and mayors. It is not just that these age-disparate events are occurring, but equally important, that society and the individual seem to be becoming more tolerant and indeed supportive of such change. Thus, when one speaks of the "on" or "off" timing of a marker event, i.e., marriage, or birth of child, the criteria for using such a label are becoming questionable. Although it is not clear at this point to what extent age and stage expectations or timetables have actually been altered, it is imperative that the therapist working with an individual understand what his internalization of a timetable is and that she not see developmental guidelines as inflexible standards.

Enabling Developmental Skills

If the developmental tasks of the life span are to be accomplished, the individual must successfully learn the broadest spectrum of enabling skills. That is, he must be able to use his senses, muscles, and skeletal system efficiently and effectively; he must be able to manipulate ideas; he needs to develop guiding philosophies; he needs to perceive himself as a meaningful, separate and influential being; and he must establish a way to communicate and cooperate with others. Just as the developmental tasks of Jung, Erikson, Levinson, and others are conceived as sequential and hierarchal in nature, so are the enabling skills viewed as logical and sequential in their development.

Mosey's Seven Adaptive Skills

As stated earlier, Mosey (1970) identified seven enabling or adaptive skills and the subskill components which must be mastered sequentially in order for the person to satisfy his needs and meet the expectations for growth by society and his environment. The skills are categorized as perceptual-motor (see end note 2), cognitive, drive-object, dyadic interaction, group interaction, self-identity, and sexual identity skills (Mosey, 1970). The skills and their subskill components are listed in Appendix H. For the most part, the adaptive skills suggested by Mosey are skills which would, normally, be integrated by the time of adulthood. Developmental difficulties arise, however, when an adult has failed to or is delayed in successfully integrating these skills, or when an adult once capable of utilizing these skills becomes unable to do so. A slip backward, developmentally, is referred to as *regression*.

As discussed by Mosey, failure to learn adaptive skills or their subskills relates to two categories of problems: (1) inadequacies in the individual's physiological makeup or in his physical maturation, or (2) deficiencies in the individual's environment and subsequent limitation in opportunities for learning (Mosey, 1970, p. 143). Of those skills delineated by Mosey, we will in this chapter focus on skills related to cognitive development, the development of moral reasoning and social perspective, and skills of sensory-motor integration. We have selected cognitive and sensory-integrative skills for discussion because occupational therapists have established identifiable developmental practice models in these two skill areas. We look at enabling skills related to the development of moral and social reasoning because we feel such skills impact on all treatment. Developmental demands and skills specific to the establishing of sexual and self-identity, and drive-object cathexis are also known to change throughout adulthood. These have been discussed in Chapter 3, and this discussion will not be repeated here.

We begin by summarizing briefly the theoretical basis for skill building in each skill area precursory to the development of skills in treatment, which is covered later in the chapter.

Theoretical Basis for Cognitive Development

Cognitive development relates to the emerging ability of the individual to understand the world around him, to conceptualize how events occur, and to manipulate ideas over time. The occupational therapy literature most often cites the work of Jean Piaget (1952, 1957, 1962, 1963, 1973) in this area, while the authors have chosen to broaden the theoretical discussion of cognitive development and refer the reader to Chapter 5, "Overview of the Cognitive Process."

The more immature the cognitive structures used in reasoning, the more difficult it is to help an individual to effectively assess his own needs, and the needs of others. The individual's ability to profit from various kinds of treatment experiences or activities may be severely hampered. For example, a patient functioning at Piaget's preoperational or concrete operational level may be unable to realistically assess the verbal feedback he is given in a patient group, as when others tell him his behavior is "inappropriate" but fail to be specific about the behaviors they find objectionable. Similarly, a patient functioning at the lowest levels may be unable to sustain interest in activities requiring a postponement of immediate gratification, or those in which cause and effect are not easily discerned. Further, cognitive development lays the groundwork for the development of moral reasoning and social perspective, as will be discussed. The way in which the individual interacts with treatment staff and his ability to reflect upon the manner and substance of his own treatment process are all influenced by his level of cognitive development, as will be discussed further in our discussion of treatment. Ultimately, the therapist will recognize that where cognitive enabling skills break down, the individual is limited in his ability to meet normative, developmental adult expectations.

Allen. The work of Claudia Allen (1982, 1985) provides another perspective on cognitive development, and one placed here with reservation. While the authors wish to summarize and comment briefly on Allen's proposals, they recognize that her model is not a developmental, skill-building model even though it is predicated on a developmental base. Allen is highlighted here in order to facilitate reader comparison with other theoretical constructs that are presented in this chapter.

Establishing Cognitive Disability. Allen's primary concern in occupational therapy is in regard to patient cognitive function. The patients whom she addresses in particular are those she describes as having a cognitive disability. Subsequently, her theory is concerned with atypical and not normal cognitive function. A *cognitive disability* is defined by Allen as "a restriction in voluntary motor action originating in the physical or chemical structures of the brain and producing observable limitations in routine task behavior" (Allen, 1985, p. 31) (see end note 3). A cognitive disability inhibits task performance, prevents goal achievement, and promotes idle behavior. All of these result in a poor adaptive response and limit independent function in the community (Allen, 1982). Allen uses membership data to conclude that a majority (or roughly 80 percent) of the patients now treated by occupational therapists have "disorders with potential for a cognitive impairment" (p. 12), and ones by definition attributable to an organic or biologic cause. Included among those 80 percent seen as having brain abnormalities are patients identified as having a neurosis, behavior disorder, psychosis, any of the schizophrenias, bipolar depressions, organic brain syndrome, or "developmental disabilities" (Allen, 1985, pp. 12-18).

Allen states that the cognitively disabled are not likely to improve; thus, for the most part they represent the chronic patient population. Those diseases discussed at length and cited as most disabling are those in which patients are identified as psychotic at some point in the disease process. These are the primary affective disorders (i.e., bipolar depression, or severe depression); the schizophrenias; and senile dementia.

Assessing Voluntary Motor Behavior. Allen proposes using careful observation of patients engaged in a specified motor task. (The Allen Cognitive Level Test has the patient do a leather lacing task; the Lower Cognitive Level Test asks the patient to imitate the therapist clapping hands. See the summary of evaluation batteries later in this chapter.) This task is used to determine the patient's level of cognitive function. The behaviors ascribed to the cognitively disabled are seen as occurring within a hierarchy of six identifiable steps or levels. In determining a patient's level of cognitive function, Allen looks at voluntary motor behavior in terms of three broad characteristics:

(1) The patient's attention to sensory cues. This includes assessing the kind of cues to which the patient responds and his ability to ignore irrelevant stimuli.

(2) The patient's ability for purposeful or goal-directed motor actions, both spontaneous and imitated.

210

(3) The extent of conscious control or awareness evident in the patient's behavior. This includes looking at the motives that compel behavior, the degree to which the patient can realistically use information to plan his actions, and his ability to attend to a task over time.

The behaviors ascribed to the cognitively disabled have some characteristics in common with the behaviors described by Piaget (Allen, 1985, p. 32) as emerging during the sensory-motor period, or the first two years of a child's life. There are important differences, however, since many of the behaviors cited by Allen are adult behaviors, not yet learned by a child and since many of the affective postures of the cognitively disabled noted by Allen are not the healthy, vigorous faces or postures of the exuberant child (see end note 4).

While Allen utilizes a developmental model in conceptualizing her hierarchy of cognitive skills, Allen takes exception with Piaget's general developmental postulates regarding the manner in which cognitive skills are built. Citing and apparently in agreement with Mounoud (1982) that the development of cognitive abilities is "a maturational process that depends only very indirectly on the interactions of the child with the environment. . . and that. . . it is strongly determined by genetic regulation" (Allen, 1985, p. 32). Allen generalizes this principle to adults and suggests that cognitive disability is primarily a matter of biology. She proposes that as therapists we can do little to build or increase cognitive skills, especially where cognitive disability is concerned. She states "changes in cognitive level are observed in acute conditions. (These changes) do not seem to be explained by the patient's experiences in the occupational therapy clinic. . . (these) changes have alternative explanations. . . such as the effectiveness of psychotropic drugs, the natural healing process, and the natural course of the disease. . . Although cognitive level changes in many acute conditions. . . it is remarkably stable in most chronic conditions" (Allen 1985, pp. 31-32). Thus, as will be further discussed in relation to treatment, Allen proposes the occupational therapist's key role is in assessment and observation and not in skill building.

There is a significant agenda in Allen's orientation in support of a medical model or biological conceptualization of psychiatric disorder, and of cognitive disorder. Beyond accepting the interrelationship of behavior and biology, the therapist is exhorted to accept a rather unidirectional relationship in which the body's biology/chemistry is believed to influence behavior more significantly than behavior influences biology. A great deal of emphasis is given to the general promise of pharmacology as a stablizing or curative agent in psychiatric disorder.

There is little discussion of the nature of the interaction between the therapist and patient, the interaction between patient and environment, or the significance, if any, seen in the therapeutic relationship. The ability of purposeful activity to influence the disease process (whether the disease is conceived of as acute, chronic, exacerbating, or stable) is challenged. Since cognition in Allen's conceptualization is defined by its outcome via a structured, voluntary motor behavior, the role of cognition in relation to self-concept, feelings, social relationships, and morality is not the concern. The cognitive hierarchy established for describing patients with cognitive disability appears to be based on the work of Piaget and on the observations of Allen in her work with psychiatric patients. Examples are provided to assist the novice reader in gaining a feel for the clinical picture that the cognitively impaired individual (as described by Allen) will present. A significant guiding premise in Allen's work appears to be the need that she identifies for occupational therapists to objectify their goals and treatment outcomes, and her criticism of the "generalist" approach taken by occupational therapists. It is, as yet, unclear to what extent Allen's cognitive levels are predictive of patients' ability to meet their general needs outside of the treatment setting. However, Allen continues to refine her framework as she works to develop the task analysis assessment process in occupational therapy in order to increase the objectivity of the cognitive evaluation.

Theoretical Base for Moral Reasoning and Development of Social Perspective

Kohlberg and Wilcox. Building on the work of Piaget, and consistent with the structural organismic approach in cognition, Lawrence Kohlberg (Kohlberg 1964, 1969, 1971, 1973, 1976, 1981, 1983; Kohlberg, Levine, and Hewer, 1983) and his associates have shown that moral reasoning and the development of social perspective follows the general pattern of cognitive development as suggested by Piaget. While cognitive-behaviorists recognize that moral reasoning may, in fact, relate to developmental changes (as discussed in the previous two chapters) they have not focused their work on identifying the ages associated with given changes in moral and social reasoning. Kohlberg and other developmentally-oriented theorists have.

Piaget's work relates primarily to logical reasoning, where *moral reasoning* relates to the decision one makes about right and wrong. *Social perspective* relates to how one perceives persons and societal structures. The understanding of moral reasoning is based primarily on the work of Kohlberg. The discussion of social perspective is based on the work of Kohlberg, James Fowler, Robert Kegan, James R. Rest, Robert L. Selman and Mary M. Wilcox, and is summarized in Wilcox's book, *Developmental Journey* (1979). The reader is referred to Wilcox's book for an in-depth discussion of moral reasoning and the development of social perspective, and to the bibliography and related readings at the end of this chapter for suggested works by the other authors.

Since Wilcox's conceptualization of social perspective follows that provided by Kohlberg, Kohlberg's developmental levels are the framework for the brief summary here. As each developmental period is summarized, the reader will note the implied and at times explicit interrelationship between moral and social perspective and the influence of these on dyadic as well as group social structures; on the role of the self in relation to authority; on the ability to empathize; and on the ability to deal with complex moral issues beyond the self.

The ages given next to each stage should be viewed as flexible and suggestive at best. As hypothesized by Kohlberg, age is less a factor than logical, cognitive development. That is, certain cognitive schemes are necessary if one is to utilize a given level of moral reasoning. Further, attaining a given age in no way ensures that a given level of moral reasoning will be employed. An adult's moral reasoning may be characteristic of any of the levels described by Kohlberg. Like Piaget, Kohlberg believes that moral development depends on the individual's experience with others, and specifically, on his being given the opportunity to "try on" new ideas related to moral decision making.

Kohlberg and Wilcox conceptualize three primary developmental levels in moral reasoning. These are termed the Preconventional Level, Conventional Level, and Postconventional Level. Within each level are two smaller steps or stages. The reader will note that the first or preconventional level does not begin until the child is somewhere in Piaget's preoperational stage of cognition. In other words, the infant and very small child are seen as totally egocentric and not capable of making moral decisions. The levels with their stages are briefly summarized as follows:

Preconventional Level. (Emerges somewhere between ages 2 to 7; may persist to adulthood.)

Stage 1: The individual is aware of good and bad, right and wrong, but decisions are made based on the expectation of punishment or reward. One respects or obeys an authority figure because he is bigger or more powerful; laws are obeyed in order to avoid punishment. There is little or no ability to empathize with or take the role of another.

Stage 2: Reciprocity may occur, but it is pragmatic. The individual is still very egocentric, and views others the same way. His philosophy might be "I'll scratch your back if you'll scratch mine." Everyone is seen as out for themselves. Society and authority are seen to function to prevent harmful acts. There is limited ability to take the role of other or to empathize; empathy is possible when a person is seen as very similar to the self.

Conventional Level. (Emerges sometime during or after the age of 6, and may persist to adulthood.)

Stage 3: The individual at this stage is most concerned with meeting the expectations of family and peer group. He tries to please others in order to win their approval and be deemed a "good boy." The individual also does what he perceives as right because it makes him feel good. The values of one's own group are considered the only right values, and group loyalty is important. An authority is viewed as positive or good because he is in an authority position. Should an authority figure behave badly, a contradiction is created that the individual cannot reconcile. The individual believes that good intention should be considered where another errs. Empathy is possible only insofar as another person has ideas and values similar to the individual's. Justice revolves about the premise that "good people" should get the best treatment.

Stage 4: The individual functions within a law and order orientation. Laws and sanctions must be followed because they maintain the societal structure. Rules, laws, traditions, and sanctions hold the individual's world together. Every individual is viewed as related to some social system; persons in a different social and value system must be persuaded to change their minds. Authority is integral to the system, and is earned, as by election. Justice is the system of maintaining the basic rules of the society. Decisions regarding right or wrong are in terms of absolutes, according to the values and laws of the society. One may be able to empathize with someone who feels differently than oneself, but will experience a need to persuade them to change their minds.

Postconventional Level. (Can emerge around the age of 11 or 12; more likely to emerge later.)

Stage 5: An effort is made to define moral values and principles which have validity apart fom the social group. The individual regulates behavior according to his own internalized ideas (after he has seriously weighed and judged the givens of his societal structure). The maintenance of individual rights and human dignity is essential, and this may give one the right to question or override "laws." Authority resides within the self; although traditional sources of authority are considered, they are evaluated. All persons are equally valuable. The individual can fully empathize with another and perceive their world through the other's eyes. The belief is held that the individual should be allowed to make decisions regarding his own life and death. Most people never truly function at this stage.

Stage 6: (See discussion in end note 5) A hypothetical stage infrequently, if ever, encountered; viewed by some as an ideal. This stage is shaped by a morality of individual principles and conscience, with a commitment to the unconditional value and rights of all persons. The individual is capable of "ideal role-taking" (Wilcox, 1979, p. 159) or the ability to empathize with and take the role of all the participants in a moral dilemma, and in such a way that each is accorded ultimate and equal respect. The individual is able to creatively resolve polarities and contradictions.

As summarized by Wilcox, the following are guiding premises in the development of moral reasoning and are reminiscent of the premises given previously as regards all cognitive development (Wilcox, 1979). (The reader is advised that many of these premises are being challenged in the recent literature, but Kohlberg's work continues, overall, to be regarded as useful for providing a conceptual, descriptive structure for understanding the direction and nature of change in moral reasoning. For further comments regarding areas of controversy, see end notes 5 and 6.)

1. Stage development is invariant; one must go through the stages in sequence without skipping any stages. (Wilcox, 1979, p. 78)
2. While the time needed to move from one stage to another may vary from individual to individual, there are no sudden jumps from a simple to a complex level. (Wilcox, 1979, p. 80)
3. Individuals tend to prefer to function at the highest stage they can understand. (Wilcox, 1979, p. 208)
4. Most individuals cannot comprehend moral reasoning that is at a stage more than one stage beyond their own. (Wilcox, 1979, p. 208)
5. An individual's moral reasoning tends to be at one stage, although he may occassionally use reasoning one step higher or lower.
6. Individuals are motivated to move from one stage to the next by cognitive disequilibrium that results from a conflict in which they must question their own reasoning and search for more adequate solutions to moral dilemmas. (Wilcox, 1979, pp. 80-81)
7. Conditions that tend to stimulate moral development are: (a) The individual is exposed

to a cognitive conflict, and to reasoning one step above his own; (b) The individual has an opportunity to engage in role-taking or situations necessitating empathy; (c) The individual functions within a social structure having higher levels of justice. (Wilcox, 1979, p. 195)

Issues of Moral and Social Reasoning as They Impact Occupational Therapy

While the occupational therapist may or may not perceive herself as concerned with increasing the level of her patient's moral reasoning, the issues of moral reasoning and social perspective have great impact, and must be conceived broadly. The individual's moral and social view will impact on the way in which he can profit from given treatment experiences, his ability to establish meaningful dyadic and large group relationships, the manner in which he looks at the treatment setting and treatment staff, and on the ability he has to function in various social and occupational roles and to successfully negotiate developmental tasks. To cite an illustration from treatment: it is quite common in mental health facilities to incorporate a milieu approach. Patients are expected to interact in a climate in which the feelings and rights of others are respected, and where persons of different ages and roles can come together and can learn more tolerance for all persons. Beyond that, activities employing role-reversals (psychodrama, sociodrama, or assertiveness training) may be used to assist the individual to understand the perspective of others. If, however, the individual patient is not conceptually capable of taking the role of or empathizing with those who are very different from himself, the therapeutic activity often serves only to increase his own sense of frustration, or to cause other patients to become frustrated and angry with him. This experience may mimic the kind of frustrating experiences he encounters in his everyday world, and that serve to heighten his sense of alienation.

The patient's ability to relate within social structures is often reflected in his manner of dealing with treatment staff: For example, frequently, the therapist-patient relationship is experienced by the patient as one in which the therapist is the "authority." This can occur much as it does in a teacher-student, doctor-patient, or parent-child relationship, even when the therapist has a firm commitment to treating the patient as an equal partner in the treatment process. The authority position is especially promoted when the treatment staff take a parental stance, i.e., determining ward privileges or restricting a patient's access to activities or persons when he has not met treatment mandates. Individual patients then respond according to their own beliefs regarding their relationship to authority. One patient may blindly follow all staff sanctions, even when constructive questioning would be appropriate. Another will look for constant proverbial pats on the back, letting him know he is doing well. Some individuals may be able to respond only to very clear, tangible reward and punishment systems. While one individual might find security in following hospital rules, and wish to adhere to them "because they are the rules," another might find such an experience very nonproductive.

It becomes the task of the staff within a treatment setting to individualize their approach to house rules, and issues of right and wrong, in order that the patient can use the social sanctions particular to treatment in a growth-producing way. This necessitates the therapist understanding her own beliefs and biases regarding authority; and depends on her ability to deal flexibly with moral dilemmas, as well as her ability to allow the individual patient to solve problems in a manner that might be very different from that which she prefers. At the same time, she cannot be so intent on challenging the patient to function at a higher level of moral reasoning that she in essence demands that he respond at a stage far beyond his own ability to conceptualize. She must meet him at his level, then provide a challenge for him to move just a little further.

The therapist must be aware, too, that the ability for a sophisticated level of cognitive, moral, or social reasoning is not dependent on formal education or training and there is nothing to guarantee that a given staff member will function at a higher level than any given patient.

Theoretical Basis for Building Sensory-Integrative Skills

Up until the early 1970s, mental health treatment and the application of developmental principles had tended to focus on skills related to intellect and insight and those accompanying specifiable tasks of work, play, and self-care. The work of Lorna King (1974), which resulted from her observation of those individuals termed process schizophrenics (see end note 7), created an interest in a much different area of enabling skills: those that have come to be termed sensory-integrative. *Sensory-integration* refers to the ability of the human organism to perceive, process, and utilize sensory data in a way that permits fluid, purposeful movement. The integrative process, while depending on the constant interaction of all systems within the whole organism, is believed to be governed by the central nervous system, and especially the noncortical or subcortical portions of that system, or those housed in the cerebellum and brain stem. The reader can easily illustrate subcortical movement to herself: think for a moment of yourself arising from your chair to tune in your favorite television program. You are (most likely) able to do this without thinking about how to get up, or how to walk. Perhaps you daydreamed about an earlier phone call, or unfinished conversation. Because you did not have to concentrate on the process of moving, or keeping your balance, one could say your action was accomplished subcortically. Subcortical regulation depends on adequate sensory stimulation from all sensory systems, telling the person where he and his body parts are in space, as well as on proper arousal. With proper subcortical regulation, the individual can move fluidly, even automatically as he thinks about other things. If you have broken a leg or strained a back muscle, you are acquainted with the disabling result of having to think about every move you make. Your movement becomes slowed, perhaps fearful, and labored.

King noticed that many process schizophrenics with whom she worked had in common a similar, ineffective posture and pattern of movement. Generally, this pattern included:

216

1. Limited mobility of the head;
2. 'S' curvature of the spine (lordosis);
3. Shuffling gait;
4. Tendency to hold arms and legs in a flexed, adducted, and internally rotated position;
5. Dominance confusion;
6. Atrophy of the thenar eminence and weak grip strength;
7. Poor balance; and
8. Lessened responsiveness to vestibular stimulation (i.e., lack of nystagmus) (King, 1974a, 1974b).

King postulated that process schizophrenics are unable to move fluidly because they have an ineffective proprioceptive feedback mechanism, the most important component of which is an *underactive vestibular regulating system*. Thus, the process schizophrenic cannot effectively at a subcortical level utilize sensory information regarding his own position in space. This leads to restricted, protective movement. In limiting his own movement, the individual tends to exacerbate the problem by decreasing vestibular and proprioceptive input. In having to corticalize movement, movement is slowed and loses it fluidity. This tends to interfere with the individual's ability to engage in normal physical activities, ultimately lessens his comfort in social situations, and increases his withdrawal.

A downward spiral of decreased movement and involvement is created, which King sought to reverse. She introduced activities designed to increase proprioceptive, and especially vestibular sensory input, and to increase the likelihood of movement regulated subcortically. Activities were selected that would also normalize movement patterns, strengthen upper trunk stability and increase flexibility, while being pleasurable and not requiring concentration. These motor changes were believed to improve body image and self-confidence, improve attentional and social response, and lay the necessary foundation for building skills related to cognition and improved daily task function.

King postulated that the same general neurodynamics might play a contributory role in autism, and she suggested the use of sensory-integrative principles in work with depression and the elderly. Since King's earliest publication (King, 1974) sensory-integrative principles and treatment approaches have been utilized by occupational therapists with other chronic, or regressed psychiatric patients (Ross and Burdick, 1981).

It should be noted that the physical posturing and movement described by King in relation to the schizophrenic is similar to the extrapyramidal or Parkinsonian-like effects of the long term use of major tranquilizers. It has been difficult in research to ascertain the extent to which medication may be responsible for the physical pattern created. Also, other chronically disturbed patients, and the elderly, while perhaps tending to limit their mobility or having attention problems, do not necessarily display the very characteristic posture and gait described by King. Subsequently, there remains a great deal to be learned about the exact nature of sensory-integrative deficits, and their relationship to the problems of those identified as psychiatrically disabled.

Current Practice in Occupational Therapy

The Person and Behavior

Innate Motivation. The individual is perceived as a physical-psychosocial being with an organismically determined press to grow and become increasingly complex. The basis for this growth and development is in the physical maturation of the individual as well as in his innate need to experience all aspects of himself and to expand his intellectual prowess. The need to experience and master the challenges in his world acts as a motivation, "nudging" the individual to "seek out environmental interactions" (Mosey, 1970, p. 140). In so doing he continually encounters new information, novel experiences, and new demands that disturb the status quo. Tension is created, provoking a process of response to change known as *adaptation*. The person must respond to (1) external requirements as well as (2) his own feelings as he integrates new information, learns new skills, reappraises his current beliefs, and makes other necessary accommodations. A history of successful adaptation increases the likelihood that future requirements for change will be successfully met. This is because the individual (1) sees the similarity between problems he now encounters and those he has dealt with previously, (2) has increased confidence in his own ability to cope with change, (3) can call upon strategies that he has employed before, and (4) has established a social support network to which he can turn (Danish, et.al., 1984).

Environmental Nourishment. While the person needs to develop in the same sense that a plant needs to grow, the environment plays an essential role in the developmental process. From society, the person gains information about what is expected from him at various stages in his life; and these expectations are internalized, thus helping to define his expectations for himself. The environment, which includes the people, objects, ideas and activities he encounters, provides the fertile ground in which learning and ultimately development can occur. The individual must have the opportunity to not only observe the actions of others, he must have the opportunity to actively participate with objects (tools, or materials), and to exchange ideas and deal personally with others. Developing this way, even when causing periods of disruption or dissonance, is ultimately satisfying to the person, and increases his sense of competence. From the persons in his social network, the individual may gain support and encouragement for his attempts at change, and finally, praise when he has succeeded in meeting their expectations.

There is general progress by the individual through identifiable life stages, which have accompanying developmental tasks. These stages have been discerned across a variety of cultures and in the life histories of those who lived long ago, as well as in contemporary man. The broad stages are characterized as *orderly*, *sequential*, and *invariant*. Skills specific to the biological, cognitive, social, and psychological development of the individual develop in a manner also conceptualized as orderly, sequential, and hierarchical, and similarly across cultures. These skills enable the individual to meet the greater demands of developmental tasks and to ultimately function in a manner seen as stage appropriate.

Readiness. Implicit in the stage concept of life and skill development is the supposition of readiness. That is, there appear to be specific normative ages or age ranges at which the individual's physical maturation, psychological need, and societal demands combine to create a climate in which certain issues are best addressed, skills developed, or commitments to change made. Trying to encourage the person to build skills before he is ready (as with "pushing" a child) is believed to either (1) be futile or (2) build skills that will prove unstable. Failure to build development skills during the time of optimum readiness may (1) impede this and future skill development and/or (2) lead to a sense of failure or lessened satisfaction with oneself.

Barriers to Development. Because all life stages and enabling skills are seen as hierarchical, no one stage or step in skill building can be skipped. Barriers to adult learning and development can be broadly conceived as:

1. Situational barriers, i.e., lack of time, lack of funds, or lack of information;
2. Dispositional barriers, i.e., biological or physical limitations, attitudes and perceptions one holds, or past experiences with previous developmental issues;
3. Institutional barriers, i.e., those that arise from policies that limit certain people from taking advantage of opportunities for advancement (Aslanian and Brickell, 1980; cited in Rodgers, 1984, p. 506).

The developmental therapist thus perceives the need to evaluate and address these barriers and to establish goals that will lead to successful skill accomplishment in accordance with the developmental priorities of the individual.

Function of Activities

There is a strong educative thrust in the developmental framework as proposed in this text. This may be in terms of laying a foundation for skill building, teaching remedial skills, or planning for anticipated skill requirements. Activities are analyzed according to their component skill requirements. Then activity selection is a match-making process in which the individual's life stage, level of function, and developmental needs are matched to activities which utilize skills already in the person's repertoire while providing a chance for him to learn new skills. There is no illness implied in the developmental framework, and activities are not predicated on diagnosis (see end note 8).

When possible, activities may be selected for their ability to increase insight and help the individual to generalize learning across past, present, and anticipated life experiences. However, the developmentally oriented therapist recognizes the individual differences in cognitive skill; and there is not the generalized emphasis on insight as is evident in the object-relations framework, or on thoughts as occurs in cognitive-behavioral treatment. The specific activities chosen and skills targeted for learning will vary according to the emphasis on the treatment program, and in this chapter have been discussed in reference to selected treatment approaches.

While sensory-integrative treatment tends to encourage novelty and spontaneity, skill building overall typically requires that there be ample opportunity within an activity format for experimentation, repetition, and practice, and finally, refinement of given schemes. Some skills, such as learning to plan a budget, learning to do basic meal preparation, or learning the skills in hand sewing, while not perfectable, can be reasonably acquired in a relatively short period. Other skills, such as being able to interact comfortably in a diverse social group, or skills specific to anticipated employment (secretarial skills, or computer skills) are not likely to be mastered in a short period of time. In the instance of an individual wishing to learn skills that are more extensive or require much practice, he often begins the process of learning component skills or practicing these in occupational therapy, and eventually is directed to other educative facilities for further skill development. In some instances within the therapy setting, information may be given in a class-like format by a therapist or appropriate agent. In such a structure, the individual is taught along with others who have similar learning needs.

Purposefulness. The therapist is always aware of the individual's need to feel a sense of purposefulness in whatever activity is selected. The purpose is understood in the developmental framework in terms of intrapsychic, interpersonal, and environmental changes that accompany life stages. Most people, regardless of their age, have a need to be a contributing member of their family or society. However, the way in which they can contribute changes. For example, little children love to help Mom sweep, polish furniture or wash the car; the school age child delights in cleaning blackboards or running errands for the teacher; the adolescent seeks to help his peers; the adult may be concerned with how to help in his church or community; and the older adult is pleased in teaching those that choose him as a mentor or in giving a helping hand to family members in need. This need to contribute is also seen with the disabled. In physical medicine and rehabilitation settings, patients often give suggestions to one another regarding wheelchairs or equipment, as well as support for enduring the pain and frustration that each experiences during the rehabilitation process. The need to contribute is evident also in those who experience emotional or psychiatric problems, and at times these individuals are baffled as to how they can contribute to anyone else when, as one patient put it "I can't even take care of myself." When the individual cannot identify activities that would seem purposeful or directions he anticipates his life will take, the therapist uses her knowledge of adult growth and development to make some educated guesses about what activities would help the individual to make necessary adaptations and accomplish meaningful tasks. To illustrate:

A 76 year old woman, never married, was being seen as a home-care patient. She was incapacitated by a series of strokes that left her unable to walk, with impaired speech, and in a generally weakened condition. She was markedly depressed, stating that she felt useless because she was unable to participate with her family in a way she perceived as helpful and normal. The therapist was called in because family caretakers felt unable to meet the incessant demands they felt this woman made on them. The therapist talked with the patient about the ways in which she, as an "elder statesman" in the family might pass on to others (in this case, grandnieces and nephews) the wisdom she had gained over a lifetime. Although she was no longer interested in pursuing a hobby that she had once enjoyed (painting greenware), she did follow up the suggestion that she could pass this skill on to a grandniece. When the therapist queried whether this woman might want to save her philosophies and knowledge of family history in a written or taped diary to be read later by younger kin, the woman could not see the usefulness of such an endeavor, calling it "presumptuous." However, in the therapist-directed process of looking at family momentos and recalling life experiences, the woman did an informal life review: evaluating what she had done in her life, and considering which decisions had been positive and where she had erred. While this woman is not cited to illustrate any magic cure (she continued to have bouts of depression), the severity of her depression appeared lessened. She was, according to family members, less demanding, slept more restfully, and seemed more accepting of her own limitations.

What is significant here is that this woman could not articulate any need to engage in a life review. She continued to perceive her usefulness in much the same way as she had 20 years prior. When those earlier avenues became closed to her, she could generate no other possibilities. It might be noted also that this woman evidenced some cognitive impairment, and her ability for insight and abstraction appeared limited. Still, the need for Erikson's "integrity" was quite evident.

In summary, as suggested by the examples given, activities are purposeful within a patient's life experiences when they utilize his skills, are consonant with the perceptions he has of himself within given roles, and allow him to meet changing internal and external expectations.

The patient may or may not be able to articulate his needs in relation to activity, but often will experience a feeling of discomfort when he tries to fulfill new challenges with old ways of doing things. With her knowledge of development, the therapist can assist the patient to select activities that will more effectively meet his changing needs.

Theoretical Assumptions

1. Human development occurs in an orderly fashion throughout the life cycle.
2. Steps within the developmental process are sequential and none can be skipped.
3. The person has an innate drive to encounter his world and master its challenges.
4. As a person proceeds through the life cycle he will encounter life events and changing internal and external conditions that will necessitate reappraisal and change.
5. Confrontation with change creates tension, disequilibrium, and stress.
6. The person's response to demands for change can result in adaptation and mastery, attempts to maintain the status quo, or regression and dysfunction.
7. The person's ability to master developmental tasks is influenced by his physical capability, learned skills, his life experiences, and the availability of resources and opportunity.
8. Successful adaptation tends to lead the individual to feel self-satisfaction and to gain societal approval.
9. A history of successful adaptation promotes future success in meeting challenges.

10. Through the use of purposeful activity in occupational therapy the individual can learn or relearn the skills requisite to coping with developmental demands.

11. Activities are purposeful when they accomodate the patient's needs, interests, abilities, and place within the life span, and when they provide sufficient opportunity for growth and change.

12. As in life, during treatment the patient has responsibility for his own growth and development.

The Role of the Occupational Therapist

As she adjusts to the developmental needs of the patient, the role of the occupational therapist is flexible and may vary from being a teacher, to a facilitator, to participant, and to supporting agent. As a teacher or facilitator, the occupational therapist selects or creates a *growth facilitating environment* (Mosey, 1970, p. 141), and provides purposeful activities that will enhance the acquisition of knowledge and skills necessary to maintain optimum function, prevent regression, and promote developmental change in the treatment and later community environment. In some instances, she may use a class-like structure to disseminate knowledge and promote skill- building activity while she remains sensitive to the uniqueness of each patient.

When the therapist identifies specific areas in which enabling skills are lacking, a key function of the therapist is to design or select experiences, or help the patient select experiences, that will provide a vehicle for him to learn and practice essential skills. In some instances, as with the building of some sensory-motor skills, the activity might be quite noncognitive, and the therapist will attempt to promote an atmosphere of relaxation or play. She might, for example, work toward increasing a patient's level of alertness by engaging with him in an improvisational rhythm band. In other instances, as with skill building in the areas of cognitive or moral development, the therapist could stimulate discussions around daily patient concerns involving the sharing of materials, mutual respect, rules and authority, and personal philosophies. As facilitator, she could enhance the exchange by asking provocative questions and posing hypothetical dilemmas designed to be within the patient's conceptual grasp, yet thought-provoking.

In order to do this, the therapist must be familiar with the developmental requirements in a range of human endeavor, as well as to hold a conceptual picture of the ebb and flow of life-span development.

While change necessitates a period of moderate disequilibrium, the therapist can assist the patient (if the patient is cognitively able) to understand his changing needs and to place his immediate stress in a larger perspective by providing him with information about life stages and developmental tasks. In so doing, she provides a conceptual framework from which the patient can assess his occupational, avocational, and social options.

In a supporting role, the therapist conveys to the patient her confidence in his capabilities and his ability to meet the demands of normal developmental stress, to accommodate to the growth changes that ensue, and to meet the challenge of life's tasks. She will serve as a resource that helps him to make the transition from the treatment setting to the community setting.

Throughout the treatment process, the occupational therapist is conscious of environmental/cultural expectations, and thus assists the patient to adopt strategies and behaviors which will promote physical-psychosocial maturity and motivate performance that meets cultural-environmental-developmental expectations.

Evaluation

Whether or not one makes a conscious effort to do so, each of us employs a developmental stance in assessment, no matter what our frame of reference. When an individual indicates that he is in distress, we ask ourselves, "How does this person function as compared to the expectations of society and himself?" For example, if a patient is 23 years old, we want to know if he is going to school, or pursuing a career, or living at home—and though we may be flexible and avoid judgments, we are nevertheless interested in this information because we know what is expected of a 23 year old. Much of what each of us consider healthy or constructive is related to the life-span expectations that all of us within a given culture hold in common. In that sense, each of us make developmentally based assessments.

However, there are emphases particular to the developmentally oriented assessment. If the reader reviews the earlier discussion of developmental theory, she will discern movement from global or broad constructs to specific, and she will see a holistic concern for all areas of function. The process of assessment can move quite naturally in much the same way. The therapist might, for example, meet a new male patient, age 37. She would ask the individual to describe what he perceived as his present difficulties. She would note the stage within the life span, as suggested by Jung, Levinson, Erikson, or other life-span theorist, and she would wonder if the individual, at age 37, was in or approaching a period of life reassessment. She would realize that societal expectations for this individual included that he have some degree of job stability, family relatedness, and peer affiliation.

She could ask for a brief history from the patient, or his family, with special emphasis on his current status regarding occupation, social affiliation, roles, and pastimes. The therapist could then determine whether or not the individual was in or out of synchronization with the developmental tasks of his stage. During the assessment, the occupational therapist is sensitive to the specific life course that the patient has experienced and to the individuality that it represents. When organizing and evaluating the data from the patient's life history to target the patient's present level of function, the therapist may seek to answer the following questions:

1. Based upon chronological age, in which life stage of development is the patient?
2. Does the patient's life history and skill performance suggest that he is adequately functioning in this stage?
3. Does the patient demonstrate the skills that suggest that he has mastered the develop-

mental tasks identified with each of the stages prior to the present developmental level at which the patient is presently functioning?

4. What are the present stresses and expectations confronting the patient to which he must respond and cope with in order to continue to grow, change, and adapt in life?
5. Is the patient's network adequate to help the patient confront stress, resolve the psychosocial crisis, and meet the challenges of his life course?
6. Does the patient demonstrate coping strategies rather than defensive patterns?
7. How does the patient respond to both stress and change? Is the patient challenged or overwhelmed by stress?
8. Can the patient identify and use personal, interpersonal, and environmental resources to respond to change or stress?

When it appears that the patient has not been able to succeed at tasks specific to life-stage expectations, the therapist will use her assessment to determine (1) which areas of or which enabling skills are deficient or weak; and which are strong; (2) what barriers (environmental or intrapersonal) are keeping the individual from developing or utilizing his skills; and (3) in what situations and under what conditions is the individual most likely to function best.

Throughout assessment, the therapist will identify areas of strength and potential means of building on available resources. She recognizes that adults (as children) do not function optimally or necessarily in a stage-consonant manner in all areas of endeavor, or equally well in all situations. We have all seen, for example, persons who are able to think clearly and effectively until they encounter a stress, i.e., an illness, or accident— at which point they become confused and childlike. The same fluctuation can be true of more dysfunctional patients.

Most therapists working with psychiatric patients can recount experiences in which individuals were able to function well within the treatment setting but not outside the setting. For instance, a patient could sit for long periods in occupational therapy cooperating with other patients to accomplish a group mural, laughing spontaneously and appearing very at ease. Once back into the community, the individual became anxious, unable to concentrate, and fearful of making mistakes.

While one can use such an example to document that higher social skills did not truly exist, one could also question if the difference in function depended largely on the degree of acceptance and support the patient felt. When he felt accepted, his anxiety was lessened and his ability to use his own skills was optimum. In an environment in which others were generally oblivious to this same person's need for encouragement, doubts set in, anxiety ensued and function declined (see end note 9).

The Developmental Profile. To identify the boundaries of performance for specific enabling skills, the therapist uses interview, observation during task performance, and interprets her observation findings. (Mosey, 1970) Based upon the patient's interview responses (verbal and nonverbal), or information from the family or significant others, the therapist will conceptualize a developmental profile. The profile which is based upon the patient's history reflects functional skill performance such as that based upon the seven adaptive skills identified by Mosey (Appendix H), the mastery of life tasks, responses to psychosocial crises, and patterns of coping.

To date, there are no standardized occupational therapy tests which accurately reflect adult skill performance based upon a continuum of normal growth and development. The tests which are available to assess enabling skills are primarily in the area of sensory-motor-integration function and have been standardized for the child population. These tests have been used by therapists as screening tools to identify adult performance problems and possible directions for treatment of the adult patient. A *screening tool* is a test, or specific activity which is used to distinguish an individual patient who has a particular skill, or more often, deficit, from those individuals who do not. It is used to identify the patient's skills, abilities, and problems in a particular area of function. Specific to the assessment of cognition as it is demonstrated in voluntary motor behavior, Allen has introduced the Allen Cognitive Level Test (ACL) and the Lower Cognitive Level Test (LCL).

Mosey provides broad general guidelines for assessment of the seven adaptive skills, and lists the following tests for perceptual-motor assessment: the Ayres tests, which have been grouped together and are now called the Southern California Integration Tests (SCIT, 1972), the Marianne Frostig Developmental Test of Visual Perception, the Winter Haven Perceptual Copy Forms Test, the Developmental Test of Visual-Motor Integration, and the Illinois Test of Psycholinguistic Abilities (Mosey, 1970). Ross and Burdick (1981) include a sensory-integrative assessment tool in their manual, and acknowledge their incorporation of Lloren's sensory-integrative evaluation for children (Llorens, 1967).

Should the occupational therapist choose to use any of the previously mentioned tests (or others that have been developed since those of the 1960s) as screening tools with adults or as standardized assessments with children, the authors recommend that the therapist research the literature that summarizes assessment protocol, reliability, and validity studies, and the neurological, psychological, and occupational therapy views and critiques of these instruments.

If the therapist chooses to assess performance of the seven adaptive skills identified by Mosey (1970), she will observe the patient's responses during activities and try to answer some of the following questions.

1. Does the patient receive adequate information from his five senses and respond to his sensations in a manner that promotes an age appropriate, physical-psychosocial response?
2. Is the patient oriented to time, place, and person?
3. Can the patient use language to communicate his thoughts and feelings?
4. Can the patient read and write?
5. Can the patient identify a goal and pursue it?
6. Can and how does the patient problem solve?
7. Does the patient initiate activities that allow him to pursue his interests, satisfy his

needs, and express his capabilities?

8. Do the chosen activities assist the patient in mastering life tasks, confronting and resolving psychosocial crises, and allow for coping and adaptation throughout life?
9. How does the patient relate to another person?
10. What is his response to the therapist during the interview?
11. Can he initiate and maintain a conversation in a variety of settings and circumstances? In the community? With a friend? In his job? With his supervisor or an authority figure? Within an intimate relationship? In a care-giving or nurturing relationship?
12. Do his social interactions meet his needs and promote adaptive functioning throughout life?
13. Does the patient participate in a variety of group situations? A small group (three to nine persons)? A large group (ten plus persons)? In a family? In religious, social, work, or community settings?
14. Does the patient work cooperatively with others to accomplish a goal?
15. Does the patient adequately communicate his views and needs to the group in order to benefit from the group experience?
16. Does the patient assume various group membership roles?
17. What is the patient's self-concept, (physical-psychosocial view of himself)?
18. Can the patient identify his strengths, abilities, and limitations?
19. Can the patient describe how others view him, his physical characteristics, his life roles, and significant life history?
20. How does the patient feel about himself and his life course?
21. How does the patient feel about his masculine and feminine characteristics?
22. Does the patient feel that he can adequately express his sexual needs?

These questions are based upon the subskill components of Mosey's seven adaptive skills. (Mosey, 1970) Given the time constraints of most interviews and task assessment sessions, the occupational therapist will not be able to answer all of these questions, but will concentrate on specific skill areas for assessment because they relate to the patient's identified problem or to the particular developmental emphasis of the program (as with sensory-integrative or cognitive developmental treatment).

As the interview progresses and the occupational therapist observes the patient's behavior during the assessment tasks, she also makes assumptions and draws inferences from the patient's verbal and nonverbal responses. These interpretations are then discussed with the patient in a manner that considers the patient's ability to understand and the therapeutic benefits of sharing. The outcome of this patient-therapist discussion can clarify the developmental profile and affirm or negate the therapist's interpretation as well as pose questions that will identify additional assessment needs. The therapist's interpretations are based upon physical-psychosocial developmental theories and the normal pattern of growth and change that occurs throughout the life span.

Assessment Batteries. In the occupational therapy literature that describes assessments used in mental health, there are no assessments specifically identified with the developmental frame of reference other than those previously mentioned for evaluating sensory-motor--integrative function and cognitive function. The authors have identified the following assessment batteries with the developmental frame because the battery tasks elicit developmental data that has been identified with this frame of reference.

The Lifestyle Performance Profile: An Organizing Frame. Authored by Gail Fidler, the assessment suggests guidelines for gathering data to describe physical-psychosocial skills that reflect adaptive performance and mastery of life tasks. Further discussion and details are available in Hemphill (Hemphill, 1982, pp. 43-47).

The Adolescent Role Assessment. The author Maureen Black states that this is not a diagnostic tool and proposes this assessment as a guide for evaluation and treatment planning. An interview format is described to elicit data to indicate past, present, and future role adjustment based upon occupational choice (Hemphill, 1982, p. 49-53).

The Adult Psychiatric Sensory Integration Evaluation. This battery is also referred to as the Schroeder, Block, Cambell Adult Psychiatric Evaluation (SBC). The SBC is used to assesss sensory-motor responses, developmental history, and various neurological soft signs. The test assesses 27 items, which vary from dominance to posture, to reflexes, to body image. The items are rated on a 0 to 3 scale and reflect behavioral performance. The test was designed to screen sensory-motor problems of schizophrenics. Data is being gathered to standardize this screening tool (Hemphill, 1982, pp. 227-253). Specific procedures, observation protocol, and scoring and work sheets are available from SBC Research Associates, Psychiatric Occupational Therapy, 8314 Paseo Del Ocaso, La Jolla, California 92037.

Sensory-Motor-Cognitive Assessment. This is an assessment developed by Mildred Ross and Brenda Smaga to be used with the geriatric-psychiatric population. It assesses 17 items which reflect sensory-motor and perceptual-cognitive function. Its tasks incorporate the work of Ayres and Llorens and also Koh block and person drawing experiences. Battery protocol, summary format, and case examples are available in the book *Sensory Integration* (Ross and Burdick, 1981).

Allen Cognitive Level Test (ACL). This is an assessment developed by Claudia Allen and refined by Josephine Moore. The patient is given leather lacing and asked to imitate one or more standard lacing patterns. It is designed to establish the level of cognitive disability. See Allen (1985) for specific instructions for administering the test, scoring, and discussion regarding validity and reliability.

Treatment Goals

As with all the treatment frameworks presented in this text, the developmental frame has been strongly influenced by the general acceptance in health care of behavioral goal setting.

Behavioral Goal Statements. Mosey speaks to the behavioral influence (referred to by her as an "action consequence" relationship), in which enabling subskills (or their components) are carefully identified and promoted through judicious and selective reinforcement by the therapist.

Danish, et al., (1984), in their discussion of life development intervention, stress that problems must be viewed in terms of "behaviorally oriented positive goal statements" (Danish, et al., 1984, p. 539), and they speak of the necessity for a delineation of "behavioral components of a skill" in skill development (Danish, et al., 1984, p. 540). However, treatment goals are selected by the developmental therapist under some guiding premises that differ from that of the behavioral therapist. The developmental therapist may find herself in the position of establishing goals that target behavior that is at a lesser developmental level than that which is ultimately desired, but seen as a necessary foundation for adult behavior. For example, a patient who is behaving in a manner that is regressed may (though not necessarily) be allowed to engage in activities that meet more infantile needs, i.e., for being nurtured, touched, or being very messy. This is on the premise that more regressive activities or interactions may be required before more age appropriate activities can be tackled. The developmentalist believes that once the more primitive need is met, or primitive skill mastered, the individual has an innate need to move to higher level challenges.

The behaviorist would be more likely to start with higher level, age appropriate goals, looking for any chance to reinforce age and stage appropriate behavior. The behaviorist would ask, "Is allowing and essentially reinforcing more primitive behavior serving to strengthen or promote lower level function?" The behavioral therapist might also question the amount of time spent and potentially wasted on reinforcing lower level behavior, when, as they believe, judicious reinforcement can work quickly to establish higher level schemes. This debate is exemplified in differing approaches to anorexia nervosa. The developmentally oriented occupational therapist might pay special attention to issues concerning a young woman's sexuality and her problems with femininity, and could institute treatment goals related to increasing the woman's understanding of her conflicted feelings regarding sexuality. Activities might be centered around selecting clothes, or wearing appropriate make-up, having fun in a heterosexual peer group, or other activities designed to help the woman deal with developmental issues related to self-image. The behaviorist might take a more controlled approach: strictly reinforcing proper eating habits and weight gain. In one behavioral setting, for example, participation in occupational therapy was a reward for an anorexic woman's weight gain. As added incentive, when a two pound gain was achieved, the patient was given individualized time with the occupational therapist working on a project of the patient's choice (see end note 10).

Thus, treatment goals are selected in accordance with the overall treatment philosophy and theory regarding growth and development. Developmental treatment goals are more likely to be compatible with those of the object relations framework in which object cathexes are believed to develop in accordance with the individual's transition through psychosexual stages, and with cognitive-behavioral treatment. In some instances, as those described, developmental treatment may conflict with what we would conceive as traditional (conditioned learning) behavioral approaches.

Whatever goals are established, they must be stated in terms of desired behavior or skills and subskills, be attainable and understood as such by the individual, and be achievable within a reasonable period. Short term goals allow the individual to recognize his own progress, increase his confidence, and may be viewed as steps to longer term goals (some of which may or may not be realized during the course of treatment).

Treatment Process

While we have throughout the text utilized a patient-treatment model, the reader will recognize that much of the discussion regarding the developmental process has focused on the normative process. Although acknowledging that there are many individuals who do not function within the norms and who become identified as needing professional assistance, not all therapists conceive of developmental skill building as a matter of treatment; some approach it rather as a process of education or re-education. This has been less apparent in occupational therapy than it has been in counseling.

In the discussion of developmental treatment, we will first discuss treatment as it has been conceived generally in occupational therapy. Within the occupational therapy profession, there has been an emphasis on remediation or stabilization with individuals identified as patients. The focus with these people has been in what might be called "catch up" skill building. We will then discuss, in contrast, some preventative treatment principles that are emerging in the realm of counseling and the community mental health system. These are presented for the reader's consideration because, in many instances, activities such as those familiar to occupational therapy are used. Rather than suggesting that remediation, stabilization, or prevention is necessarily a better treatment goal (all may have their place for given individuals, in given situations), it may be that as treatment progresses the therapist and patient will profit by changing their treatment emphasis. Also, while prevention or preventative medicine has not been the predominant arena for occupational therapy practice, prevention is an area that is being given increasing attention in health care. No one is certain just how committed, in terms of dollars, the government or the public are to preventative care. It seems important, however, for occupational therapists to assess what role they can or wish to play in the area of prevention.

Skill Building in Occupational Therapy. Developmental skill building follows logically given the postulates presented thus far. The therapist provides an environment which enhances the opportunity for the individual to follow a normal developmental pattern and selects activities that bridge the gap between the individual's present skill level and the skills he needs to learn and master. Once new skills have been attained, the next, successively higher step in skill development is approached. While enabling skills across all areas are interdependent, the person often presents an uneven developmental picture: that is, he has achieved some age appropriate developmental tasks, but not others; or he has strong skills in some areas, but not in others. The process of developmental skill building is one of maximizing strengths and building upon previous accomplishments while developing new skills.

Depending upon the specific nature of the deficits or delays, projected learning needs, and the treatment philosophy of the therapist, skill building may be approached quite differently in one treatment center than in another, even where the clinicians all espouse a developmental

229

approach. We will discuss briefly several approaches to skill building evident in occupational therapy, then present an evolving, preventative posture.

Cognitive Developmental Treatment

Allen. As described earlier, Allen's treatment model is designated for the severely or chronically cognitively disabled. Once a determination is made regarding a patient's cognitive level, activities are provided in occupational therapy that are compatible with the patient's limited abilities and at which he can succeed. Allen (1985) provides a guideline for task analysis to assist the therapist in matching the cognitive demands of voluntary motor tasks with the cognitive capabilities of the patient.

As stated previously, Allen asserts that the cognitively disabled are not likely to improve, or, if they do improve, do so because of the natural healing process or positive effects of pharmacology. This would be especially likely to occur with acute psychotic episodes. Thus, according to Allen the goals of occupational therapy are best conceived as "*measurement* and *management* as alternative to *improvement*" (Note: the emphases are Allen's; Allen, 1985, p.32). The measurement to which Allen refers is the measurement of cognitive levels, to ascertain the severity of the disease; and careful observation of change to assess if medications are taking effect (Allen, 1985, p. 22). The primary emphasis is on the role of the therapist as an observer, helping to establish a medical diagnosis, watching for changes in cognitive function, and helping to determine the extent of a patient's residual disability and accompanying potential need for post-treatment care. The therapist will select tasks that take into account the patient's interests, abilities, and limitations (Allen, 1982). The therapist is advised to be supportive, for example, reassuring the patient that his medication will soon help him to feel more comfortable, and providing activities that the patient can succeed with. Skill building is not a goal (see end note 11).

The therapist who is aware of Allen's theory and proposals regarding psychiatric dysfunction, has a clearly identified purpose that guides her interactions with cognitively disabled patients, and her approach seems best suited to assisting the lower functioning patient. Allen's proposals serve to caution the therapist against having unrealistic expectations for the patient, the therapist, or the treatment process. The therapist utilizing this approach must be aware of what she has deliberately omitted, as well as that to which she has attended.

Once the decision is made in favor of this approach, the parameters in regard to assessment and intervention become quite circumscribed. On the one hand, this may facilitate concise and objective documentation and keep the therapist from trying to be "all things to all people." On the other hand, this approach may limit the therapist's ability to address other needs that are experienced as pressing to the individual, and may fail to utilize potential for improvement that continues to exist. (An example of the application of Allen's theory is provided in the following.)

In her book, Allen provides the brief case example, then poses the questions that follow it. Finally, she provides answers that would be consistent with her cognitive approach.

Case Example—Depressive Episode

History

Mabel is a 66 year old woman who was admitted because of severe depression, which has been worsening for the last two years since the death of her husband. One year ago she retired, having worked successfully as a special education teacher for 30 years; nine months ago she was forced to admit her mother to a nursing home, about which she feels guilty. During the last two years she has lost 40 pounds, has had intermittent difficulty sleeping at night, and has been progressively unable to manage at home. She has been seeing a psychiatrist as an outpatient; the psychiatrist has been treating her with antidepressants and chlorpromazine, but there is some question of her reliability in taking medication.

OT Interview

When seen, Mabel sat huddled in her chair in a wrinkled dress, hair half-combed, with slight perspiration, probably caused by her constant leg and hand movements. Her response to questions was minimal, with no identification of interests or goals. Mabel stated that she wanted out of "jail," but knew the name of the hospital. She made a vauge effort to do the ACL but then stopped. listing a number of reason: "I can't do anything anymore. I never will. You'd better try someone else. My eyes are too bad to see this. They'll never let me out of this place".

Questions

1. List the diagnostic symptoms of depression that are identified in the history and OT interview (DSM III criteria).

2. Cite examples of task behavior that you can anticipate.

3. After two weeks, the therapist notices that Mabel is showing some improvement; she has been smiling, and her personal appearance is better. Mabel completes the steps in level 4 tasks, but shows no initiative in varying her actions or in exploring the relationship between objects. Her task behavior is limited to 30 minutes. The physician must evaluate the effect of medication at this point.

a. Write your observations of Mabel's performance; include observations and terminology useful to the physician.

b. Write an interpretation of the observations.

c. Write your plan (Allen, 1985, p. 206). The answers to these questions are also provided by Allen and reproduced with permission.

Case Example XI

1. DSM III criteria for depression in this case are weight loss, sleep disturbance, diminished ability, and loss of interest or pleasure.

2. Anticipate OT observations: loss of energy with slow movements; indecisiveness in making choices; and resistance to, or reluctance to attend OT activities.

3. a. Mable's functional performance corresponds with the improvement in her personal appearance. She is able to sustain performance for about 30 minutes and shows interest in completing tasks selected by the therapist.

b. Current level of function is typical of level 4. Level 5 behaviors were not observed. Her functional history indicates that her quality of performance should improve to at least a level 5 and probably a level 6.

    c. Plan. Continue to observe for higher level performance as her medication is titrated (Allen 1985, p. 217).

    The preceding is from pages 206 and 207 of Claudia Allen's *Occupational Therapy for Psychiatric Diseases: Measurement and Management of Cognitive Disabilities,* Boston, Little Brown and Company, 1985 and is reproduced with permission.

Some thought-provoking issues raised by Allen's work, and not easily resolved concern the questions:

1. To what extent, do the rules of normal development continue to apply where disability (be it emotional, cognitive, physical, or social) is present?
2. How does one determine that a person biologically limited is no longer capable of growth or positive change?
3. If one accepts that most, perhaps all psychiatric or emotional problems have a biological counterpart, how can the mental health treatment community respond to the biological part of the whole person in an optimally healing manner?

Since skill building is not a goal, nor growth through the developmental process anticipated, this treatment model will not be discussed further here.

    The interested reader is referred to Allen's *Occupational Therapy for Psychiatric Diseases: Measurement and Management of Cognitive Disabilities* (1985) for a complete discussion of this cognitive approach.

    Leva. Leva (1984) describes a therapeutic approach based upon Piagetian principles that expands beyond the sensory-motor period and which is applicable to multiple functional levels besides the psychotic or more chronic problem to which Allen refers.

    When applying Piagetian theory in treatment, the therapist assumes that the process of change in therapy follows the same developmental line as the one that occurs during normal growth and development. Thus, the treatment process as discussed by Leva is conceptualized upon a developmental framework.

    Leva identifies problems that exist when an adult primarily functions within the sensory-motor, preoperational, concrete-operations, or formal operations periods. In the *sensory-motor* phase the individual is characterized by reflexive behavior rather than planned or controlled behavior, i.e., he exhibits poor control of behavior patterns such as that seen in perseveration, overeating, or excessive smoking and drinking; he is unable to set achievable short term goals, i.e., giving up cigarettes for a day, getting to work on time; he misinterprets reality and feedback that he receives, i.e., he may hallucinate or he may personalize comments that are not intended for him; and he has difficulty in coordinating internal and external cues, i.e., the patient who is unable to postpone his need for a cigarette and disrupts a group meeting by leaving for a cigarette break (Leva, 1984).

    The treatment response to these problems is one which helps the individual set short term goals which are accomplished through motor and environmental (concrete) interactions and which provides outcomes which give immediate feedback (Leva, 1984). A sample short term goal may be "work on a project for one half hour in occupational therapy before a ten minute break."

When functioning at the *preoperational level* or period of preconceptual thought, the individual may demonstrate one or more of the following: a limited view, a static view or a distorted conception of reality, i.e., "tunnel vision"; a rigid view or confusion due to distorted or unrelated perceptions, i.e., the patient may be convinced that someone dislikes him or that comments addressed to others are intended for him; knowledge of what needs to be done and a cognitive ability to respond, but inflexible or inadequate responses; inability to set realistic, accomplishable short term goals; lack of understanding of his own capabilities; and inability to use experience to gain an understanding of the environmental and personal relationships that exist (Leva, 1984).

In response to these problems the therapist would seek to (1) broaden the patient's view of reality (the situation); (2) assist in the identification of changes that need to occur; (3) expand the individual's knowledge and skill base that he uses to cope and problem solve; and (4) identify his abilities to increase the individual's self-understanding and esteem (Leva, 1984).

Problems identified with the *concrete operational period* include an overdependence on objective reality, that is the individual bases his perceptions, values, goals, and behavior upon the views of others and their expectations. He often has unrealistic short term goals, goals based upon inaccurate views of the future, his own abilities, and possible behavioral outcomes; and he has a scattered focus on the problems identified. One might see a patient who can identify many problems, but is unable to set priorities and begin problem solving; his plans for problem solving are rigidly implemented, or he is incapable of flexibility and adapting to an unexpected, unplanned event or response. For example, the patient may become confused or feel overwhelmed in new situations or when confronted with life's daily traumas, such as his automobile stalling, or having to cope with an ill family member (Leva, 1984).

During treatment, the therapist would cooperatively work with the patient to (1) gain an objective view of the situation or problem and see the existing variables in social and environmental relationships; (2) set goals which he could meet with his given capabilities; and (3) identify and coordinate plans to resolve or cope with problems and to increase his ability to respond flexibly (Leva, 1984).

An individual who functions at the *formal operations level* may experience the following difficulties: he perceives reality but may misinterpret social interactions and behavioral codes; he lacks personal standards and may not have clearly identified his interests, values and goals; his ability to problem solve is sporadic; he has knowledge and skills but does not know how to apply these principles and concepts to respond to daily life situations. The treatment response to these problems strives (1) to increase the individual's knowledge of natural and scientific laws, i.e., the need for rest and adequate nutrition in order to maintain health; (2) to identify the relationships that form concepts, i.e., the patient's tardiness and poor social skills are interfering with his job performance; (3) to verbally retrace plans, images and concepts, i.e., the patient's ability to make a plan and verbalize the plan of action (Leva, 1984).

In general, treatment based upon Piagetian-developmental theory introduces task and social experiences compatible with the patient's current level of function. Where possible, the therapist will help the patient conceptualize problems and understand their negative impact as well as how they can provide a challenge to grow and an opportunity for coping. By using activities as well as having the patient talk about his experiences, the therapist tries to help the patient gain more control over his own actions.

Each developmental period is identified with characteristic means of problem solving, and each can be associated with characteristic limitations in being able to meet daily needs. Leva's work suggests that patients at all cognitive developmental levels are potentially accessible to treatment, and one does not perceive the split between lower and higher cognitively functioning patients. Her proposals are traditionally Piagetian in that they suggest that cognitively attuned experiences can be used to improve an individual's function, regardless of developmental level.

Building Cognitive Skills Related to Moral Reasoning and Social Perspective

Kohlberg and Wilcox. Kohlberg and Wilcox address the normative process of cognitive development in childhood and adulthood. Kohlberg's work has been applied frequently in the field of elementary and higher education. The occupational therapist utilizing the principles of Kohlberg or Wilcox is most likely to do so with the individual judged to be reality oriented, nonpsychotic, and evidencing some mature adult behaviors. For example, the authors have used Kohlberg's strategies with disturbed (nonpsychotic) adolescents who were experiencing multiple problems with parents, school, and the law.

As discussed earlier, Kohlberg and Wilcox do not view lower level cogntive function as necessarily indicative of illness or disability, and in their works they cite examples of normal adult behavior in which lower stages of cognitive, moral, and social reasoning predominate. Kohlberg, like Piaget, does, however note the importance of central nervous system maturation (and we can assume, continued adequate function) and opportunity as requisite for development. It is not clear to what extent such emotional factors as stress, anxiety, and depression might interfere with the individual's ability to truly learn from the experiences provided in the environment. Thus it is uncertain how the emotional attributes of psychiatric problems as well as the potential physiological limitations addressed by Allen, might affect moral development.

Creating Cognitive Dissonance. Utilizing the principles of these developmentalists, the occupational therapist would observe her patient's predominant manner of cognitive and moral processing. If the patient seems limited in his ability to act upon a range of useful and socially acceptable ways of reasoning, the therapist would try to create situations designed to stimulate cognitive growth. She would (1) expose the patient to reasoning at a level just slightly higher than that he was employing; (2) encourage role-taking or role-reversal to the extent that he was cognitively capable; and (3) be aware of the importance of the manner in which rules and authority were handled within her own setting. A major aim of these actions is to create an internal conflict in the individual's reasoning. Jerome Bruner (as cited in Wilcox, 1979, p. 192) emphasizes the importance of both enactive or physical experience in cognitive learning as well as the opportunity to talk about the learning experience. The combination of enactive learning and the opportunity to reflect upon and reason about an activity or interaction has been found to be much more useful in promoting social and moral development than physical activity or verbalization in isolation.

An example that demonstrates enactive learning around a social issue is one that occurs often in practice:

A patient leaves an occupational therapy activity group because, as he insists, the patient group has "intentionally ignored me" and "doesn't like me."

The occupational therapist can use the experience to help the patient de-center. The therapist might state that she did not sense that anyone in the group was angry with the patient. She then asks the patient to generate other explanations for the slights he felt. If he is unable, the therapist might interrupt the patient group and ask the group members to respond briefly to the concern.

The therapist does not insist that the patient is wrong, nor demand that he accept alternative explanations. Rather, she tries to create dissonance in the patient's accepted way of interpreting this kind of social interaction.

As another illustration, we can consider the patient who pilfers materials from the occupational therapy clinic because, as he reasons, "There's so much stuff there, how can it hurt?"

Recognizing that the patient is using a preconventional level of moral reasoning, the therapist might try to increase the patient's ability to empathize by asking what his response would be if someone went into his room and took "just a few" of his belongings. In this instance, the therapist is trying to both create cognitive dissonance as well as increase the ability for empathy. This would be in contrast to a response that emphasized that such a behavior necessitates punishment.

Summary

As demonstrated in the examples from practice, the occupational therapist who is trying to enhance cognitive development related to moral reasoning and social perspective does not see her role as one of "giving knowledge"; but rather, of helping the patient to educe, or draw from himself, new ways of interpreting information to create his own knowledge.

The therapist who takes such an approach recognizes that learning of this kind does not occur quickly (although there may be flashes of insight or recognition), and she knows the patient will need to engage in many such experiences in his life to bring to actual fruition a movement from one development stage to the next. But she believes that unlike information that is handed to a person, learning that has been gained through a person's reasoning out an activity or interaction is more likely to become a permanent, meaningful, and integrated part of himself.

Sensory-Motor-Integration Treatment

We will now ask the reader to switch gears and consider a developmental treatment approach very different from the ones just discussed. Stated very simply, a cognitive-developmental theorist holds that an individual who can think and reason effectively is better able to interact with others, has increased confidence, and ultimately, his physical being will reflect this increased confidence, judgment and skill. The sensory-integrative therapist believes that the ability to utilize cognitive information and interact effectively with others is built upon a sound body image, the ability to interpret sensory data easily and correctly, and the facility to move through three-dimensional space comfortably. If a person has to think about moving across a room, then there is not much thinking that can be diverted elsewhere. The result may be the individual who appears awkward and inept, unable to concentrate and out of touch with the general milieu.

As discussed, in occupational therapy the sensory-integrative approach in mental health has been postulated and applied by King (1974) in her work with process, nonparanoid schizophrenics, and suggested for autism, geriatrics, and depression. Ross and Burdick (1981) suggest sensory integration for any long term psychotic, regressed, or elderly patients as a means to maintain or improve movement, attention span, and general skills. Ross and Burdick give extensive guidelines for carrying out a sensory integration treatment program, and provide a model assessment tool, as well as specific recommendations for selecting activities and structuring group sensory-motor-integrative experiences. However, Ross and Burdick provide a treatment plan that includes the building of cognitive skill. For the sake of clarity, we will summarize the treatment principles of King, which emphasize noncortical or noncognitive activities. A therapist might, in practice, use sensory-integrative treatment as a prelude to other aspects of skill development, such as the cognitive skills addressed by Ross and Burdick.

As stated by King, activities are selected according to their ability to do one or more of the following: (King, 1974a; 1974b)

1. Normalize patterns of excessive flexion, adduction, and internal rotation, i.e., activities involving reaching up and out, such as balloon volleyball, or painting a large mural;
2. Incorporate maximum vestibular stimulation (movement of the head through many planes), i.e., swinging, twirling, and rocking;
3. Make bilateral use of tonic muscles against resistance (as in heavy work patterns), e.g., tug of war, digging in a garden, folding larger sheets;
4. Involve deep pressure touch, e.g., being "rolled up" in a parachute or sheet;
5. Give proprioceptive feedback (by stimulating joints and tendons), e.g., clapping, jumping rope, and jogging;
6. Incorporate eye pursuit, e.g., catching a ball, and "Nerf©" ping-pong;
7. Stimulating a range of senses, i.e., utilizing taste, sounds, smells, and rhythms;
8. Adduce smiles and pleasure, as with noncompetitive games, surprises, and recreation;

236

9. Provide a sense of mastery, where activity is task-oriented.

An essential purpose in using activity is that the patient's attention be on the pleasure of the activity so that he is not consciously planning his motor movements. The therapist is also exhorted to recognize the potential alerting effect of some activities and calming effects of others, and to select an appropriate continuum of activity as based on a patient's or patient-group's needs. The therapist is encouraged to be involved, to have fun, and to encourage spontaneity rather than competition (see end note 12). The time allotted for a typical sensory-integrative treatment session as discussed by King and Ross and Burdick is 30 to 45 minutes.

Although the sensory-motor-integrative approach is not the preferred one for all mental health populations, it has influenced occupational therapy by heightening the therapist's awareness of the physical component of the psychiatric disability. Occupational therapists use exercise, fitness, relaxation, and aerobic experiences to maintain muscle function, endurance, and an attractive, healthy body image. These exercise-fitness groups can be adapted to the patient's age, ability, and needs. The occupational therapist designs exercise groups to incorporate popular television exercise sessions, aerobic records, and inexpensive equipment.

Building Other Adaptive Skills

Ann Mosey gives general treatment guidelines for developing the seven adaptive skills in her presentation of a developmental frame of reference (Mosey, 1970). In agreement with other developmental theorists, Mosey states that the therapist needs to begin with the most primitive subskill a patient has not learned yet needs to learn, and create a learning experience in which this can occur. It becomes the therapist's task to identify what skills are lacking, and to envision experiences in which these skills might be learned and well-practiced.

We can cite, for example, the new mother who seeks treatment because of extreme depression or anxiety following the birth of her first child, and describe a typical (though abbreviated) developmental approach:

Upon assessment, the therapist finds that the young woman has limited experience with infants, and lacks both basic skills and information related to meeting the physical and emotional needs of an infant. The developmental therapist would note the particular skills and areas of knowledge that were lacking, and would provide learning experiences in which these could be acquired. She might have the woman practice "feeding," dressing, and bathing a doll; or the woman's own infant, if that were possible, until such time that the patient felt comfortable with her own skills. Further, the therapist would identify resources (literature, or individuals expert in the area of child care) that could be used to help the patient learn more about children's growth and developmental needs.

The therapist would also recognize the importance of the patient identifying resources and learning means to meet her own need for recreation or time away from the child.

Mosey offers a model in which given subskills are conceived as behavioral goals, and suggests using the behavioral method of giving positive or negative reinforcement to promote skill building. Although the use of behavioral goal setting is not particular to Mosey, and is suggested by other therapists also, it should be noted that her conceptualization of an external, therapist-given reward is not consistent with the developmental postulates of Piaget and Kohlberg, who state that the need for development is innate, satisfying, and self-regulating, and does not need behavioral reward to be sustained.

One area in which Mosey's discussion of enabling skills and developmental treatment has seemed to especially impact current occupational therapy practice are those guidelines she has proposed for the delineating developmental levels of group process. These are described briefly in Appendix C.

As noted by Briggs, et al. (1979), "Few therapists have the opportunity to follow a client through developmental stages or adaptive skill learning, over an extended period of time" (Briggs, et al., 1979, p. 144). Thus, when one speaks of developmental skill building, there is often only a speculative movement through developmental stages. Actual treatment may focus on demonstrable, shorter term goals, and is more often conceived as maintaining function, building remedial skills, and offsetting remission.

However, the life developmental model, to be discussed, adds another perspective on skill building.

Life Development Intervention

Coming from the counseling literature, the life development intervention model of treatment has a strong educative and preventative component.

Life development intervention (LDI) works to "help people encounter routine and unexpected life circumstances by developing their personal competence in life planning and their interpersonal competence in developing a caring social network. The intent is to encourage individuals to be producers of their own development, to be active problem solvers and planners and to develop a sense of self-efficacy" (Danish, et al., 1984, p. 531)

A "generic" model of LDI is suggested by Danish, et al., for dealing with a variety of life events. They delineate six stages in the helping process:

1. Goal Assessment — Translating problems or inadequacies into positive, attainable goal statements as well as analyzing barriers to goal attainment.
2. Knowledge Acquisition — This may include formalized information given by the helper or designated others.
3. Development of Decision-making Skills — A hierarchy of steps for successful decision making is taught, and emphasis is given to the fact that indecision is a decision in favor of inactivity.
4. Risk Assessment — This is a planned review of alternatives and roadblocks, and a weighing of benefits as well as potential costs of a selected plan of action.
5. Creating Social Support — Especially important for future problem solving is the ability to recognize, gain access to, and make use of social and community resources.
6. Planning Skill Development — This includes developing a rationale for learning a given skill, determining the behavioral components of a skill, developing criteria to

establish when a given skill is accomplished, determining how the skill will be learned, evaluating skill attainment, and considering how the skill development model might be applied to other, perhaps future goals (Danish, et al., 1984, pp. 538-540).

The individual who seeks assistance may be initially helped to deal with the particulars of a given, stressful situation. Special attention will be paid to his manner of problem solving, and he may be taught a more successful problem-solving strategy. Specific goals will be determined, and skills will be targeted or taught to attain these goals. Once a current stress is handled, the therapist works to draw analogies between this stress and its demands for change (or adaptation) and past as well as future events.

Empowering the Individual. The therapist believes that when a future crisis necessitating change is encountered, the individual will more likely handle it effectively if he can (1) see similarities between this and past, successfully accomplished problem solving and (2) generalize problem-solving skills. As more and more changes are accomodated successfully, new events are approached with increasing confidence (Danish, et al., 1984, p. 533).

Serving as a guiding superstructure to skill building, the individual is assisted to look at his life through a life-stage format. As proposed by Danish, et al. (1984), LDI becomes the ability to identify and set life goals. The issue for the individual is not "Where have I failed," but "What do I want to learn," and "What course do I wish to set" (Danish, et al., 1984, p. 532). This approach is described as "proactive," not "reactive" and is believed to be one that gives a sense of empowerment (Danish, et al., 1984, p. 532).

We can refer to the example given earlier of a classically developmental approach designed to teach necessary skills to a young mother with a newborn. In LDI, the mother would be taught skills related to child rearing, as indicated. Then, however, the occupational therapist would help her to look ahead to anticipate future needs. The patient might be asked to think about such questions as, "What will I want to be doing when the child is two or five years old and no longer needs constant care?" Goals of LDI might, for this woman, relate to her wish to increase her level of education or gain occupational skills that can be used three years hence.

LDI Used in a Group Context. Much of the discussion of life development intervention is as regards to its use with several individuals or more, all encountering or expecting to encounter similar life changes. For example, young persons graduating from high school and lacking specific career plans; mothers of toddlers; or older persons anticipating retirement might be contacted through a community outreach program. The ensuing process is viewed as one of helping through education, not through "treatment." If we use prospective retirees (and their spouses) as an example, they might be brought together in an informal classlike structure. They would be:

1. Asked regarding their expectations for change;
2. Given information regarding the more common changes they could expect to encounter, i.e., changes in the amount of leisure time, changes in spendable income; change in status; and changes in the amount of time spouses are together;
3. Given a rationale for learning new skills or learning new ways to balance their time;
4. Helped to select desired skills;

5. Taught specific skills, i.e., how to utilize community resources; avenues for volunteerism; or skills specific to a new hobby, avocation, or potential source of supplementary income;

6. Provided a chance to practice new skills under supervision;

7. Given a support group where they can compare notes and gain encouragement as new skills are put into action. Cantor (1981) also gives an example of a proactive program for retirees.

As in the example just given, looking at expected life changes appears to interface effectively with an occupational behavior orientation (see discussion of Occupational Behavior Frame of Reference in this text), and is similar to the educational modules discussed with cognitive-behavioral treatment, the difference being here that the emphasis is on prevention and not on treatment.

LDI and Dollars. When such prevention or proactive programs are made available through community mental health centers, this occurs because the community health system is seeking to identify members of the population more likely to experience problems. Not only by helping individuals avert a crisis, but also by helping to familiarize them with nontreatment community resources, the teaching agency expects to take some of the demand from the health care system while facilitating community involvement of a much more positive nature.

It requires foresight to envision the positive outcome of LDI programs, and research dollars to substantiate their effectiveness. With the competing demands of individuals already identified as in extreme stress, the occupational therapist might have difficulty finding or even creating an opportunity to offer LDI programs. Additionally, there are other professional groups, including recreational therapists, nurses, and education specialists who, in given agencies, provide this kind of service. Yet, with LDI emphasizing, as it does, choices regarding one's use of time in activities — be they social, individual, vocational, or avocational, principles of life development intervention could add another dimension to occupational therapy practice.

Life development intervention, as described by Danish, et al. (1984) is used with individuals who have had at least some success in coping with previous life events, who have some ability for insight, and have demonstrated motivation. However, it should be added that programs similar in principle to LDI have been instituted by community agencies for the chronically dependent patient. The "chronic" patient (one who appears frequently at a mental health facility for treatment) is assisted to recognize his own strengths and limitations, plan for his future, and helped to meet his needs through a network of community based but nontreatment providers.

Life development intervention for the physically, cognitively, or emotionally limited person might involve helping the individual determine reasonable and attainable goals: resources within the community, and avenues for goal achievement. While many of the normal developmental tasks, as identified by Erikson, Jung, et al., might or might not be attainable, goals appropriate to the limited abilities of the individual would be established, and also could serve for him to increase his sense of dignity, worth, and empowerment.

Chapter Summary

As has been evident with other frameworks of therapy presented in this text, the adult developmental framework incorporates some values and practices that are consistent with alternative frames of reference. One finds, for example, a general acceptance of many premises of object relations theory (a theory which is, in itself, developmentally organized); incorporation of behavioral goal setting and program assessment; and a basis of knowledge in the area of cognitive theory that is shared by cognitive behaviorists. While one can use this as evidence of eclecticism, it will become clear to the reader that there exists information shared in common by theorists and practitioners from all theoretical models, as well as certain common values and expectations. We address here the significant beliefs and guiding priorities that distinguish the developmental frame of reference.

Contributions

1. The developmental frame of reference provides a logical way to understand the whole person from birth to death. It treats with equal consideration the individual's subjective experiencing, objective behaviors, responsibility to self, and interdependence with the environment.

The occupational therapist may choose to focus on a particular aspect of development or skill in treatment; but by appreciating the interrelatedness of all skills, and the overriding needs and concerns the individual experiences, she can better make treatment relevant. Further, the therapist with such an understanding can more effectively work with other disciplines in a well- integrated treatment approach.

2. The developmental approach provides a sound basis for preventative or proactive intervention. It gives the individual and the therapist guidelines by which they can prepare for general kinds of anticipated change, while not claiming to predict the particulars of events.

When treatment seeks to assist the individual in generalizing his learning across the past, present, and future, the individual gains confidence that he will be able to cope effectively with both expected and unexpected future events. As a result, preventative programming, while still a relative newcomer in mental health care, offers the hope of reducing the severity of crisis related to stress, and a reduction in patient readmission to inpatient programs.

3. Seeing the human need to grow and learn as innate, and viewing mastery as satisfying to the individual, the developmental therapist does not perceive her role as one of orchestrating reinforcements, as might occur in a behavioral treatment model.

Skills and actions maintained by personal (internal) satisfaction as well as naturally occurring social encouragement are more likely to be continued after treatment has discontinued than behaviors that have been sustained by therapist contingencies (see end note 13).

4. The developmental framework is a growth (skill-building) model and does not depend on labels of health and illness. While physical barriers to development may be addressed by medically oriented treatment, skill building depends on providing opportunities for learning. The necessity for the constant updating of skills is endogenous to all of us, and does not connote illness. There are differing views regarding the suitability and benefit of conceptualizing psychosocial dysfunction according to a medical or illness model; however, for those individuals who are intimidated by the connotation of mental illness, seeking assistance within a developmental framework may be more tenable and personally acceptable.

5. Developmental (sequential) skill building contrasts with behavioral skill building and avoids the potential problem with the establishment of unstable "splinter skill." One could expect, therefore, that skills built according to a developmentally based hierarchy will be durable, and provide a firm foundation for those skills that will be added to meet future demands.

This assumption represents an area of considerable debate between developmentally and behaviorally oriented helpers, and not one adequately verified by research.

The opposite, or behavioral stance, as discussed earlier in the chapter, is that needless and valuable treatment time will be spent building skills that are no longer appropriate, and reside in the "no man's land" of skills. Behavioral therapists would be more likely to identify skills and subskills (or skill components), all of which represented age-appropriate behaviors.

6. The developmental framework has been described as especially suited for the treatment of those individuals who come into therapy with a low level of function. (Levy, 1974; Briggs, et al., 1979; Mosey, 1970; Allen, 1985). As proposed in this text, and as suggested by adult developmental programs in counseling, the authors see the adult developmental framework as versatile and applicable across a broad range of individual function. The nature and emphasis of programs will, of course, vary according to the developmental needs of the individual patient.

Limitations

1. As conceived in this text, the adult developmental frame of reference needs extensive application, assessment, research, and documentation to clarify its utility. The current frames of reference in occupational therapy that are developmental in origin have been too exclusionary in emphasis to serve as adequate tests of an adult development frame of reference. They do serve, however, as input into the larger knowledge base and represent compatible practice theories within the greater framework.

2. There is seldom, if ever, an opportunity to see the individual's progression from one life stage to another, or to see the completion of a developmental task during treatment. Thus, while one can establish the efficacy of skill building, it is not possible to verify that skill building has led (or necessarily will lead) to satisfying transitions through life stages. These stages must be understood as hypothetical constructs that aid in determining priorities in treatment.

3. The rules of normal development are being used to establish treatment guidelines for individuals whose life courses have often traveled far from the norm. Developmental theory does address the problem of failure to achieve developmental expectations, identifying such failure in general terms as a matter of physical inability or limited opportunity. However, it becomes difficult in practice to determine why given individuals, physically able, have been seemingly incapable of or unwilling to take advantage of opportunity. While these may be the individuals blocked by the "dispositional barriers" cited by Aslanian and Brickell (1980; cited in Rodgers, 1984), they nevertheless present seemingly intractable treatment dilemmas; and their development needs may be best served by an alternative treatment approach.

4. It is not yet clear what specific skills are necessary to enable one to perform the various developmental tasks, what subskills comprise these skills, or how to determine best if these subskills exist. For example, what skills enable an individual to satisfactorily pursue a career? Given a patient who has not been able to settle on a career, how does one determine which enabling skills are deficient? In a closely related problem, even where it is clear that given skills are lacking and must be learned, it is not always clear how these needed skills can most successfully be taught or enhanced.

Using her knowledge of occupation and observing the behaviors of her patient, the occupational therpist will need to use her judgment in deciding which skills and subskills are deficient, which would reasonably represent initial and latter goals for treatment, and what constitutes an optimum learning environment. It should be added that this lack of precision in knowledge about the skill components of given tasks is not particular to the developmental framework. It can be seen as especially problematic in this frame, however, because of the perceived need to build skills in a stepwise fashion.

5. There is a danger that an overly rigid interpretation of life stage concepts will lead to unreasonable expectations for conformity. When the individual expresses dissatisfaction with his own life, then that may be sufficient cause to pursue treatment. When the individual expresses satisfaction with his life courses, but society or significant others indicate disapproval of his conduct, the problems posed in treatment may be quite different.

We have emphasized throughout the chapter the importance of using a life stage concept as a flexible construct, while appreciating the wide diversity in individual experiencing. When life stage constructs are rigidly applied, we believe they lose their utility.

6. Some in the human sciences believe that adult developmental theory has been built upon a lopsided structure in which more has been learned about the experience of men than of women. While we cannot develop this discussion further here, the interested reader is referred to sources identified in end notes 5 and 6 for a presentation of this concern.

As we leave this frame of reference, we reiterate that an understanding of human development can only enhance the therapist's practice, regardless of the frame of reference that she embraces. The extent to which an adult development frame of reference will be chosen as a guiding structure for occupational therapy practice in mental health is as yet uncertain.

End Notes

1. An example of this movement toward transcendence is found in the story of *Siddhartha*, by Herman Hesse (Bantam Books, 1977) which abounds with Jungian metaphors and allegory, as do all of Hesse's novels. The reader interested in gaining a "feel" for Jungian philosophy and symbolism in an enjoyable way is encouraged to read Hesse's works. It should be noted that Hesse and Jung were contemporaries in Europe, and Hesse was at one time in analysis with Jung.

2. Since this publication, the terms "sensory motor" and "sensory integration" are terms currently used. In this text we refer to sensory-motor-integration.

3. While all health professions are becoming more aware of the ability of the physical body, i.e., brain and chemical hormones to influence a person's ability to think and feel, and conversely, of feelings, i.e., anger, and sadness to influence physical well-being, it is not nearly so clear how the two interrelate. Meltzer (1979, p. 114) in his discussion of schizophrenia refers to the as yet unresolved "critical issue of identifying the interaction between psychological and social factors which may contribute to the pathogenesis of cerebral dysfunction as well as be their consequence."

4. There remains in the authors' mind, the question of what to do regarding individuals who exhibit scattered, higher cognitive skills, such as those reflected in verbalization. While a two year old has never been capable of adult behavior, an adult now demonstrating a predominantly lower level of cognitive function may have integrated many adult experiences, memories, and behaviors into his learning repertoire. Are all of these forgotten, or unavailable? What kind of internal cognitive or emotional dissonance may be created when these are ignored?

5. The description of these six stages of moral development and the development of social reasoning represents a summary of the work of Kohlberg, as cited in the bibliography, plus, the work of Wilcox (1979). Since it is based on the writing and proposals of Kohlberg, the reader should be aware of some of the more recent views regarding Kohlberg's stage theory.

In the current literature (see especially Kohlberg, Levine, and Hewer, 1983; and Kohlberg, 1983) it is proposed that while stages one through five may represent "hard," empirically definable changes in moral reasoning, there exist also "soft stages" of adult development. These stages cannot be formalized or proven empirically, but involve the increasing ability of the adult to reflect upon and integrate ideas of metaphysics, religion, love, justice, and those related to the understanding of the nature of reality. Among these is hypothesized a seventh stage, which describes the further development of an ethical and religious perspective. Since Kohlberg acknowledges that reasoning by Stage 6 has not been empirically defined (Kohlberg, Levine, and Hewer, 1983, p. 8) one might question if Stage 6 also belongs to the category of soft stage.

6. The reader is advised of two additional areas of controversy:

(a) Kohlberg's contention that once the person has achieved a higher level of moral function he will not abandon it for a lower one has been challenged by Henry (1983, pp. 1-19),

Locke (1979), and Kohlberg himself. As stated by Henry, " . . .in practice, people are not fully consistent, and do maintain a range of views representing different 'stages'" (Henry, 1983, p. 11).

(b) Gilligan (1982) suggests that Kohlberg's theses regarding moral development are more valid for and more descriptive of male than female experiences and therefore are biased against women. Gilligan states that to understand morality, one must look at not only the morality of justice (as stressed by Piaget and Freud), but also the ethics of "care and response which is more central to understanding female moral judgment" (Kohlberg, Levine, and Hewer, 1983).

Kohlberg (Kohlberg, Levine, and Hewer, 1983) does not refute Gilligan's contention that ethics related to caring need to be viewed as a part of the greater morality of justice, but does refute her claim that standard Kohlbergian moral dilemmas and test scoring systems have an inherent biased down-scoring of female reasoning (Kohlberg, Levine, and Hewer, 1983, pp. 121-141).

7. King cites the categories discussed by Sullivan (1947) regarding schizophrenia. The *process schizophrenic* is the individual who beginning in childhood gradually became increasingly "different," eventually to require treatment. This is in contrast to the *reactive schizophrenic*, who has functioned at least marginally adequately, until a breakdown occurred during a period of recognizable stress. The process schizophrenic tends not to respond well to treatment, and comprises a large part of the chronic patient population (King, 1974, p. 531).

8. An exception would be Allen's correlation of diagnostic categories with function.

9. This same situation may also be viewed in behavioral terms as an overreliance on external, behavioral reward, or a failure to generalize learning.

10. The interested reader might wish to contrast these two approaches to anorexia with the cognitive-behavior approach of Giles (*American Journal of Occupational Therapy*, 1985).

11. Pharmacology has a long history in mental health treatment, and may indeed offer increased hope for psychiatric patients in the future. That it is not a magic cure is evidenced by the large number of long-standing patients who continue to require care. The position we found most often presented in medical literature and most consistent with our experience is that medication, when successful, helps reduce psychotic thinking and alleviates severe symptoms, but that it is not the end-all in treatment. Rather, individuals with chronic or recurring psychiatric problems have a need to adjust to social, occupational, and emotional demands; and tend to lack the skills or confidence to do so. Skill building is seen as an important element in shortening the length of inpatient treatment, and helping to avoid unnecessary future hospitalizations. This is especially significant with those patients identified as schizophrenic. But, even with the bipolar, affective disorders known to be highly responsive to lithium or a similar derivative, it has not been the authors experience that once the acute episodes of psychotic thinking cleared, the individuals necessarily felt ready to go home and resume their lives as before.

12. The *New Games Book*, edited by Andrew Fluegelman (1976), is a frequent reference for noncompetitive play.

13. We are aware that in Mosey's discussion of developmental treatment (Mosey, 1970) she describes the judicious application of positive and negative reinforcement by the therapist. However, we do not find this aspect of behavioral therapy to be consistent with the basic tenets of developmental theory.

References

Allen C: Independence through activity: The practice of occupation therapy (psychiatry). AJOT 36: 731-739, 1982.

Allen C: Occupational Therapy for Psychiatric Diseases: Measurement and Management of Cognitive Disabilities. Boston, Little Brown and Company, 1985.

Aslanian C, Brickell H: Americans in Transition: Life Changes as Reasons for Adult Learning. New York, College Entrance Examination Board, 1980.

Ayres J: Sensory Integration and Learning Disorders. Los Angeles, Western Psychological Services, 1973.

Baily D: The effects of vestibular stimulation on verbalization in chronic schizophrenics. AJOT 32(7): 445-450, 1978.

Beck M, Callahan D: Impact of institutionalization on the posture of chronic schizophrenic patients. AJOT 34(5): 332-335, 1980.

Blakeney A, Strickland R, Wilkinson J: Exploring sensory integrative dysfunction in process schizophrenia. AJOT 37(6): 399-406, 1983.

Briggs A, Duncombe L, Howe M, Schwartzberg S: Case Simulations in Psychosocial Occupational Therapy. Philadelphia, F. A. Davis Company, 1979.

Buhler C: The curves of life as studies in biographies. J Appl Psychol 19: 405-409, 1953.

Buhler C: Meaningful living in the mature years. In Leemeir RW (Ed): Aging and Leisure. New York, Oxford University Press, 1961.

Buhler C: Genetic aspects of the self. Ann NY Acad Sci 96: 730-764, 1962.

Buhler C: The developmental structure of goal setting in group and individual studies. In Buhler C, et. al. (Eds.): The Course of Human Life. New York, Springer, 1968.

Campbell J: (Ed): The Portable Jung. Hull RCF (trans). New York, Viking Press, Incorporated, Penguin Books, Incorporated, 1971.

Cantor S: Occupational therapists as members of pre-retirement resource teams. AJOT 35(10):638-643, 1981.

Chickering A, Havighurst R: The life cycle. In Chickering AW (Ed). The Modern American College. San Francisco, Jossey-Bass, Incorporated, Publishers, 1981.

Cutler Lewis, S: The Mature Years: A Geriatric Occupational Therapy Text. Thorofare, NJ, Slack, Incorporated, 1979.

Danish S, D'Augelli A, Ginsberg M: Life development intervention: Promotion of mental health through the development of competence. In Brown SD, Lent RW: Handbook of Counseling Psychology, 1984.

Endler P, Eimon M: Postural and reflex integration in schizophrenic patients. AJOT 32(7): 456-459, 1978.

Eimon M, Eimon P, Cermak S: Performance of schizophrenic patients on a motor-free visual perception test. AJOT 37(5): 327-332, 1983

Erikson E: Childhood and Society. New York, W.W. Norton, and Company, Incorporated, 1950.

Erikson E: Identity and the Life Cycle: A monograph: Vol. 1, 1959, pp 1-171, New York, International Universities Press. Psychological Issues.

Erikson E: Identity, Youth and Crisis. New York, W.W. Norton, and Company, Incorporated, 1968.

Farrell M, Rosenburg S: Men at Midlife. Boston, Auburn House, 1981.

Fiorentino M: Reflex Testing Methods for Evaluating C.N.S. Development. Springfield, IL, Charles C. Thomas Publisher, 1965.

Fluegelman A (Ed): The New Games Book. Garden City, NY, Headlands Press Book, Doubleday and Company, Incorporated, 1976.

Giles G: Anorexia nervosa and bulimia: An activity-oriented approach. AJOT 39(8): 510-517, 1985.

Gilfoyle E, Grady A, Moore J: Children Adapt. Thorofare, NJ, Charles B. Slack, Incorporated, 1981.

Gilligan C: In a Different Voice — Psychological Theory and Women's Development. Cambridge, MA, Harvard University Press, 1982.

Gould R: The Phases of Adult Life: A Study in Developmental Psychology. Am J Psychiatry 5: 521-531, 1972.

Gould R: Adult Life Stages: Growth Toward Self-Tolerance. Psychology Today. February:26-29, 1975.

Gould R: Transformations. New York, Simon and Schuster, 1978.

Havighurst R: Developmental Tasks and Education. New York, David McKay Company, Incorporated, 1972.

Hemphill B: The Evaluative Process in Psychiatric Occupational Therapy, Thorofare, NJ, Slack, Incorporated, 1982.

Henry R: The psychodynamic foundations of morality. In Meacham JA (series ed): Contributions to Human Development. Basel, S. Karger, 1983, vol 7.

Hesse H: Siddhartha. New York, Bantam Books, Incorporated, 1977.

Huddleston C: Differentiation between process and reactive schizophrenia based on vestibular reactivity, grasp strength and posture. AJOT 32(6):438-445, 1978.

Jung C: Memories, Dreams, Reflections, Jaffe A.R. (record-ed), and C. Winston (trans). New York, Pantheon Books, 1963.

Jung C: Man and His Symbols. New York, Doubleday and Comapany, Incorporated, 1964.

Jung C: The Stages of Life. In Modern Man in Search of a Soul. New York, A Harvest/HBJ Book, Harcourt Brace Jovanovich, 1933.

King L: A sensory integrative approach to schizophrenia. AJOT 28(9):529-536, 1974(a).

King L: Information from author's notes taken during a workshop on sensory-integration, given by Ms. King at Colorado State University (Ft. Collins, CO), May 19, 1974 (b).

Kohlberg L: Development of moral character and moral ideology. In Hoffman ML, Hoffman LW: Review of Child Development Research, vol.1. New York, Russell Sage Foundation, 1964.

Kohlberg L: Stage and sequence: The developmental approach to socialization. In Hoffman ML: Symp: Moral Character and Moral Processes. Chicago, Aldine Publishing Comapny, Incorporated, 1969.

Kohlberg L: From is to ought. How to commit the naturalistic fallacy and get away with it in the study of moral development. In Mischel T (Ed): Cognitive Development and Epistemology. New York, Academic Press, Incorporated, 1971.

Kohlberg L: Stages and aging in moral development: Some speculations. Gerontologist 13: 497-502, 1973.

Kohlberg L: Moral stages and moralization: The cognitive-developmental approach. In Lickona T: Moral Development and Behavior: Theory, Research and Social Issues. New York, Holt, Rinehart and Winston, Incorporated, 1976.

Kohlberg L: Essays in Moral Development. Vol. I.: The Philosophy of Moral Development. New York, Harper and Row Publishers Incorporated, 1981.

Kohlberg L: Essays in Moral Development. Vol. II: The Psychology of Moral Development. New York, Harper and Row Publishers Incorporated, 1983.

Kohlberg L, Levine C, Hewer A: Moral stages: A Current Formulation and Response to Critics. Vol. 10: Contributions to Human Development. Veacham J (series ed): Basel, S. Karger, 1983.

Levinson D: The Seasons of A Man's Life. New York, Ballantine Books, Incorporated, 1978.

Leva L: Cognitive-behavioral therapy in the light of Piagetian theory. In Reda M, Mahoney M: Cognitive Psychotherapies. Cambridge, MA, Ballinger Publishing Company, 1984.

Levy L: Movement Therapy for Psychiatric Patients. AJOT 28(6): 1974, pp 354-357.

Llorens L: An evaluation procedure for children six-ten years of age. AJOT 21(2):64-69, 1967.

Llorens, L: Application of a Developmental Theory for Health and Rehabilitation. Rockville, MD, American Occupational Therapy Association, 1976.

Locke D: Cognitive Stages or Developmental Phases. A Critique of Kohlberg's Stage-Structural Theory of Moral Reasoning. J Moral Educ 8: 168-181, 1979.

Meltzer L: Biochemical studies in schizophrenia. In Bellak L (Ed): Disorders of the Schizophrenic Syndrome. New York, Basic Books, Incorporated, 1979.

Moore J: Concepts from the Neurobehavioral Sciences. Dubuque, Iowa, Kendall/ Hunt Publishing Company, 1973.

Mosey A: Three Frames of Reference in Mental Health. Thorofare, NJ, Slack, Incorporated, 1970.

Mosey A: Recapitulation of Ontogenesis. AJOT 22(5):426-438, 1968.

Mounoud P: Revolutionary periods in early development. In Bever T (Ed): Regressions in Mental Development: Basic Phenomena and Theories. Hillsdale, NJ, Lawrence Earlbaum Associates, 1982, pp 119-131.

Neugarten B and associates. Personality in Middle and Late Life. New York, Atherton Press, 1964.

Neugarten B: Continuities and discontinuities of psychological issues into adult life. Hum Dev 12:121-130, 1969.

Neugarten B: Time, age and the life cycle. Am J Psychiatry 136(7): 887-894, 1979.

Newman BM and Newman PR: Development Through Life: A Psychosocial Approach. Homewood, IL, 1979.

Piaget J: The Origins of Intelligence in Children. New York, International Universities Press, 1952.

Piaget J: Logic and Psychology. New York, Basic Books, Incorporated, 1957.

Piaget J: Play, Dreams and Imitation in Childhood. Gattegno C, Hodgsen F (trans). New York, W.W. Norton and Company, 1962.

Piaget J: The Psychology of Intelligence. Patterson, NJ, Littlefield, Adams and Company, 1963.

Piaget J: The Child and Reality. Arnold Rosin (trans). New York, Grossman Publishers, 1973.

Reed K: Models of Practice in Occupational Therapy. Baltimore, Williams and Wilkins Company, 1984.

Rider B: Sensorimotor treatment of chronic schizophrenics. AJOT 32(7): 451-455, 1978.

Rodgers R: Theories of adult development: Research status and counseling implication. In Brown SD and Lent RW: Handbook of Counseling Psychology. New York, John Wiley Sons Incorporated, 1984.

Ross M, Burdick D: Sensory Integration. Thorofare, NJ: Slack, Incorporated, 1981.

Sheehy G: Passages. New York, E.P. Dutton, 1976.

Sullivan H: The Conceptions of Modern Psychiatry. Washington, DC, William Allen White Psychiatric Foundation, 1947.

Vaillant G: Theoretical hierarchy of adaptive ego mechanisms. Arch Gen Psychiatry 24:107-118, 1971.

Vaillant G: Adaptation to Life. Boston, Little Brown and Company, 1977.

Wadsworth B: Piaget's Theory of Cognitive Development. New York, David McKay Company, Incorporated, 1971.

Wilcox M: Developmental Journey. Nashville, Abingdon Press, 1979.

Zemke R, Gratz R: The role of theory: Erikson and occupational therapy. Occupational Therapy in Mental Health 2(3): 45-63, 1982.

Additional Readings

Bruner J: Toward A Theory of Instruction. New York, W.W. Norton and Company Incorporated, 1966.

Bruner J, Olver R, Greenfield P, et al. Studies in Cognitive Growth. New York, John Wiley and Sons Incorporated, 1966, chap 10.

Fowler JW: Stages of Faith. The Psychology of Human Development and the Quest for Meaning. San Francisco, Harper and Row Publishers Incorporated, 1981.

Perry W: Forms of Intellectual and Ethical Development in the College Years — A Scheme. New York, Holt Rinehart and Winston Incorporated, 1970.

Rest J: New approaches in the assessment of moral judgment. In Lickona T (Ed): Moral Development and Behavior. New York, Holt Rinehart and Winston Incorporated, 1976.

Rest J: Development in Judging Moral Issues. Minneapolis, University of Minnesota Press, 1979.

Selman R: Taking another's perspective: Role-taking development in early childhood. Child Dev 42:1721-1734, 1971.

Selman R: Social-cognitive understanding: A guide to educational and clinical practice. In Lickona T (Ed): Moral Development and Behavior:Theory, Research and Social Issues. New York, Holt Rinehart and Winston Incorporated, 1976.

Chapter 8

Occupational Behavior Frame of Reference

A movement developed during the late 1960s and throughout the 1970s to endorse the original philosophical base of the profession, and one result in the 1980s was the emergence of the occupational behavior frame of reference. The authors view this frame of reference as an emerging one, still in the process of development. It is summarized here to acknowledge the frame of reference as part of the existing body of knowledge in occupational therapy and to identify its present state of development.

Definition

Occupational behavior is described as a generic frame of reference for occupational therapy (see end note 1) (Rogers in Kielhofner, 1983, p. 95; Reed, 1984, p. 97), which is drawn upon the principles of general systems theory, the philosophical basis of the profession as elucidated by Meyer (1922/1977) and Slagle (1933) and the expansion of the occupational behavior principles posed by Reilly (1969, 1974). The occupational behavior frame of reference views man as an open system that changes and functions dynamically through a circular process of *input, throughput, output,* and *feedback* (see end note 2). This system (man) emphasizes, achieves and maintains a state of health through the balance of work, play, and self-care activities (collectively known as occupation). Occupation, an inherent need, promotes the effective use of time, assists in the fulfillment of life's roles, and facilitates man's competent function in and adaptation to his environment.

The theorists contributing to this frame of reference and in the literature emphasize that this framework can meet the challenges of physical and psychosocial dysfunction, as well as meet the needs of individuals of all ages. Some emphasis is given to its suitability for those considered chronically disabled. (Rogers in Kielhofner, 1983, pp. 95-96; Barris, Kielhofner, Watts, 1983, p.279; Matsutsuyu in Hopkins and Smith, 1983, p. 130.)

Theoretical Development

In 1966, the term "occupational behavior" was used by Reilly in a discussion of psychiatric occupational therapy. This discussion was based upon the work of Meyer and Slagle who expressed their belief in the need for a balance of work, play, rest, and sleep occupations. Three years later, in 1969, Reilly outlined a theoretical framework of occupational behavior (Reed, 1984, p. 97). This framework served as the foundation for the curriculum at the University of Southern California and acted as the focus of research for its graduate program. The goal of the framework was to build an open theoretical system that could respond to changes in the medical and behavioral sciences. Reilly suggested that we "not turn our backs on medicine" but make a "distinction between the tasks of medicine and the tasks of occupational therapy" (Reilly, 1969, p. 300).

Throughout the 1970s, Reilly's framework was studied by graduate students and some clinicians, and further developed by Reilly. These studies of graduates and clinicians, and the work of Reilly, resulted in a text edited by Reilly, titled *Play as Exploratory Learning* (1974).

Reilly's work served as the foundation for the occupational behavior frame of reference that emerged in the 1980s. Her work is amplified and in some cases modified and represented in numerous articles that identify the theoretical principles of occupational behavior and propose or exemplify its application in practice. Among the contributors to the occupational behavior literature are: Rogers (J), Shannon, Barris, Watts, Burke, Bloomer, Takata, Heard, Webster, Kielhofner, Pezzuti, Mack, Matsutsuyu, Florey, Lindquist, Parham, Moorehead, and Gregory.

In 1983, two textbook publications that presented the occupational behavior frame of reference became available: *Health Through Occupation: Theory and Practice in Occupational Therapy*, edited by Kielhofner (1983), and *Psychosocial Occupational Therapy — Practice in a Pluralistic Arena*, co-authored by Barris, Kielhofner, and Watts (1983).

In the edited text, Kielhofner supports the suggestion made by Shannon (1977) and others that the occupational therapy profession adopt one *paradigm* for the profession that would serve all areas of practice, rather than continue to support multiple frames of reference, which he believes promote specialization and could fragment practice. According to Kuhn, a paradigm is a structure which defines the values and beliefs shared by the members of a profession (Shannon, 1977, p. 230) (see end note 3). Kielhofner states that a single paradigm would allow the occupational therapist to keep and reorganize the profession's body of knowledge and "view it in a new light." The paradigm could also give continuity to current theory and practice, and maintain traditional principles (Kielhofner, in Kielhofner (Ed), 1983, p. 56). Occupational behavior as a basis for a professional paradigm is supported also by Rogers (in Kielhofner (Ed), 1983, p. 95), and Reilly (1971), to whom Rogers refers. In the literature this use of the term "paradigm" evolved to the description of occupational behavior as a "frame of reference" or "model" of human occupation. With this change in terminology came some changes in the direction taken by occupational behavior's proponents.

Kielhofner proposes that the occupational therapy profession adopt a paradigm (and frame of reference) that is based upon general systems theory. In *general systems theory,* one attempts to organize all phenomena (human or nonhuman) according to its nature and complexity in order to establish how all phenomena interrelate. It is a holistic concept in so far as it is believed that a single phenomenon cannot be understood in isolation, or apart from its relationship to all other phenomena. Kielhofner proposes using Boulding's hierarchical levels as the means for organizing occupational therapy knowledge. Boulding's hierarchical levels include frameworks, clockworks, cybernetics, open systems, differentiated systems, iconic systems, and social systems. (The reader is referred to Kielhofner in Kielhofner (Ed), 1983, pp. 60-66, for an elaboration of this hierarchy.)

The concept of a general systems approach, and especially the workings of an open system, were adopted for use in occupational behavior. As evidenced in the co-authored text, *Psychosocial Occupational Therapy — Practice in a Pluralistic Arena* (1983), the goal of organizing occupational therapy's body of knowledge begins with the critique and selection of knowledge. According to Rogers, "While the process of knowledge development is eclectic, or draws from many sources, it is also highly selective. Knowledge entering the occupational behavior framework is filtered for its direct relevance to human occupation (Rogers, in Kielhofner (Ed), 1983, p. 115). In *Psychosocial Occupational Therapy—Practice in a Pluralistic Arena,* much of the profession's body of knowledge in psychosocial practice is either bypassed, minimized, or negated in terms of its relevance to this emerging framework, rather than acknowledged for its contribution to the understanding of human occupation. In accordance, Barris, Kielhofner, and Watts suggest limiting the practice of psychosocial occupational therapy to practice within an occupational behavior frame of reference. This limitation is justified by Barris, Kielhofner, and Watts in their text when they state, ". . . it is not only not confining to set limits on the scope of practice, but it can serve to strengthen and ensure the professional survival of the field" (Barris, Kielhofner, and Watts, 1983, p. 314). Thus, one sees a shift in emphasis from occupational behavior as a paradigm, or means to organize existing knowledge, to its function as a frame of reference, from which guiding assumptions will organize practice.

The knowledgeable reader will recognize in the theoretical constructs and principles of application of the occupational behavior frame of reference social and role theory; behavioral, humanistic-existential, and developmental principles; and, as will be pointed out further on in the chapter, there is also a significant influence of Neo-Freudian "ego-psychology," in addition to what may be an influence from Murray's theory of personality.

The occupational behavior literature frequently refers to articles from the *American Journal of Occupational Therapy* or to unpublished master's theses. In some cases it becomes difficult to identify the origination of some of the data presented. However, some of the consistent citings in occupational behavior are from the following: Boulding and von

Bertelanffy, in the area of systems theory; RW White, in the areas of competence, adaptation and motivation; Ginzberg, in the area of occupational choice; Smith, in the area of role competence and socialization; Bruner, in the area of play skills and coping; and Kuhn, as noted regarding paradigm building. Additionally, there are multiple references to Erikson, Havighurst, and Piaget. The consistent occupational therapy citations are from Meyer, Slagle, and Reilly.

While doing the theoretical search, the authors encountered numerous articles that note the application of occupational behavior theory. Occupational behavior theory has been applied with the developmentally delayed, (Webster, 1980; Kielhofner and Takata, 1980; Kielhofner, 1979), in psychiatric assessment, (Oakley, Kielhofner, and Barris, 1985; Neville, 1980; Cubie and Kaplan, 1982; Florey and Michelman, 1982; Bloomer, 1982), in pediatric practice, (Takata, 1980; Mack, Lindquist, and Parham, 1982; Kielhofner, Barris, Bauer, Shoestock, and Walker, 1983), with adolescents (Pezzuti, 1979), with the older adult retiree, (Gregory, 1983), in hospice care (Tigges and Sherman, 1983), and for pain management (Gusich, 1984).

It should be noted that the occupational behavior literature often cites the work of Clark (1979) in which she focuses on human development through occupation (HDTO). In her articles, Clark analyzes theoretical frameworks and proposes the integration of these frameworks within general systems theory to form the framework of human development through occupation (HDTO). The theoretical works investigated are those of Fidler, Mosey, Wilbarger, Llorens, and Reilly, and are depicted in Table 8-1. Clark's work is the most vivid attempt to incorporate the existing body of occupational therapy knowledge into a contemporary framework that uses systems theory and that integrates some of the multiple theoretical views that exist in occupational therapy. The reader should be aware that Clark's "Development Through Human Occupation" and the "Occupational Behavior Frame of Reference" (and its use of the term "model of human occupation") represent two separate frameworks and are not synonymous terms.

An effort to integrate occupational behavior principles and another body of knowledge in occupational therapy is made in 1982 in the work of Mack, Lindquist, and Parham. In their synthesis of occupational behavior and sensory integration theories, which is published as a two part series of articles in the *American Journal of Occupational Therapy*, Mack, et al. note the compatibility of the two frames of reference as well as some differences. The commonalities they recognize are in the use of a developmental perspective, the use of play to facilitate adaptive behavior, and the goal of competence in life tasks. The differences they see are in the underlying concepts, the assessment and treatment procedures, and the emphasis in research (Mack, Lindquist, and Parham, 1982).

Current Practice in Occupational Therapy

In presenting the occupational behavior frame of reference as it is applied in current practice, the authors were confronted with multiple or brief definitions of terms, theoretical assumptions, concepts, and principles. Thus, the material presented is derived from multiple

Table 8-1

Analysis of Four Theoretical Frameworks for Occupational Therapy

| Theory | Art of Occupational Therapy | | | | Science of Occupational Therapy |
	Focus of Intervention	State of Function	State of Dysfunction	Actions	Research Validation
Adaptive Performance	Adaptive skills of doing Self-care Intrinsic gratification Service to others	Balance between skills and subskills Promotes competence and efficacy	Imbalance due to influence of internal processes or external environment causes subskill deficits and problems of doing	Identify levels of functions in skills and subskills Provide shared learning experiences in life-work situations Promote subskill development	Descriptive Analytical Criterion-referenced measurements program plans
Biodevelopment	Developmental sequence of human biological processes	Integrative use of biological processes Promotes adaptive skills Conceptualization Manipulation Socialization	Impairment of ability to process and act upon information received from the environment	Identify process deficits Use developmentally sequenced sensory motor activities, special techniques and equipment to normalize biological processes	

Table 8-1 (con't)

Analysis of Four Theoretical Frameworks for Occupational Therapy

Theory	Art of Occupational Therapy				Science of Occupational Therapy
	Focus of Intervention	State of Function	State of Dysfunction	Actions	Research Validation
Facilitating Growth and Development	Physical, social, and psychological parameters of human life roles, tasks, and relationships	Mastery of tasks and relationships necessary to engage in life roles	Stress, trauma, or disease affect performance or achievement of necessary behaviors	Role of change agent Controlled use of purposeful activity to stimulate role behaviors Developmental analysis of problems	Quasi-experimental Descriptive/Analytical Criterion-referenced measurements Standardized measurements Program plans Program modalities
	Acquisition and performance of work and play behaviors	Self-directed achievement of role requirements	Internal and/or external forces impair capacity for participation and adaptation	Promote exploration and competency of role requirements through identification and development of functions, habits, skills, and task performance	Descriptive/Analytical Criterion-referenced measurements Program plans

Reprinted with permission from Nuse Clark, P. Human development through occupation: Theoretical Frameworks in Contemporary Occupational Therapy Practice, Part 1 *AJOT* 33(8):509, 1979.

sources to provide a basis for a discussion of current practice. The discussion may appear as a collage of ideas without clear boundaries that can be seen and interpreted from multiple perspectives.

The Person and Behavior

Based upon Kielhofner's application of Boulding's hierarchical schema from general systems theory, the patient is seen as an open system. An open system with its constituent subsystems is the self maintained by a dynamic (cybernetic) process of input, throughput, output, and feedback. When the system functions competently, "order" exists, the patient initiates activity out of his need to explore, displays competent skills in fulfilling life roles, adapts to his environment and feels in control of his life situation (Kielhofner, 1983).

The Person As An Open System. The open system functions according to a cybernetic cycle. The cycle begins with *input*, which is information that comes from the environment, or from within the patient. The occupational behaviorist believes that the system is intrinsically motivated. That is, the system grows, changes, and works because of its need to explore and be active. It is not motivated by external rewards. The view of motivation which is based upon the views of Berlyn, White, and DeCharms (see end note 4), is summarized by Burke and Kielhofner. They state that motivation based upon a neurological and intrinsic need to explore and master the environment is compatible with the concept of occupation as conscious, planned, and pleasurable actions which are goal directed and result in "active engagement" (Burke and Kielhofner in Kielhofner (Ed), 1983, pp. 128-129).

Information or "input" enters the system, and is processed by the "throughput" process (which reflects the organization and interrelationships of the subsystems) to produce "output," or the person's occupational behavior. The output or the patient's behavior gives information to the patient, which begins the cycle anew. Thus the system maintains itself through its own action (Fig. 8-1).

Order. When the cycle functions optimally, order exists. *Order* means that the individual "competently performs everyday tasks and behaviors of life and gains satisfaction from his performance in work, play and self-care (Barris, Kielhofner, and Watts, 1983, p. 189). Therefore, order is manifested in the system's "output." Order has also been defined as the "ability to engage in a healthy pattern of occupation. . . a balance between inner needs and external requirements" (Barris, Kielhofner, and Watts, 1983, p. 217). When order exists, there is a state of health which is developed, restored, and maintained through an active process of occupation. Health and the promotion of health rather than illness, pathology, and dysfunction have priority in occupational behavior theory.

Disorder. Disruption in this cybernetic cycle is considered disorder. *Disorder* is defined as "order not existing" or the lack of order which is the "ability to engage in a healthy pattern of occupational behavior." Disorder exists when the person fails to explore and master his environment, and when he does not meet daily expectations of society (Barris, Kielhofner, and Watts, 1983, p. 217).

Disorder may also be referred to as occupational role dysfunction, "insufficient rules,

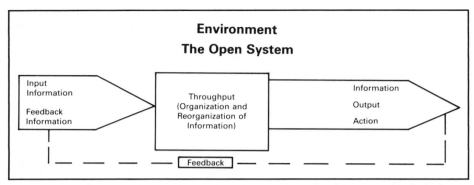

Figure 8-1. Occupational Behavior. Reproduced with permission from Kielhofner, G and Burke, J: "A Model of Human Occupation," part 1. *American Journal of Occupational Therapy,* 34(9):575, 1980.

skills and habits that contribute to role performance (Rogers in Kielhofner, (Ed), 1983, p. 107); or as problems in daily living (Kielhofner, (Ed), 1983).

A Classification System for Disorder. Medical or psychiatric diagnoses are believed to give little information about occupational disorder. In lieu of such diagnostic categories, the proponents of occupational behavior classify disorder according to the following:

1. Open system dysfunction — The basic cycle is interrupted; output shows extremes in activity or inactivity;
2. Disruption of intrinsic motivation — Decreased interest and involvement in occupation which results in a sense of failure, self-doubt, and efficacy and an increased sense of being controlled, which leads to a lack of meaning;
3. Dysfunction of decision making capacity — Decreased interests, interest and value conflicts, and a sense of meaninglessness, which causes stress, despair, decreased performance and diminished satisfaction in occupation and vocational experiences;
4. Role dysfunction — Loss or change in role, or role stress that results in decreased need satisfaction, lack of skill, poor time management, or inability to meet social expectations;
5. Temporal dysfunction — Poor perception and conception of time, a decreased sense of future; being "stuck in time" and exhibiting poor management of time;
6. Disorder in environmental interactions — Conflict between the patient's ability and environmental expectations. The impact of institutionalization and its support of learned helplessness, with the lack of opportunity for occupation and the lessened control over one's life also causes disorder; and
7. Disorder of performance components — Lack of social skills and process skills, poor problem solving and planning, inability to anticipate consequences, poor organization, inability to sequence behavior, and poor perceptual-motor skills (Barris, Kielhofner, and Watts, 1983 pp. 218-226).

Occupational Behavior. The state of order or disorder is evident in the patient's occupational behavior. When viewed collectively, work, play, and self-care are titled occupational behavior or occupational performance (Barris, Kielhofner, and Watts, 1983, p. 189). In the occupational therapy literature and even in that which discusses theory, "occupation," "occupational performance," and "occupational behavior" seem to be used interchangeably, but with variation in definition and interpretation. Occupation may refer to the way in which a person occupies time, one's career, one's adaptive behavior, or purposeful activity. In the edited text of Kielhofner (1983) occupation is defined as follows:

Occupation is "behavior which is motivated by an intrinsic, conscious urge to be effective in the environment in order to enact a variety of individually interpreted roles that are shaped by cultural tradition and learned through the process of socialization" (Burke and Kielhofner, in Kielhofner (Ed), 1983, p. 136).

Occupation is "culturally defined and organized activity which when performed by a person, engages the person's mind and body in purposeful, meaningful, organized and self-initiated action" (Wolfe, cited by Mailloux, Mack, and Cooper in Kielhofner (Ed), 1983, p. 287).

Some other definitions include:

Occupation is "observably conscious, planned and pleasurable" actions which are goal directed and result in "active engagement" (Burke and Kielhofner in Kielhofner (Ed), 1983, p. 131).

Occupational behavior is "the performance of daily work, play, and self care tasks" (Barris, Kielhofner, and Watts, 1983, p. 298).

Occupational performance — The same as that cited for occupational behavior (Barris, Kielhofner, and Watts, 1983, p. 298).

Occupation . . . "consists of those behaviors with which people fill the majority of their time . . . all forms of work, play and self care are types of occupation" (Barris, Kielhofner, and Watts, 1983, p. 278).

What appears to be the common emphases among these definitions, especially as they are used throughout the cited texts, are the component of consciously motivated action rather than any that might be conceived as unconsciously motivated; an emphasis on observable action as contrasted, for example, with thinking, feeling, or reflecting; and the aspect of organized rather than random activity. There is implied also in the literature the idea that occupation is constructive, or positive, and brings satisfaction to the self. Therefore, activity which brought the self into discredit with others (i.e., intentionally destructive behavior) would presumably not be occupation.

The Subsystems of the Open System. Man as an open system has three subsystems: (1) the volition, (2) habituation, and (3) performance subsystems which are hierarchically ordered and presented here from "highest" to "lowest" order (see end note 5). The three interact to determine how the system functions in the environment, and their interrelationship reflects the throughput of the dynamic cycle. (Oakley, Kielhofner, and Barris, 1985).

The occupational behavior literature does not explain how the subsystems function throughout the life span within the context of work and play. However, the terms that describe the subsystems have been defined and refined and are presented here.

Volition Subsystem. The highest subsystem in the hierarchy is the volition subsystem. *Volition* is the individual's decision to engage in occupation (Oakley, Kielhofner, and Barris, 1985, p. 148). The decision to interact or the motivation to act comes from the internalization of images that have been identified as "personal causation," "valued goals" and "interests" (Oakley, Kielhofner, and Barris, 1985).

Personal causation refers to the individual's belief that he has skills which he can use effectively, that he is personally in control, and that he will succeed in the future in whatever he chooses to do; thus he is capable of achieving competence and maintaining his own "emotional well being" (Oakley, Kielhofner, and Barris, 1985, p. 148).

Values are defined as "the individual's internalized images of what is good, right and desirable to do." The individual's values will reflect society's values, and influence how the individual sets priorities and uses time. The concepts of past, present, and future time, and the use of time is referred to by the occupational behaviorist as *temporal orientation*. Temporal orientation influences the person's ability to set goals. To set goals, the patient must have a concept of the future which depends on adequate temporal orientation (Oakley, Kielhofner, and Barris, 1985, p. 148).

Interests are the "propensity to derive pleasure from objects, people or events." They organize behavior by "prioritizing choices of activity" (Oakley, Kielhofner, and Barris, 1985, p. 148).

Habituation Subsystem. The middle subsystem of the hierarchy is the habituation subsystem. This subsystem is composed of habits and roles which organize, regulate, and maintain behavior in everyday routines to meet socially approved standards, help the individual to pursue his interests and values, and allow the individual to adapt to his environment (Rogers in Kielhofner (Ed), 1983, pp. 100-101).

Habits are "instantaneous automatic choices of action throughout the day. . . that organize temporal behavior to meet societal requirements for competence. . . serve to organize a person's skills into regular sequences and to order them in the context of day and week. . . along with roles they maintain the output or behavior of a person. . . organizing behavior so that it fulfills both the demands of the external environment and the internal needs of the individual. . . they function as collections of performances organized into coherent wholes that serve the larger daily routine" (Barris, Kielhofner, and Watts, 1983, p. 203). Habits are learned through trial and error, and "become patterned through repetition" in a consistent environment. Habits are believed to allow an easy flow of activity. They guide behavior by providing a set of "rules that are 'not conscious processes' and that serve to 'monitor action and make needed adjustments'" (Barris, Kielhofner, and Watts, 1983, p. 204). An habitual activity would be combing one's hair, walking a familiar path, or driving a car.

The concept of roles has been influenced by the social sciences and the work of R. W. White, and cited from introductory sociology and social psychology texts. Since 1969, the concept has been discussed and developed by Heard, Kielhofner, and others. Presently (March, 1985), it is defined as follows:

Role is a "position in society that contains a set of expected responsibilities and privileges" (Black cited in Barris, Kielhofner, and Watts, 1983, p. 198). Roles have an internal and external component. The external one consists of the status given a role by society, and the expectations identified with a role by society. The internalized component is incorporated into an individual's behavior and self-perception, and pertains to how the person experiences and acts on his or her roles (Barris, Kielhofner, and Watts, 1983, p. 198).

The occupational behaviorist believes that there must be a balance of roles; that is, that the individual must have a variety of activities and a sufficient number of roles and activities to fill his time meaningfully. (Barris, Kielhofner, and Watts, p. 199). Other general beliefs regarding roles include:

1. Roles prescribe the use of time;
2. Roles provide the standards for behavior and competence;
3. Roles change over time throughout the life span;
4. Roles are learned through socialization;
5. The history of role performance influences the individual's success in roles; (Barris, Kielhofner, and Watts, 1983).
6. Failure to internalize roles results in maladaptation;
7. Conflict or inconsistency of roles results in maladaptation;
8. Maladaptation can result when there is a conflict between internalized roles and the individual's values, interests, and personal causation (Oakley, Kielhofner, and Barris, 1985, p. 149).

There are three broad classes of roles generally believed to interface: personal-sexual, familial, and occupational. Some occupational behaviorists have identified occupational roles as the primary concern for the occupational therapist in evaluation and treatment (Barris, Kielhofner, and Watts, 1983, p. 201).

A taxonomy of occupational roles is also identified in the literature and is listed as follows:

1. Participant in an organization;
2. Hobbyist/amateur;
3. Friend;
4. Family member;
5. Care giver;
6. Home maintainer;
7. Student;
8. Religious participant;
9. Worker; and
10. Volunteer (Barris, Kielhofner, and Watts, 1983, p. 202).

This taxonomy is presented by Oakley in an unpublished master's thesis; therefore, the influences and possible origination within the social sciences is not easily identified by the reader. Heard's discussion of role theory (1977) and its application in occupational role acquisition identifies Chapple, Meyer, and Reilly as influences in role classification and Linton, Turner, Bruner, Koestler and a social psychology handbook as providing a basis for role theory.

Performance Subsystem. The third subsystem, lowest in the hierarchy, is the performance subsystem which houses the skills responsible for producing action (Rogers in Kielhofner (Ed), 1983, p. 100; Oakley, Kielhofner, and Barris, 1985, p. 148). *Skills*, sometimes referred to as occupational performance components, are "abilities to produce purposeful action in the world" (Oakley, Kielhofner, and Barris, 1985 p. 149). Rather than use Mosey's adaptive skills classification system, Barris, Kielhofner, and Watts propose a new system which they feel relates to occupational function and the occupational therapy domain of concern. The three types of skills identified are perceptual-motor, process, and communication-interaction skills. These three skills each have constituents identified as neurological, musculoskeletal, and symbolic components (see end note 6). Competent behavior exists when the three types of skills are integrated (Barris, Kielhofner, and Watts, 1983, pp. 207-208).

The three skills have been defined as follows:

1. Communication-interaction skills — The skills to interact with others and to engage in "collaborative and competitive activities."
2. Process skills — "Involve planning, problem solving, and similar cognitive performances that organize action in time and space" and which are used to respond to and function in every day life.
3. Perceptual-motor skills — Skills that "range from simple perceptions and movements to complicated tool use abilities" (Barris, Kielhofner, and Watts, 1983, p. 207).

Information is not provided to indicate how these skills and their constituent parts would be used in assessment or treatment, or in the grading of activities.

The Person-Environment Interaction. An important aspect of understanding the person within the occupational behavior framework is to appreciate his interaction within his environment. Environmental variables noted as important are physical space, persons, and tasks: components of which include "press" (see end note 7), population density, types of objects available (see end note 8), and the extent and type of sensory stimuli (Barris, Kielhofner, and Watts, 1983, pp. 204-206).

The person is believed to enter the environment when he is sufficiently aroused by it, when it evokes his interest, and when he perceives it as offering an opportunity to engage in activities that he values.

The Role of the Occupational Therapist

The role of the occupational therapist is identified as an environmental manager, a mutual problem solver, and co-planner. In these roles the therapist uses herself therapeutically, and uses occupations and task oriented groups as therapy. During therapy, she engages the patient in activity to help the patient problem solve, improve his compatibility with his environment, and to elicit, maintain, and restore order to the system (Barris, Kielhofner, and Watts, 1983, pp. 264-265).

The occupational behaviorists' concept of the therapeutic use of self is a broad one which supports the occupational therapist assuming the roles of teacher, supervisor, coach, player, role model, and craftsman (Barris, Kielhofner, and Watts, 1983, p. 276).

As an *environmental manager*, the therapist promotes a healthy atmosphere which will motivate the patient to use his abilities and strengths to develop the skills needed to have a balance of work, leisure, and self-care occupations. The occupational therapist conveys an attitude of respect for the patient, acknowledges his abilities and capabilities, identifies her expectations for his behavior, and communicates that she values work, self-care and leisure activity as ends within themselves and the means to elicit growth, change, and learning. As an environmental manager she might, for example, reduce demands within the environment, increase or decrease structure, or make available increased resources (Barris, Kielhofner, and Watts, 1983, p. 265). She will also try to create a psychosocial climate which communicates her caring and hope. The occupational therapist is identified as an environmental manager in both health and community settings (Barris, Kielhofner, and Watts, 1983).

As a *co-problem solver and co-planner*, the occupational therapist works in three areas of counseling; (1) time management and problem solving, (2) leisure counseling, and (3) occupational choice counseling. In the three areas of counseling, the occupational therapist and the patient mutually identify problems and strengths, set goals and plan courses of intervention, and use tasks that will result in healthy participation (Barris, Kielhofner, and Watts, 1983).

During *time management counseling*, the occupational therapist focuses on the use of time and the patient's view of time. The therapist will help the patient identify the proportion of time spent in work, play, and self-care activities, the patient's satisfaction with his use of time, and the changes that need to occur in present activities and the use of time in order to accomplish future goals (Barris, Kielhofner, and Watts, 1983). Thus, time management is conceived to include both the external adjustments to "societal time clocks" and the internal satisfaction with one's own use of time.

During *leisure counseling*, the patient and occupational therapist identify values and leisure interests, and plan time for leisure interests (Barris, Kielhofner, and Watts, 1983). In some settings, this is an area which has been identified by the therapeutic recreation specialist as his area of expertise.

During occupational choice counseling, the occupational therapist helps the patient to choose activities which will help him fulfill his occupational roles. Occupational choice is a developmental process which follows a progression: (1) fantasy period, (2) tentative period, and (3) realistic period (Barris, Kielhofner, and Watts, 1983, p. 199). During the fantasy period, the young child (or adult engaged in occupational reappraisal) imagines the pleasurable aspect of an occupation. During the tentative period, the older child (or adult further along in his reappraisal) evaluates more realistically the ability of an occupation to meet both his self-interests and values, along with social expectations. During the realistic period, the individual selects an occupational role. As a part of occupational choice counseling, the therapist may use values clarification exercises or skill training or both to help the individual determine and meet his occupational goals (Barris, Kielhofner, and Watts, 1983, pp. 272-273).

The Function of Activities

It is through the "art and science" of occupational therapy that an activity becomes an occupation that promotes health and becomes meaningful to the patient (Barris, Kielhofner, and Watts, 1983, p. 281). Recent occupational behavior literature describes the art and science of occupational therapy as a "competency oriented practice" in which the occupational therapist helps the patient to initiate and complete an activity in order to heighten his sense of accomplishment and control.

The goal is the completion of a culturally and personally acceptable action or end product. The merit of activity lies in the end product not in the activity process. The use of an activity as a "bridge" for the therapeutic relationship (as supported by humanistically-oriented therapy) is believed to "denigrate" the value of occupation (Barris, Kielhofner, and Watts, 1983, p. 276). The use of activities as a means to explore feelings in occupational therapy is described as at odds with goal achievement. As elaborated by Barris, Kielhofner, and Watts (1983) there is "a time and place for everything" (p. 280). In occupational therapy, it is "the time and place for performance where negative feelings are tolerated and controlled while the person works toward the positive feelings of accomplishment, satisfaction, control and self worth." (Barris, Kielhofner, and Watts, 1983, p. 280). The analytic approach is described as the one in which activity is seen as a product of "unconscious and negative" forces; the occupational behavior theorist purports that bringing the patient's attention to his "unconscious" will "risk undermining (his) sense of accomplishment" (Barris, Kielhofner, and Watts, 1983, p. 280) (see end note 9).

In summary, process orientation to activity is viewed generally as incompatible with production or task completion; negative feelings are controlled and (by inference) their clarification or resolution not pursued by the occupational therapist. Product or task orientation is seen as positive for the individual.

Activities are occupations used as therapy and are used in the context of a person's normal routine. Occupations include all forms of work, play, and self- care and must be currently part of the culture (Barris, Kielhofner, and Watts, 1983, p. 278). Specific activities mentioned are play, games, sports, performing arts, arts and crafts, activities of daily living, and work (Barris, Kielhofner, and Watts, 1983, pp. 281-289).

Activities are graded according to developmental principles and generally according to the principle whereby demands in activities match performance abilities (Barris, Kielhofner, and Watts, 1983, p. 267). Graded activities are used to build the patient's ability to exert self-control within his environment, to promote competence in work, play, and self-care, and to provide optimum conditions for adaptive performance (Barris, Kielhofner, and Watts, 1983, p. 267).

The occupational behaviorist may use activities to restore morale, decrease stress, provide habit training, develop roles, increase the individual's sense of accomplishment and control, organize time as a vehicle for social interaction, and as a means for the individual to positively relate to and within the larger culture. Further, activities may be used as a means to correct attention and behavior, and as a means of substitution for nonconstructive use of time (Kielhofner, 1983; Barris, Kielhofner, and Watts, 1983).

Evaluation

As has been previously identified in the profession, the occupational behaviorist identifies two components of the occupational therapy assessment process: screening and evaluation. Screening has been traditionally done through the physician's referral. The occupational behaviorist suggests that the occupational therapist screen for occupational dysfunction or occupational disorder (Barris, Kielhofner, and Watts, 1983, p. 233). This suggestion is based upon the view that not all patients have both medical problems and occupational dysfunction; therefore, the need for services should be identified separately, using different criteria. The occupational behavior literature suggests that this already occurs in school, residential, and community settings (Barris, Kielhofner, and Watts, 1983).

After the need for occupational therapy services has been identified, the occupational therapist assesses occupational disorder, which has been classified into seven categories: (1) open system dysfunction, (2) disruption of intrinsic motivation, (3) dysfunction in decision making, (4) role dysfunction, (5) temporal dysfunction, (6) disorder in environmental interaction, and (7) disorder in performance components (Barris, Kielhofner, and Watts, 1983).

Barris, Kielhofner, and Watts state that there are two aspects of evaluation: (1) the occupational therapist must select the instruments and procedures for identifying the patient's strengths and weaknesses; and (2) the occupational therapist must then organize and interpret the evaluation data using a conceptual framework. The suggested conceptual framework is "logistic and conceptual." The occupational therapist logistically considers her caseload and the scope of the occupational therapy program and patient demographics and treatment history. Conceptually, the occupational therapist considers the nature of the disorder which is reviewed using the case analysis method of Cubie and Kaplan (Barris, Kielhofner, and Watts, 1983, p. 256). The reader is referred to the Occupational Case Analysis Interview and Rating Scale which is briefly summarized in this chapter.

Evaluation Instruments. To assess occupational disorder, the occupational therapist uses tests, interview, observation, and history taking (Barris, Kielhofner, and Watts, 1983). In *Psychosocial Occupational Therapy — Practice in a Pluralistic Arena,* the authors list the assessment instruments identified with occupational behavior based upon their compatibility with the views of order and disorder as defined in the framework (Barris, Kielhofner, and

Watts, 1983, p. 247). Many of the assessments are based upon the work of graduate students in unpublished master's theses. Here, the authors have chosen to list only those which are available in text or juried publications. They include the following:

Bay Area Functional Performance Evaluation (BaFPE). The BaFPE was designed by Judith Bloomer and Susan Williams to assess performance in general activities of daily living. It consists of two subtests: the Task Oriented Assessment (TAO) and the Social Interaction Scale (SIS). The assessment is based upon a functionalist view and the acquisitional (behavioral), occupational behavior, adaptational, and functional restoration frames of reference (Hemphill, 1982, p. 262). Assessment tasks, which include sorting shells, completion of a bank deposit slip, drawing a house floor plan, drawing a person, and completion of a block design, are used to assess the patient's ability to paraphrase, make decisions, and organize. Patient motivation, self-esteem, attention span, and ability to abstract, as well as possible evidence of mood or thought disorder can be determined with the tasks. A comprehensive manual for the administration of the BaFPE is available from Consulting Psychologists Press, Inc., 577 College Ave., Palo Alto, CA 94306 (Bloomer, 1982).

The Occupational Case Analysis Interview and Rating Scale. This case analysis method was developed in 1982 by Cubie and Kaplan. The analysis consists of 14 interview questions, ten of which are derived from the model of human occupation, and four of which give a global assessment of the system. Questions assess personal causation, goals, interests, roles, habits, output, the physical and social environment, and feedback. The global systems analysis seeks to identify the dynamics of the system, its compatibility with the environment, and past, present and future related issues (Cubie and Kaplan, 1982).

The Occupational Role History. The occupational role history is an evaluation designed by Florey and Michelman, and is based upon the occupational behavior frame of reference and Moorehead's work on occupational role. It is used to elicit data based upon the patient's occupational role history, not the patient's diagnosis. During a semistructured, one-half hour interview, 34 questions are used to determine the patient's comfort, satisfaction, and competence in work, homemaker, and school roles; to determine the areas of skill and problems; and to determine the degree of balance between work, chores, and leisure. The interview also elicits demographic data, information regarding the sequence and continued development of occupational roles, and information about the patient's interests and the tasks he does alone or with others which lead to satisfaction or dissatisfaction with his occupational roles. The data is interpreted upon the basis of quality of performance in one's roles over time (Florey and Michelman, 1982).

Developmental Task Level of Adolescent Girls. This is an assessment questionnaire designed by Pezzuti that includes an interest check list, based upon the one originated by Matsutsuyu, and a personal data sheet. The 28 questions are used to assess emotional independence, the existence of a feminine social role, acceptance and use of one's physical image, the ability to select and prepare for an occupation, one's value system, and one's concept and use of time (Pezzuti, 1979).

Inventory of Occupational Choice Skills. This paper and pencil self report was developed by Shannon to assess adolescents who are trying to make an occupational choice. It identifies play, work, and chore activities (Reilly, 1974, pp. 295-301).

Environmental Questionnaire. This is an interview guide designed by Dunning to assess physical, social, and task environments. The guide is based upon the semistructured interview of Berelson and Steiner (1964). It is used to gather data regarding the individual's life space and life style through the identification of the relationships that exist between the patient's behavior and his community, his economic constraints, extrinsic environmental factors, and intrinsic personality factors (i.e., anxiety about change, or broad perspective of change), objects and personal possessions, availability and proximity of social stimulation, others in the social environment, expectations of task outcome, ability to see alternatives, and use of community resources. Dunning notes the limitations of the assessment and suggests its use in conjunction with other instruments that measure task, time, and patient interests, and states that this questionnaire needs refinement in order to be made valid and reliable (Dunning, 1972).

Comprehensive Evaluation of Basic Living Skills (CEBLS). Casanova and Ferber combined several basic living skill evaluations from physical medicine to form the CEBLS. The assessment has three sections: personal care and hygiene, a practical evaluation, and a written evaluation. Each section is rated on a four point scale. The skills assessed include the patient's ability to wash, clothe and groom himself, plan and prepare a meal, use public transportation, use the telephone, read, write, understand time, solve math problems, and manage money (Casanova and Ferber, 1976).

Inventory of Depersonalization and Occupational Skill Loss During Hospitalization. This assessment has been influenced by the work-play model of Reilly, Shannon, and Meyer and developed during the author's graduate work. It identifies the conditions that promote the decreased use of daily living, work-play or occupational skills. The skills assessed include: (1) self-care, (2) motor, (3) social, (4) general work habits, (5) specific work skills, (6) use of time, (7) play, recreation or leisure skills, and (8) decision making (Gray, 1972).

The Interest Check List. This interest check list is a paper and pencil questionnaire usually used in combination with an interview designed by Matsutsuyu to assess the patient's interests, past, present, and future. The categories assessed include: manual skills, physical sports, social recreation, activities of daily living, and cultural/educational interests. In addition to completing the check list, the patient is asked to write a narrative that describes his interests and hobbies, and to identify how he has used his leisure time from "grammar school to the present" (Matsutsuyu, 1969, pp. 326-327).

The Evaluation Process. As the occupational therapist uses the assessment instruments, she trie to identify the following: (1) the patient's pre-onset occupational role; (2) the patient's current occupational role; (3) the clinical status; (4) the relationship between clinic status and role; and (5) the patient's values and expectations regarding recovery of occupational role (Kielhofner, 1983, p. 289).

Throughout the evaluation process, she assesses the adaptive relationship between the patient and his environment, the past role behavior in relation to the present, and the patient's abilities and strengths as well as the problems that impair his capacity to perform in his occupational roles (Barris, Kielhofner, and Watts, 1983).

The Treatment Process

Patients are viewed as having occupational role dysfunction, and treatment is directed toward building or restoring the habits and skills needed to lead to occupational role function and competence, and ultimately a more satisfying quality of life (Kielhofner, 1983; Barris, Kielhofner, and Watts, 1983).

In Pursuit of Competence. Competence and its essential elements are described by Kielhofner and Miyake (1983). *Competence* is relative to one's particular situation in life. It is the ability of the system to interact in the environment, to maintain itself, to grow and to make choices that increase the control one has of one's environment and to see oneself positively. The elements of competence are: the person's abilities, the person's self-assessment, the expectations for performance communicated by the environment, and the available opportunities and resources in the environment (Kielhofner and Miyake, in Kielhofner (Ed), 1983, pp. 260-261).

Mack, Lindquist, and Parham state that competency is critical for adaptation (1982, p. 369). Florey and Michelman use the *Diagnostic and Statistical Manual of Mental Disorders III,* (DSM III), as a guide to define and determine adaptive function. *Adaptive function* according to DSM III is a composite of three major areas: (1) social relations (with emphasis on breadth and quality of interpersonal relationships, especially with family and friends); (2) occupational functioning (the amount, complexity, and quality of work accomplished as a worker, student, or homemaker); and (3) the use of leisure time (range and depth of involvment and pleasure derived from recreation activities and hobbies) (DSM III, 1980, pp. 28-29).

The DSM III discusses, defines, and prioritizes these three areas for the therapist to use when assessing the patient's level of function during the past year. Greater weight is given to social relationships and occupational function. Leisure time is considered only when there is no apparent deficit in social or occupational functioning, or when the opportunity for work is limited or unavailable (DSM III, 1980, p. 28). This weighted guide should be considered as the occupational therapist implements evaluation, plans treatment, and implements treatment strategies.

Goal Setting. Goal setting is a cooperative process between the patient and the therapist. The occupational therapist tries to help the patient learn, use, and internalize the goal setting process. Both short and long term goals are established. Long term goals may include the more "global" objectives of maintaining function and of establishing function in new areas, while short term goals may describe daily or weekly activity (Barris, Kielhofner, and Watts, 1983, p. 234). As with other treatment frameworks, goals are reviewed periodically to establish the efficacy of treatments. Occupational behaviorists indicate it is important that the patient be an active participant in goal setting, and that he be able to recognize his own progress toward the goals he has established.

The Treatment Program. Treatment based upon occupational behavior frame of reference is described as developmentally based treatment (Kielhofner, 1983) and methods which facilitate age appropriate occupations and enhance normal development are used. Normal developmental opportunities are sequenced according to developmental principles. Sequential treatment is used because skill and habit deficiencies at an earlier stage of occupational development are believed to influence development of later roles and their component skills and habits (Kielhofner, 1983). Rogers proposes the following developmental guides for structuring treatment experiences:

1. "A client's interests may be used to engage participation;
2. Play, arts and crafts, games, chores, and educational and cultural activities provide opportunities for self-discovery of values, attitudes, aspirations, and abilities;
3. Play, arts and crafts, games, chores, and educational and cultural activities provide opportunities for decision making;
4. Work and leisure skills may be reprogrammed through play;
5. The teaching of skill begins with a playful phase and proceeds through structured learning and achievement phases;
6. Skills of daily living are learned through repetition;
7. A repetitive environment and skill mastery promote habit formation;
8. Novel tasks evoke new behaviors;
9. An overall sense of success in task performance is needed to promote skill acquisition; and
10. Time management is a skill, and must be practiced to provide balance in work, rest, and leisure roles" (Rogers, in Kielhofner (Ed), 1983, p. 113).

Principles of Hierarchy. Within the treatment environment, the therapist attempts to incorporate or simulate as much as possible the patient's expected environment, postdischarge (Rogers in Kielhofner (Ed), 1983, p. 113). Treatment principles are referred to as principles of restoring order and are listed in Table 8-2. They are considered general strategies for treatment, and not specific recipes for intervention (Barris, Kielhofner, and Watts, 1983, p. 235). The underlying principles that govern these strategies are based upon rules of hierarchy and are identified by Kielhofner, Mailloux, Mack, and Cooper. They are:

1. Treatment should focus on higher levels of the hierarchy because the higher levels mediate changes in the lower systems;
2. The higher levels of the system maintain the system, therefore they maintain change;
3. Lower level functioning affects higher level function;
4. The higher level system can change to compensate for lower level dysfunction; (Kielhofner in Kielhofner (Ed), 1983, p. 85);
5. Graded activities use and adapt the environment to increase output of the system; and
6. Individualized activities increase the meaningfulness of the activity (Mailloux, Mack, and Cooper, in Kielhofner (Ed), 1983, p. 291).

The occupational behavior frame of reference supports the use of play, games, hobbies, chores, work, cultural, and educational activities in a milieu that supports occupation.

Table 8-2

Principles of Restoring Order

Decision Making

Provide opportunity to discover and develop interests.

Facilitate development of new interests and values to correct faulty patterns of occupational behavior.

Foster interests and values consistent with the person's everyday settings.

Enable discovery of values by providing a value system in occupational therapy.

Help people to identify ways to actualize interests, values, and goals in their lives.

Provide opportunity to identify and assess occupational choices and to pursue new choices.

Role

Provide opportunities to enter responsible active and productive roles.

Make expectations for performance clear to facilitate socialization.

Use groups as a context for performing various roles.

Use therapy to precipitate or facilitate role transition as appropriate.

Temporal Adaptation

Provide schedules that replicate time use in the larger culture.

Enable people to acquire the temporal perspective of their settings.

Guide people with maladaptive patterns of time use to identify change needs and to develop schedules of time use.

Provide opportunities to implement and practice new routines (habits) of time use.

Environment

Provide appropriate levels of arousal (challenge).

Opportunities for decision making should be present.

The atmosphere and physical environment must be consistent with expectations for performance.

Understaff settings to evoke performance.

Allow performance in a range of settings to increase flexibility of performance.

Performance Components

Provide skill training relevant to the contexts of daily life.

Follow a developmental sequence in skill training.

Acknowledge roles, interests, and values in choosing skills to be learned.

Consider the symbolic, neurological, and musculoskeletal constituents in regenerating skills (Barris, Kielhofner, and Watts, 1983, p 245-247.

Reproduced with permission from *Psychosocial Occupational Therapy — Practice in a Pluralistic Arena*, RAMSCO Publishing Company, Laurel, MA, 1983.

(Rogers, in Kielhofner (Ed), 1983, p. 109). Occupations which are valued and popular in society should be used in conjunction with activities that are graded and made purposeful to promote an adaptive response between the patient and his environment (Barris, Kielhofner, and Watts, 1983).

The Socialization Process. Occupational therapy provides a socialization process to promote the acquisition of occupational behavior, to improve role function, to promote competent behavior, and facilitate the person-environment adaptative relationship.

Burke and Kielhofner note some of the early views of the socialization process in occupational therapy which suggested (1) that the therapist give explict expectations for behavior; (2) that she communicate the expectation that the patient participate in occupational therapy activities; (3) that there is value in activity; (4) that the patient be allowed to choose activities, but that idleness is not an option; (5) that disability is not an excuse for refusal to participate in activity; (6) that "patients not be allowed to talk about their problems in therapy" (Fuller, 1912); and (7) that treatment occur in a normalized hospital environment in which natural rhythms of time are incorporated to generate habits (Kielhofner and Burke, in Kielhofner (Ed), 1983, p. 21).

Today, the socialization process occurs in an atmosphere which is organized to stimulate the patient's interests, facilitate his exploration, and promote his competence through a structure that matches the patient's abilities. In this atmosphere, the therapist conveys an attitude that values activity and its therapeutic benefits, identifies role expectations and the skills necessary to fulfill these roles, and provides order to develop and regulate habits and temporal adaptation (Barris, Kielhofner, and Watts, 1983). Occupational group experiences (i.e., groups organized around such tasks as play, ADL, and work) are seen as a vital component of occupational behavior therapy, providing a means by which social skills can be enhanced and roles, habits, and skills developed.

Chapter Summary

Before looking at the contributions and limitations of the occupational behavior frame of reference, we will summarize very briefly what we see as its emphases.

Occupational behavior seeks to combine general systems theory with select principles of ego psychology, development, behaviorism and humanism-existentialism, and role theory. While not identifying itself with ego psychology, the frequent references to White and his theories regarding the conscious, intrinsic motivation of the individual to explore and master his environment serve as an important cornerstone of occupational behavior that can be identified as originating in the 1950s and 1960s with ego psychology. Due in part to this emphasis on conscious choice and conscious motivation, the occupational behavior framework deals with the portion of habits, skills, and roles that are deemed to be within the patient's conscious awareness, and does not choose to focus on extrinsic motivation.

One can, however, discern a strong "field" emphasis, with the environment and the person-environment interaction perceived as a significant force in not only sanctioning or discouraging appropriate activity, but in also acting as the arena for role prescription and development, habit development, and skill acquisition. The person cannot be understood apart from his environment; and the therapist actively seeks to modify the treatment environment when necessary to enhance its ability to support successful occupation.

In accordance with general systems theory and principles of cybernetics, the individual is viewed as a self-initiating, self-perpetuating, and self-regulating system that functions according to a four-part cycle of input-throughput-output and feedback. Output (or occupation) is cited as the most critical component, and output is the part of the cycle that is most thoroughly developed in occupational behavior literature.

What constitutes input (both in terms of input as information and the process of information being taken in) is not of primary emphasis. The process of throughput, or the "how" of the cycle, relates to the ability of the volitional, habituation, and performance subsystems to function in accord. The individual must recognize his own values, and be able to make active, meaningful, occupational choices. The background for this, in part, is created by the existence of adequate everyday habits, which allow for ordinary tasks to be accomplished without undue difficulty. There must exist, also, adequate skills related to the multitudinous components of daily life tasks. What constitutes feedback or how it is best given or received is not elaborated. However, feedback in the system is described as a necessary component that both gives the individual information about the success of his performance and helps him make necessary performance adjustments. When anything disrupts the four-part cycle, disorder results. Assessment and remediation, or the restoration of order, is directed toward the "output" or occupational portion of the cycle.

The occupational portion of the cycle is most generally conceived in terms of work, play, or self-care. Throughout his life, the individual must engage in given occupations. The choices he makes in this regard will be determined by environmental sanctions and opportunity in concert with the individual's own values and interests. Understanding his own values and interests can help the individual make satisfying occupational choices. However, it is the demonstrable success within these occupations and not his feelings or understanding that are of primary concern. Occupational accomplishment is believed to bring about a sense of self-worth and to enhance the sense the individual has that he is in charge of his own life.

Helping to organize the individual's participation in occupation are components of temporal orientation. That is, the individual operates within a time schedule that is both environmentally defined and personally or internally held. Proportionately too much or too little time given to selected activities, or a failure to have a solid internalization of a sense of time, diminishes the ability of the individual to engage successfully in occupation.

Occupation, in the broad sense, is organized by means of roles. The individual must be able to function successfully in several roles, must recognize the societal expectations within a role, and must be able to conceive of himself within a role. The roles the individual takes on will depend in part on life-stage changes, societal expectations, and his own values and interests. Roles both shape and are shaped by given occupations. If roles are to be adequately performed, the individual must have an adequate and sound functioning repertoire of habits and skills. When habits and skills are inadequate, role function and occupation are disturbed, output is diminished and disorder ensues.

Treatment is directed to restoring order; order which will be made evident via output or occupation. Treatment principles are general in nature, and directed toward habit and skill building. As the individual perceives his own accomplishments, he becomes increasingly satisfied, senses his own empowerment, and gains confidence in his ability to function within his environment.

Contributions

Occupational behavior theorists have been outspoken in their criticism of much of previous occupational therapy practice, and their negation of knowledge gained through this practice. The result has been the stimulation of controversy and discourse. One outcome may be that more professionals will examine their own values, biases, and beliefs in relation to psychosocial occupational therapy, and as regards changing priorities within the occupational therapy profession.

Occupational behavior proponents have sought to return professional focus to the action aspect of man's being, and have thus returned attention to what is special about occupational therapy within the psychosocial science field. Further, they have provided a conceptual structure by which information can be organized and duplication of services avoided.

Occupational behavior reiterates the basic tenets of occupational therapy that the individual has power within his own domain to achieve purpose and well-being through his active participation on his own behalf. It presents a positive posture, emphasizing what can be, rather than cannot be, accomplished.

Occupational behavior does not require a connotation of ill health to be utilized, and can be viewed as appropriate to medical and nonmedical settings, reactive and proactive courses of treatment, and to understanding changes throughout the individual's life cycle.

The occupational behavior framework has been identified as the most viable option for the chronic populations which are increasingly referred to occupational therapy. In relation to this, occupational behaviorists recognize the existence of practical limitations in what can reasonably be accomplished during the duration of treatment.

Limitations

It is not clear to what extent occupational behavior seeks to function as a paradigm, and to what extent as a frame of reference. As occupational behavior assumptions are crystalizing, they do not appear to be moving in the direction of organizing knowledge that already exists, since a great deal of the profession's knowledge about occupation and man's engagement in activity as provided through the perspective of alternative frames of reference has been negated in the occupational behavior literature. If the information proposed exclusively within occupational behavior parameters is to serve as the foundation of knowledge about man's involvement in activity, the practitioner is left with a great many conceptual and practical gaps.

The terms and assumptions used to describe basic tenets of this framework lack clarity and consistency, and their origin is not always clear, making it difficult for the reader, practitioner, or researcher to orient themselves to the framework and evaluate the assumptions presented.

Theoretical assumptions are scantily developed, and their relationship to each other not made clear. While references to role, environmental press, population density, intrinsic motivation, temporal adaptation, and time management are potential avenues for exploration and new learning for the reader, these concepts are given limited development. Further, it is very difficult to surmise how all of these aspects of the whole system work in concert to bring about meaningful activity.

While it is the prerogative of the theorist to pick and choose among theoretical components, it is necessary that the relationship of theoretical assumptions be precise and consistent.

There appear to be inconsistencies, as for example, when exclusive attention is paid to intrinsic motivation, yet great emphasis is given to the role of external (or environmental) forces in shaping expectations, creating opportunity, and rewarding success. It is not that seeming contradictions are not resolvable, but an important role of the theorist would be to illustrate how seeming contradictions are reconcilable within the broader conceptual structure.

The split created between the activity process and product (with occupational behavior choosing a product-orientation), may, on the one hand, serve to enhance the ability of the occupational behavior approach to demonstrate the value of activity; or may ultimately lessen the opportunity for broadening the patient's (and other's) understanding of how and why occupation can be meaningful and therapeutic. This issue is one of conjecture.

There are many absolutes or dichotomies created in the presentation of occupational behavior tenets. Many assumptions are presented as matters of "black or white." On the one hand, this may, as noted, be provocative and stimulate discussion. On the other, this may "turn off" students or practicing therapists who might otherwise seek to gain knowledge in the area of occupational behavior.

Occupational behavior is a frame of reference that strives to return professional emphasis to the action portion of man's being. As it seeks to assert itself within the broader scope of occupational therapy theory and practice, it has disavowed much of the information gathered via the perspective of alternate theoretical frames. This can be understood as not dissimilar to the path taken in the development of other theoretical frames, as the proponents of each emerging framework struggle to establish the essential veracity and uniqueness of their own perspective. We would, however, echo the sentiments of Hall and Lindzey, who caution against "theoretical imperialism," as they state simply:

"Let the theorist present his theory in the most forceful manner possible but let him respect the fact that there is no such thing as theoretical certainty" (Hall and Lindzey, 1970, p. 599).

Note: The authors are aware of the recently available text edited by Kielhofner in which some of the terms discussed in this chapter have been modified and theoretical concepts further developed. These most recent developments are not reflected in this chapter.

End Notes

1. A "generic" model is one of the three types of models identified by Reed (1984) which gives a broad definition of the concepts which explain the philosophy, values and beliefs of occupational therapy. The broad definitions allow the model to be applied in any of the specialty areas of the profession (Reed, 1984, p. 97).

2. The reader will recognize the terms input, throughput, output, and feedback as deriving from the field of technology, and analogous to the systems function of a computer. The metaphor is established of "man as machine." However, beyond being an open system, man is viewed as also having a symbolic component which allows him to imagine and speculate upon his own process, or to have consciousness. Thus, he becomes more than machine.

3. The reader interested in becoming better acquainted with Kuhn's conceptualization of a paradigm is referred to T.S. Kuhn, *The Structure of Scientific Revolutions*, Chicago: University of Chicago Press (1st. ed. 1962; 2nd. ed. 1970).

4. Berlyne believes that the person engages in activity for its own sake, experiences pleasurable conflict and arousal when he encounters his environment, and will seek activity that meets his interests. See K.E. Berlyne, *Conflict, Arousal and Curiosity*, New York: McGraw-Hill Book Co., 1960.

R.W. White states that the individual has urges for activity of all kinds, and that the ego gains satisfaction from exploration and competence, thereby serving as a motivation for the person to encounter his world. White is described by Hall and Lindzey (1970) as a neo-Freudian "ego psychologist." An ego psychologist does not deny the basic Freudian constructs of id-ego-supergo, but chooses to focus on the autonomy of the ego in its being able to consciously determine avenues of exploration and to gain (for the individual) conscious satisfaction in his own accomplishments (Hall and Lindzey, 1970, p. 63). See R.W. White, "The Urge Towards Competence," *AJOT*, Vol. 25, 1971, p. 271; also R.W. White, "Ego and Reality in Psychoanalytic Theory: A Proposal Regarding Independent Ego Energies," *Psychological Issues* Vol. 3, No. 3, 1963, pp. 1-210.

DeCharms proposes that the individual's primary motivation is to be effective and produce change in the environment. See R. DeCharms, *Personal Causation*, New York: Academic Press, 1968.

5. The basis for organizing these subsystems as higher or lower is not entirely clear. It would seem, however, reasonable to suggest that these subsystems interrelate and have a continual and reciprocal effect on each other, and ultimately must function in relative accord if the open system is to operate properly.

6. In Barris, Kielhofner, and Watts, 1983, one reads that the symbolic "constituents of skills refer to the internal images that coordinate and interpret incoming sensory information;

formulate internal ideas, intentions and plans of action; and trigger and guide nervous system activity. These symbols are internal maps of external reality that inform the individual about the potential for and the constraints on action" (p. 208).

This use of the term symbolic is not to be confused with the object-relations perspective in which one object or action comes to represent another or stand for more than itself; this is a perspective in which symbols may be conscious or unconscious in the individual's awareness.

One is reminded, however, of Tolman's discussion of the internalization of "maps" or images as a part of learning, something he calls "sign learning." See F.C. Tolman's *Purposive Behavior in Animals and Man* which is discussed in end note 2, Chapter 4, "Behavior Frame of Reference," in this text.

7. "Press" refers to "the demands that the environment places on the individual for behavior" (Barris, Kielhofner, and Watts, 1983, p. 206). Although the concept is not developed by these authors, it is reminiscent of the work of Murray, as presented in his personality theory, which he termed "personology." As summarized by Hall and Lindzey, to Murray "press" represented the "effective or significant determinants of behavior in the environment. In simplest terms a press is a property or attribute of an environmental object or person which facilitates or impedes the efforts of the individual to reach a given goal" (Hall and Lindzey, 1970, p. 180).

Thus, the press of an object in the environment relates to how the person perceives that a given aspect of the environment can or cannot meet his needs, and thereby helps determine whether a person will seek out or avoid objects within his environment.

Murray generally ascribed to the Freudian conception of id-ego-superego, and placed importance on unconscious motivation in behavior. The reader may recall that Murray developed the Thematic Apperception Test (TAT), a commonly used projective instrument.

8. Objects are described as connoting "use-expectations" (Barris, Kielhofner, and Watts, 1983, p. 206). This would refer to the conscious and cultural connotations of objects; personally symbolic or unconscious associations are not of concern.

9. It should be noted that the concept of "nonconscious" phenomena is approached in several ways in the occupational behavior literature. Habits are described as "not conscious" organizers of activity that to a positive end organize and promote function and represent a primary concern of the therapist. However, the unconscious emotions related to activity are generally described as negative, and are not the concern of the therapist.

References

American Psychiatric Association: Diagnostic and Statistical Manual of Mental Disorders, (DSM III). Washington, DC, American Psychiatric Association, 1980.

Barris R, Kielhofner G, Watts J: Psychosocial Occupational Therapy — Practice in a Pluralistic Arena. Laurel,Maryland, Ramsco Publishing, 1983.

Berelson B, Steiner G: Human Behavior: An Inventory of Scientific Findings. New York, Harcourt Brace Jovanovich, Incorporated, 1964.

Black M: The adolescent role assessment. AJOT 30(4):73-79, 1976.

Black M: The occupational career. AJOT 30(4): 225-228, 1976.

Bloomer J, Williams S: The Bay Area functional performance evaluation. In Hemphill B: The Evaluative Process in Psychiatric Occupational Therapy. Thorofare, NJ, Slack, Incorporated, 1982, p.255-308.

Brokema M, Danz K, Schloemer C: Occupational therapy in a community aftercare program. AJOT 29(1): 22-27, 1975.

Burke J: A clinical perspective on motivation: Pawn versus origin. AJOT 31(4): 254-258, 1977.

Burke J, Kielhofner G: Defining occupation: Importing and organizing interdisciplinary knowledge. In Kielhofner G (Ed): Health Through Occupation — Theory and Practice in Occupational Therapy. Philadelphia: F.A. Davis, 1983, pp. 125-145.

Casanova J, Ferber J: Comprehensive evaluation of basic living skills. AJOT 30(2): 101-105, 1976.

Clark P: Theoretical frameworks in contemporary occupational therapy practice. Part 1 AJOT 33(8): 505-514, 1979.

Clark P: Human development through occupation: A philosophy and conceptual model for practice. Part 2 AJOT 33(9): 577-585, 1979.

Cubie S, Kaplan K: A case analysis method for the model of human occupation. AJOT 36(10): 645-652, 1982.

Dunning H: Environmental occupational therapy. AJOT 26(6): 292-298, 1972.

Florey L, Michelman S: Occupational role history: A screening tool for psychiatric occupational therapy. AJOT 36(5): 301-308, 1982

Fuller D: The need of instruction for nurses in occupations for the sick. In Tracy S: Studies in Invalid Occupation. Boston, Whitcomb and Barrows, 1912.

Gray M: Effects of hospitalization on work-play behavior. AJOT 26(4): 180-185, 1972

Gregory M: Occupational behavior and life satisfaction among retirees. AJOT 37(8): 548-553, 1983.

Gusich R: Occupational therapy for chronic pain: a clinical application of the model of human occupation. Occupational Therapy in Mental Health 4(3): 59-73, 1984.

Hall K, Lindzey G: Theories of Personality. Ed 2. New York, John Wiley & Sons, Incorporated, 1970.

Heard C: Occupational role acquisition: A perspective on the chronically disabled. AJOT 31(4): 243-247, 1977.

Hemphill B: The Evaluative Process in Psychiatric Occupational Therapy. Thorofare, NJ: Slack, Incorporated, 1982.

Kaplan K: A short-term assessment: The need and a response. Occupational Therapy in Mental Health 4(5): 29-45, 1984.

Kielhofner G: Temporal adaptation: A conceptual framework for occupational therapy. AJOT 31(4): 235-242, 1977.

Kielhofner G: General systems theory: Implications for theory and action in occupational therapy. AJOT 32(10): 637-644, 1978.

Kielhofner G: The temporal dimension in the lives of retarded adults. AJOT 33(3): 161-168, 1979.

Kielhofner G: A model of human occupation, part 2. Ontogenesis from the perspective of temporal adaptation. AJOT 34(10): 657-663, 1980.

Kielhofner G: A model of human occupation, part 3. Benign and vicious cycles. AJOT 34(11): 731-737, 1980.

Kielhofner G, Burke J: A model of human occupation, part 1. Conceptual framework and content. AJOT 34(9): 572-581, 1980.

Kielhofner G, Burke J, Igi C: A model of human occupation, part 4. Assessment and intervention. AJOT 34(12): 777-788, 1980.

Kielhofner G: A paradigm for practice: The hierarchical organization of occupational therapy knowledge. In Kielhofner G (Ed): Health Through Occupation: Theory and Practice in Occupational Therapy. Philadelphia, F. A. Davis, 1983, pp. 55-92.

Kielhofner G, Takata N: A study of mentally retarded persons: Applied research in occupational therapy. AJOT 34(4): 252-258, 1980.

Kielhofner G, Barris R, Bower D, et al: A comparison of play behavior in nonhospitalized and hospitalized children. AJOT 37(5): 305-312, 1983.

Kielhofner G, Burke J: The evolution of knowledge and practice in occupational therapy: Past, present, and future. In Kielhofner G (Ed): Health Through Occupation —Theory and Practice in Occupational Therapy. Philadelphia, F. A. Davis Company, 1983, pp. 3-54.

Kielhofner G, Miyake S: Rose colored lenses for clinical practice: From a deficit to a competency model in assessment and intervention. In Kielhofner G (Ed): Health Through Occupation — Theory and Practice in Occupational Therapy. Philadelphia, F. A. Davis Company, 1983, pp 257-280.

Lindquist J, Mack Wl, Parham D: Occupational behavior and sensory integration concepts in theory and practice, part 2: Clinical applications. AJOT 36(7): 433-437, 1982.

Mack W, Lindquist J, Parham D: A synthesis of occupational behavior and sensory integration concepts in theory and practice, part 1: Theoretical foundations. AJOT 36(6): 365-374, 1982.

Mailloux Z, Mack W, Cooper C: Knowing what to do: The organization of knowledge for clinical practice. In Kielhofner G (Ed): Health Through Occupation — Theory and Practice in Occupational Therapy. Philadelphia, F. A. Davis, 1983, pp 281-294

Matsutsuyu J: The interest checklist. AJOT 23(4): 323-328, 1969.

Matsutsuyu J: Occupational behavior approach. In Hopkins H, Smith H, Willard, et al.: Occupational Therapy. Ed 6. Philadelphia, J. B. Lippincott Company, 1983, pp 129-134.

Meyer A: The philosophy of occupational therapy. J Occup Ther 31(10): 639-642, 1977. (Reprint of Meyer's original article. Archives of Occupational Therapy 1: 1-10, 1922.)

Moorehead L: The occupational history. AJOT 23(4): 329, 1969.

Neville A: Temporal adaptation: Application with short-term psychiatric patients. AJOT 34(5): 328-331, 1980.

Oakley F, Kielhofner G, Barris R: An occupational therapy approach to assessing psychiatric patients' adaptive functioning. AJOT 39(3): 147-154, 1985.

Pezzuti L: An exploration of adolescent feminine and occupational behavior development. AJOT 33(2): 84-91, 1979.

Reed K: Models of Practice in Occupational Therapy. Baltimore, MD, Williams & Wilkins Company, 1984.

Reilly M: A psychiatric occupational therapy program as a teaching model. AJOT 20(2): 61-67, 1966.

Reilly M: The educational process. AJOT 23(4): 299-307, 1969.

Reilly M: Occupational therapy — A historical perspective: The modernization of occupational therapy AJOT 25(5): 243, 1971.

Reilly M (Ed): Play As Exploratory Learning. Beverly Hills, CA, Sage Publications, Incorporated, 1974.

Rogers J: The study of human occupation. In Kielhofner G (Ed): Health Through Occupation — Theory and Practice in Occupational Therapy. Philadelphia, F. A. Davis, 1983, pp 93-125.

Shannon P: Occupational choice: Decision-making play. In Reilly M (Ed): Play As Exploratory Learning. Beaverly Hills, CA, Sage Publications, Incorporated, 1974, pp 285-317.

Shannon P: The derailment of occupational therapy. AJOT 31(4): 229-234, 1977.

Slagle EC: Habit training. In Syllabus for Training of Nurses in Occupational Therapy. Ed 2. Utica, NY, State Hospital Press, 1933. Takata N: Introduction to a series: Occupational behavior research for pediatric practice. AJOT 34(1): 11-12, 1980.

Tigges K, Sherman L: The treatment of the hospice patient: From occupational history to occupational role. AJOT 37(4): 235-238, 1983.

Webster PS: Occupational Role Development in the Young Adult with Mild Mental Retardation. AJOT 34(1):13-18, 1980.

Wolfe R: Defining occupation. Unpublished manuscript, University of Southern California, 1981. Cited in Kielhofner G: Health Through Occupation — Theory and Practice in Occupational Therapy. Philadelphia, F. A. Davis, 1983.

Additional Readings

Berlyne D: Conflict, Arousal and Curiosity. New York, McGraw-Hill Book Company, 1960.

Boulding K: General systems theory — A skeleton of science. In Buckley W (Ed): Modern Systems Research for the Behavioral Scientist. Chicago, Aldine Publishing Company, 1968.

Boulding K: The Image. Ann Arbor, MI, University of Michigan Press, 1961.

Bruner J: On coping and defending. In Toward A Theory of Instruction. Cambridge, MA, The Belknap Press of Harvard University Press, 1966.

Bruner J: The Skill of Relevance or the Relevance of Skills. Saturday Review April 18, 1970, pp 66-73.

Bruner J: Nature and uses of immaturity. In Bruner J, Jolly AL, Sylva K, (Eds): Play: Its Role in Development and Evolution. New York, Basic Books, Incorporated, 1976.

Caplow T: The Sociology of Work. New York, McGraw-Hill Book Company, 1954.

Erikson E: Childhood and Society. New York, W. W. Norton & Company, Incorporated, 1963.

Fiebleman J: Theory of integrative levels. In Coleman J (Ed): Psychology and Effective Behavior. Boston, Little Brown and Company, 1968.

Ginzberg E: Toward a theory of occupational choice. In Peters H, Hansen J, (Eds): Vocational Guidance and Career Development. New York, Macmillan Publishing Company Incorporated, 1971.

Kahn R, Wolfe D, Quinn R, et al.: Organizational Stress: Studies in Role Conflict and Ambiguity, New York: John Wiley & Sons, Incorporated, 1964.

Kaplan A: The Conduct of Inquiry. New York, Thomas Crowell, 1964.

Koestler A: Beyond atomism and holism — The concept of the holon. In Koestler A, Smythies JR (Eds): Beyond Reductionism: New Perspectives in the Life Sciences. Boston, MA, Beacon Press, Incorporated, 1969.

Kluckltohn C: Values and value orientation in the theory of action: An exploration in definition and classification. In Parsons T, Shils E (Eds): Toward a General Theory of Action. Cambridge, MA, Harvard University Press, 1951.

Smith M: Competence and socialization. In Clauser J (Ed): Socialization and Society. Boston, MA: Little Brown and Company, 1968.

Super DE: Career Development: Self Concept Theory. New York, College Entrance Examination Board, 1963.

Super D: The Psychology of Careers. New York, Harper & Row Publishers, Incorporated, 1957.

White RW: Competence and the Psychosocial Stages of Development. Nebraska Symposium on Motivation, Lincoln, NE: University of Nebraska Press, 1960.

White RW: The Urge Towards Competence. AJOT 25(6): 271-274, 1971.

White RW: Strategies of adaptation: An attempt at systematic description. In Colhlo G, Hamburg D, Adams J (Eds): Coping and Adaptation. New York, Basic Books, Incorporated, 1974.

Chapter 9

Organic
Mental Disorder

A group of students was asked to point to that part of their body they felt most represented "them," their "essence," so to speak. Three, perhaps the romantics in the group, pointed to their hearts. The rest pointed to their heads.

For most of us, our thinking and feeling self is localized in our head or brain. The prospect of our losing control of our ability to accurately perceive the environment, or to manipulate our own thoughts, is perceived as an assault on our integrity. By *thinking*, we refer to the ability to select, analyze, and intentionally act upon objects and events in a meaningful way. Beyond this, we are able in thinking to reflect about ourselves; we are able to experience our sense of "I-ness." How frightening and overwhelming it could be to realize that this thinking function was being compromised, because with it goes our power and meaningfulness within our world.

There are millions of individuals who face to varying degrees a compromise of their thinking function due to a metabolic or mechanical brain insult. Such brain impairment may be due to a variety of causes — ingestion of toxic substances; a compromise of oxygen intake; acute disease; meningitis, encephalitis, multiple sclerosis; trauma; as well as chronic, currently irreversible neuropathologic atrophy from the presenile and senile dementias, Pick's disease, or Korsakoff's syndrome.

In the most recent DSM III (1980), the manual to which clinicians turn when a diagnostic label in mental health needs to be given, the term "organic mental disorder" is the broad term given to thinking, behavioral, and affective dysfunction attributable to brain disease. To

281

further describe the exact nature of these dysfunctions, the DSM III describes six constellations of impairment, one or more of which may exist within an organic mental disorder. These are referred to as the "organic brain syndromes" and include (1) delirium and dementia, (2) amnestic syndrome and organic hallucinosis, (3) organic delusional syndrome and organic affective syndrome, (4) organic personality syndrome, (5) intoxication and withdrawal, and (6) atypical or mixed organic brain syndrome (DSM III, 1980, pp. 103-104).

In common usage, the therapist can expect to hear the term "organicity" used to describe a variety of brain-related dysfunctions, and will often hear that a given individual is "organic." This is a term that is vague and often misleading, and even dehumanizing to many laypersons. The global use of the term "organic" may serve, for some, to mask their lack of specific information about brain dysfunction and may reflect a discomfort with dealing with the brain impaired. Especially in the psychosocial treatment setting, the brain impaired individual may be an anomaly within a patient group. The staff may feel unprepared, fearing that the problems of brain impairment are very different from nonorganically based disorders; or, the staff may believe that brain damage implies that there is no hope for a patient's improvement.

When the brain impaired individual appears in the psychosocial setting, he may or may not be recognized initially as having central nervous system (CNS) damage. Because brain insult can result in significant behavior changes, loss of control, anxiety, and other so-called psychiatric symptoms, the brain injured individual may be brought into a traditional psychosocial treatment setting on the belief that his affective and behavior change is psychological in origin. In some instances, individuals having some brain impairment but evidencing a good functioning ability, i.e., those with mild retardation, those in the early stages of vascular or arteriosclerotic change, or individuals with residual damage from brain trauma, may be in treatment with other nonorganically impaired individuals to deal with behavior or affective problems. For example, brain injured individuals frequently need to learn to control episodes of anger or depression, to learn or relearn effective problem solving strategies, to deal with altered feelings about the self and self-image, or to improve their ability to interact socially.

It is also a common occurrence among therapists engaged in home health treatment that older, homebound patients present with a primary or secondary problem of mild to severe brain impairment. Whenever the brain injured individual is encountered in treatment, he presents a challenge to be understood in terms of CNS and physiological change, cognitive, emotional, and affective parameters, and in his ability to function with success and dignity. When the brain impairment is due to exogenous factors that are remediable, i.e., when the intake of toxic substances is at cause, all concerned treatment staff will mobilize to interrupt the destructive process. When a diagnosis of organic mental disorder has not been established, the occupational therapist may be able to assist in establishing the presence of an organic etiology. When brain impairment is irreversible or progressive or both, the occupational therapist seeks to help the individual cope at the highest functional level, to exert as much control as possible over his own decisions, to maximize his independence, and to maintain his self-respect. While traumatic head injury, stroke, and other acute episodes of physical trauma would not be treated in the psychosocial setting, the psychosocial occupational therapist might see these individuals post-trauma as they seek to adjust to the frustration of diminished problem solving ability.

Whatever the etiology of brain impairment, the psychosocial occupational therapist can expect to encounter individuals with organic mental disorder. She needs to be conceptually familiar with the problems posed by brain injury so that she is able to respond effectively in planning and implementing a treatment approach. In this text, the reader will be oriented to the problems of and treatment principles for dealing with brain impairment from a holistic stance. While no one aspect of neurology or rehabilitation can be extensively developed, the reader will be given guidelines for conceptualizing brain dysfunction and treatment goals.

Holism

In understanding the brain impaired individual from the holistic vantage, the therapist is always cognizant that every part affects the whole organism. The holistic view has implications for evaluating and conceptualizing deficit as well as for pursuing compensation, remediation, and optimum function. There are three holistic principles that should be highlighted:

1. "A part not functioning within the whole tends to be brought into harmonious function within the system" (Wolanin and Phillips, 1981, p. 14).

In other words, the organism mobilizes to restore equilibrium. This reflects in the use of compensation or "functional adaptation" (Luria, 1966, p. 73) by covert sensory-perceptual, motor, and cognitive systems within the brain, as well as in the overt compensations demonstrated by the individual. For example:

An 86 year old home-health patient being treated for a hip fracture also had moderate arteriosclerotic brain impairment. When the occupational therapist asked about the patient's husband, now deceased, the patient responded, "Now, what was his name? I was married to him for 50 years; you'd think I could remember his name!" The patient then laughed heartily. The laugh was repeated many times during the interview, and appeared genuine.

This woman compensated for her memory loss by laughing about it, allowing herself to deal with her memory dysfunction without a loss of emotional equilibrium.

2. "If a portion in the whole is perceived by the organism as unfilled, the organism will tend to fill it" (Wolanin and Phillips, 1981, p. 14).

On a sensory level, the individual will attempt to fill a sensory vacuum. If, for example, there is sensory deprivation, hallucinations (a kind of sensory self-stimulation) may result. If an individual is blind, sensations coming in via the other sensory modes will be perceived as relatively louder, or stronger. In terms of behavior sense, one sees *confabulation* as a frequent reaction to memory deficit. In confabulation, an individual with memory gaps will construct his own story to fill in the gaps.

A young woman suffering from acute brain hypoxia was an inpatient at the treatment center. When asked what she had for breakfast that day she could not remember. But, after only a brief pause, she answered with animation "Pancakes. . . and eggs. . . and bacon. My but it was delicious — I ate everything!" The occupational therapist, knowing oatmeal and fruit was breakfast fare, recognized this as confabulation.

3. There is an innate need by the organism to give structure or meaning to chaos.

For example, unable to find the correct word, a patient with visual agnosia (the inability to name objects viewed) will frequently describe the object's purpose, properties, or use. Unable to understand why misplaced articles at home are "lost," the confused individual will often become convinced that visitors in the home are stealing from him.

The authors will address these three aspects of holism in exploring the parameters of brain dysfunction. These are: (1) the holistic interaction of functional systems within the brain and brain stem; (2) the mutual reactions between physiological change and personality; and (3) the holistic relationship between the brain impaired individual and his environment.

Holistic Relationship of Functional Systems in the Brain

There has been a tradition of looking at the CNS in terms of discrete units and functions. As every student will remember, each portion of the human body is represented geographically on the brain's cortex and each functioning system, i.e., vision, audition, smell, taste, speech, fine movement, gross movement, vestibular-proprioceptive sense, and all of the autonomic functions are represented in specialized areas and developed through specified pathways or patterns throughout the nervous system. Most of us have seen film demonstrations in which a portion of the living brain is electrically stimulated and the patient's right toe wiggles, or he complains "I'm hungry."

On behalf of increasing the knowledge of how the brain functions, there is increased understanding of the specialized extrapolation by each hemisphere in the brain (Sperry, 1964; Gazzangia, 1967, 1970; Luria, 1963, 1966, 1973; Williams, 1979; Franco and Sperry, 1977; Ornstein, 1972). The left hemisphere, which is usually dominant, is connected motorically to the right side of the body and is primarily devoted to analytical or logical thinking, especially in verbal or mathematical functions. The left hemisphere in most right-handed individuals is dominant for the learning of fine skilled motor movements, and usually dominant for the development of language. The right hemisphere processes information more simultaneously than the left; it deals holistically with information and intuitions, and has a primary responsibility for spatial orientation.

Students are frequently taught of the split between sensory and motor function. Not only are separate sensory and motor centers identified within the brain, but also texts conceptualize afferent "ascending" sensory nerve tracts bringing information into the brain, with efferent "descending" motor pathways leading to the musculature.

While such a reductionist approach to neurology serves to simplify and clarify the understanding of a complex system and aids in the differential diagnosis of brain lesions, what is too often lost is an appreciation for the functional sharing and ultimate plasticity.

Plasticity

Plasticity within the central nervous system refers to the ability of other portions of the brain to take over function when one part is damaged, and is especially striking in the cortex. In recent literature, the work of the late Aleksander Luria (1963, 1966, 1973) is most consistently cited in support of the concept of CNS plasticity. Josephine Moore (1980), whose investigation of functional anatomy has significantly influenced occupational therapy theory and practice, also supports this concept of plasticity. These two investigators plus the very persuasive exposition of the holistic position by Miller in *Meaning and Purpose in the Intact Brain* (1981) have influenced the selection of material included in this chapter.

As demonstrated by Luria, (1963, p. 36) and reiterated by Moore (1980), at different stages of development, brain organization changes and the "same" task can be carried out by different neural constellations. Moore notes that "old" pathways, perhaps replaced by newer cortical constellations, retain the latent ability to integrate a task. Fundamental to Luria's observations about brain function is the conceptualization of functional systems. He contends that no one formation within the central nervous system is responsible for a single function or behavior (Luria, 1963, p. 28). Rather, all behavior and "thinking" is made possible by the extensive interaction between a diversity of structures thoughout the brain — structures that work together as a functional unit. Luria assails the premise that vision, hearing, tactile sense, or any other function is mediated by one zone or lobe. He further stresses that what we call higher cortical function (or conscious thinking) is mediated thoughout the brain. In relation to this, when one cortical pathway is derailed, it is possible for another pathway, in a non-traumatized area, to take the same information. Luria applied the term *functional adaptation* to this ability. This is a concept that has significant implication for rehabilitation, as will be discussed.

Moore (1980) furthers the understanding of how specific structures within the brain can assume a diversity of roles. She describes the development of interneurons (nerve cells confined within the CNS), pointing out that CNS interneurons are not exclusively sensory or motor; they do not carry pain, or touch, or motor information, per se. Rather, interneurons carry "coded messages" that are modified and changed at every synapse (Moore, 1980, p. 27). Thus one can speak of the "polysensory" capability of neurons. This suggests that when a specific informational tract is damaged, others have the potential to carry the same message.

Bilaterality

In a final comment, one can easily challenge the emphasis given to brain specialization through laterality. While it is true that each hemisphere of the brain tends toward a unique approach to comprehension and function, there remains a strong tendency for bilateral function within the nervous system. This is especially evident when assessing those functions maintained at the subcortical level, i.e., those substrates that, without conscious effort by the individual, maintain body tone and balance, and keep the body always aware of its position in three-dimensional space (Moore, 1980, p. 36). Not only is the CNS structured to provide constant feedback and relatedness of both sides of the body to both brain hemispheres and all dimensions of the environment, but when one side of the brain is injured, the other hemisphere also becomes functionally impaired. Moore describes this in terms of the impaired hemisphere losing some of its ability to send information to the noninvolved side. The so-called "good" hemisphere suffers from "sensory deprivation" (Moore, 1980, p. 29). Again, we are reminded that the brain, as a holistic organ, cannot but be affected as a whole to an assault on any part.

Because all brain structures and systems interrelate, a so-called focal problem impacts the entire organism's ability to comprehend and adapt. This principle is evident when working with brain impaired individuals. Even with localized insult, one encounters a group of functionally related symptoms or what Luria calls a *symptom complex* (Luria, 1963). As an illustration, a lesion in the left (dominant) parietal lobe produces some combination of the following symptoms: diminished ability to read and write; right-left disorientation; finger agnosia; difficulty with calculation, loss of pain appreciation (pain asymbolia); ideomotor apraxia; and various aphasic disorders (Strub and Black, 1981, p. 240).

Central Nervous System Re-organization

It is also because the brain structures are interrelated, and because discrete portions of the CNS are capable of carrying out a variety of functions, that where there is an assault to one part — be it a single cortical path, or a larger portion of brain mass — the brain will reorganize in response in a compensatory effort to maintain its integrity. When the brain impairment is gradual and the brain has time to deal with the insult, a great deal of function may be carried out by intact tissue. This is demonstrated repeatedly in the practice of physicians who have patients come in with minor symptomatology despite the existence of extensive neural damage from slow growing tumors. When the brain assault is sudden, as from a car accident, the brain has not had this opportunity to compensate and the results of the trauma are immediately evidenced. However, given the period post-trauma, the intact portion of the brain can often reorganize to restore much function.

Nowhere is the brain's reorganizational ability more strikingly illustrated than in the follow-up of hemispherectomy (or the surgical removal of one hemisphere of the brain). Glees (1980) cites the longitudinal study of three individuals who had hemispherectomy (two had a right hemisphere removed, one had a left). All three had a rather remarkable recovery. They were able to walk, read, write, and maintain a relatively normal social life. While one individual needed to work within a sheltered workshop setting, another of the three was able to complete his university studies and hold down an administrative position.

While all hemispherectomies could not be expected to be compensated for so well, Glee's discussion highlights dramatically the ability for functional adaptation by the central nervous system. It is well-known that CNS neurons, once destroyed, cannot regenerate. Thus, while function may be less precise and performed more slowly, one is still faced with the remarkable plasticity of the human brain.

Holistic Relationship of Physiology to Personality

The integral holism between brain and emotion is one of those things that is obvious, and yet not so obvious. Clearly, the ability to feel emotion, or to put conceptual parameters on those sensations we experience when we know we are about to encounter an unexpected quiz, or when someone says, for example, "Will you marry me?" — achieves meaning through intergration within the central nervous system. How this happens and where this occurs is not so clear.

The Reticular Activating and Limbic Systems

The *reticular activating system* (located at the core of the brainstem, just above the spinal cord and below the thalamus and hypothalamus, and having direct connection with the limbic system, cerebellum, and cerebral cortex) has been frequently cited in its ability to deflect or stimulate feelings of arousal and excitability (Luria, 1963, 1966, 1973; Moore, 1980; Malec, 1984; Williams, 1979; Golden, 1984). The reticular activating system, which consists of activating and inhibiting neural tracts, plays a significant role in screening out irrelevant stimuli, in inhibiting inappropriate response, and also in "charging up" the individual for action. The *limbic system* (the central part of limbic activity being in the hypothalamus) is believed to serve as the substrate for innate drives (i.e., eating, sexual desire, fear), memory, and emotional behavior (Strub and Black, 1981, p. 21). As with the reticular activating system, the limbic system has complex interrelationships with other aspects of the brain, including the cortex, thus enabling the learned or volitional expressions of mood, drive, and utilization of memory. Compromise in any part of the reticular activating or limbic systems, themselves a closely interrelated system, may result in altered consciousness, altered moods, aggressive behavior, anxiety or lethargy, disorientation, inappropriate sexual response, confabulation, and memory disorders (Golden, 1984, p. 86; Strub and Black, 1981, pp. 10-27). It is generally suggested that focal lesions not affecting arousal or limbic centers are less likely, but not necessarily unable to cause emotional and personality change. Considering our discussion of functional systems, it would be the authors' bias to underscore the "not necessarily" since even a so-called focal lesion ultimately affects so much of the brain, and has the potential to disrupt vocational and social behavior. A great deal of brain impairment assaults brain tissue in diverse brain areas, and not necessarily in an easily interpretable way. It therefore seems useful to broaden the understanding of emotional response in brain disease.

Depression

Brain injury, when it is recognized by the individual as such, represents a significant loss.

There is frequently loss of function; loss of control; the individual may "look" different; he may be infantilized by others. There is frequently a loss of dexterity in cognitive processing, and with it, a lessening of self-esteem. Finally, there is frequently a disruption of vocational and family roles. The reactions of grief, shock, and dismay by the individual are to be expected and may, indeed, need to be facilitated as a part of aiding the individual to move toward a gradual acceptance of his loss. When brain assault is progressive (as with the presenile and senile dementias) the grief issue may need to be approached several times as more and more function is lost. There will be a relationship between the individual's ability to deal effectively with his loss and potential depression and the following: (1) his personality before the brain impairment (called the premorbid state), i.e., was he a person prone to depression previously? (2) his expectations for himself in therapy: are his expectations too high, too low, or reasonable? (3) the support provided by his family and the promise of what is awaiting him after therapy, i.e., will his employer seek to keep his job open?

The environmental considerations will be discussed later in this chapter. What is especially important in the initial response to depression and grief is that the patient be encouraged to express his feelings, and that he be given accurate information about what can be hoped for in therapy. While the therapist can communicate her knowledge about the brain's ability to compensate, she need also be honest in stating that most frequently the premorbid state of function will not be achieved. While the brain can compensate, usually efficiency is lost; problem solving may take longer; motor function, if retrainable, may not be as precise; and memory deficits tend to continue to be problematic. Creating false expectations will serve to ultimately decrease trust and increase depression.

Depression is influenced by other factors also. As an individual adjusts to his disability and seeks to build compensatory patterns, he encounters frequent frustration. As one patient said, in disgust, "Things just don't work right!" Attempts at compensation are fatiguing, and the individual may be exhausted after 20 minutes of work. Especially when brain impairment is of a progressive nature, the patient has many concerns about himself and the foreboding unknown. He wonders, "How will I take care of my family?" "Will I be institutionalized?" and "Will my family love me, or pity me?" Depression may be reflected as self-deprecating comments, withdrawal from activity or others, passivity, loss of self-esteem, and as sad afffect. Frequently, the real loss of peer contact and social relationships is not evident until three to six months after the patient returns to the community (Rosenthal, 1984, p. 231). The list of worries can become seemingly unmanageable. Suicidal ideation becomes quite common and is an important concern with brain impairment.

Emotional Lability

Loss of emotional control is a second frequent adjunct to brain assault. When an individual moves quickly from laughter to tears without apparent cause or without control, the term *lability* of affect is frequently applied. Certainly, compromise to the normal regulation of arousal centers can have a significant role in this lability. When cortical control of arousal and limbic centers is damaged through assault in the frontal lobes, there may be an inability to suppress inappropriate response, a lack of goal directedness, apathy or euphoria, irritability, or a lessening of moral constraints (Rosenthal, 1984, p. 230; Strub and Black, 1981, pp. 242-244; Walsh, 1982, p. 36). Again, there are other influences to consider. One concerns any general loss of cognitive function. When this occurs, there is less ability to accurately assess a problem or situation; thus, a behavioral response may appear quite out of skew because the individual has been unaware of important cues within a situation. Second, with a cognitive compromise there is frequently lessened ability to postpone immediate gratification and to be aware of and regard the feelings of others. In Freudian terms, one could say the individual loses some ego and superego function; in developmental terms, one might say he seems more child-like or has regressed. He becomes more concerned with meeting his own desires, and less concerned with social politeness. The result may be a more primitive emotionality, i.e., temper tantrums with frustration, raucous laughter or giggling with pleasure. Too, one must consider the bombardment of problems brought on by brain impairment. The emotionality may be, understandably, a reaction by the individual to feeling overly taxed. The individual coping with brain insult may, by necessity, become very focused on his own struggles, and on his own process. A loss of perspective results: victories and setbacks may loom much larger when the sphere of interaction is restricted.

Apathy

Another frequently encountered emotional aspect of brain impairment is described as apathy or lethargy. The individual appears to lack motivation or drive. If the arousal centers or medial frontal cortex are insulted, the difficulty may be a physiological problem with self-arousal; that is, once external stimulation is removed, the individual is unable to sustain attention. He may be inaccurately assessed as "resistive," "stubborn," or "depressed" (Walsh, 1982, p. 36). As with other personality components, apathy may be related to the individual's style of responding to stress before his brain insult. Further, the individual may have "learned" to be helpless as a means to gain attention in treatment centers (Sufrin, 1984, p. 199).

When an individual perceives his own situation as hopeless, acceptance may turn to resignation to less than optimal function: the individual may give up. The therapist's ability to communicate reasonable expectations, provide rest breaks, and to break up therapy into manageable units in which success is apparent, may be helpful in dealing with apathy. Ultimately, however, the individual must draw from within himself the motivation to sustain effort towards therapeutic ends.

Suspiciousness

Depending on the nature and extent of CNS damage, suspiciousness, or its extreme, paranoia, may result from an individual's inaccurate assessment of the environment (as with cortical damage), disturbance in mood, or may be due to organically induced hallucinations. Diminution in sensory-perceptual processing also frequently results in suspiciousness. In a range of sensory-related dysfunctions termed *agnosias* (i.e., tactile, visual, and auditory) the individual may have a severely restricted ability to recognize objects or faces, to distinguish or localize sounds, or to comprehend what is said to him or about him. When he cannot trust his own senses to give accurate and meaningful information about his environment, he is in a tremendously vulnerable position. This can only be compounded when, as in expressive aphasias, there is interference with the ability to verbalize one's own needs. In such instances suspiciousness may be viewed as an understandable exaggeration of the organism's attempt to protect itself; it may serve as a mechanism by which the individual slows down a social process in order to gain extra time to understand it. Some simple steps taken by the therapist to communicate through those senses that are intact, i.e., to approach the individual from a visual field from which he will not be surprised, or to assist him in identifying scrambled sensory data, to communicate slowly, and to allow sufficient time for cognitive processing, can all act to increase the individual's confidence in his own ability to understand and be understood, and ultimately to increase his trust. Also, anything the therapist can do to increase the patient's sense of power and control over his own circumstances may serve to decrease his concern about what is going to be done "to" him and move the focus to what he can learn to do for himself.

There is also an element of paranoia that may have a realistic component. Even when an individual's cognitive processing is slowed, and at times, situations misjudged, there may remain an ability to respond, perhaps on a more primitive or intuitive level, to the feelings of those around him. Thus, the brain injured individual may be aware that others are uncomfortable around him, or regard him as "strange." The following example is cited because similar situations have been encountered frequently by the authors:

Marguerite was rendered homebound by her severe emphysema. The visiting nurse suspected that she had moderate organic impairment though this had not been formally tested. Nursing notes described her as "unduly suspicious," citing Marguerite's comments that "My neighbors don't like me . . ." and "They gossip about me." Following an initial visit by the occupational therapist, the OTR chanced to be in the hallway, where she was seen by a neighbor who invited her in for coffee. Sensing an opportunity to gain perspective, the therapist chatted briefly with the neighbor, who immediately barraged her with comments about Marguerite's "unseemly" behavior and her "lack of character." Marguerite's suspicion that her neighbors did not like her and took advantage of any opportunity to talk about her was, in fact, accurate.

The therapist may have little influence over the reaction of neighbors, but she does have jurisdiction over her own attitudes. Care and respect play as important a role with the brain impaired as with anyone else; and, one could argue they have an even more important role. For while some communications depend on higher functioning to be perceived or processed, caring is communicable and receivable at the most basic level.

This leads us to consider the third aspect of holism that needs to be addressed when working with the brain impaired: the holistic interaction between the individual and his environment.

The Individual in His Environment

All of us cannot but impact upon our environment, and be impacted by it. In the ultimate analysis, the environment, being plastic, will either respond in a helpful way, or in a way antagonistic to our growth.

For the brain injured individual, his ability to perceive, selectively disassociate from, or process environmental information may be diminished. In that case, those concerned with helping him to gain access to information may place considerable effort in influencing the environment to simplify messages in order to increase their perceptibility or clarity. As with "reality-oriented" approaches, remediation may be geared towards making visual, auditory, or tactile data bolder; or in helping to rearrange tasks in order that alternate (intact) sensory systems will be emphasized, or alternate or simplified problem solving strategies viable. When the patient has difficulty responding effectively within his present (or premorbid) environment, the environment (including the family, job, or avocation setting) can be restructured to meet the patient "more than half way." This principle will be more closely examined in the later discussion of treatment.

Emotional Environment

We cannot, in therapy, separate the environment from those care-givers and significant others who will relate to the individual. In addition to our attitudes as therapists — attitudes that may include optimism, or pessimism, concern, or oversolicitousness, and that will undoubtedly affect the outcome of therapeutic intervention — the patient rebounds against the attitudes of family, work associates, and friends. With the initial diagnosis of organic dysfunction, family members may experience as much grief, confusion, and even chaos as the individual himself. Assessing the nature of family roles and the extent to which family members might be able to provide support is important. Providing information and support to the family is equally critical. Understanding the patient's job and his avocational interests may be helpful in determining constructive avenues for therapy and may give clues for motivating the patient. Therapy is devoted to increasing functional capabilities and emotional consonance within the expected, or everyday environment. It is always helpful for the patient to be aware of how a therapeutic task is related to his ability to function optimally outside of the treatment setting. This helps provide meaning, and when necessary, the therapist may need to be very explicit or creative in communicating this information in a way that can be truly understood.

The therapist needs to be aware that she, as well as involved family and acquaintances, will be affected by their investment with the individual. Family members may be overwhelmed by new experiences that seem so removed from anything they have experienced previously. They may be frightened by a loved one who behaves so unpredictably, or who seems to get angriest at those who love him most. They may be distraught with concern about how they will care for the individual. Anything the therapist, along with other health personnel, can do to help family members to understand the nature and expected progress of the disease process and treatment approach may assist family members to "get a handle" on their own feelings, and be potentially more helpful to the patient.

Summary

To conclude, the reader has been oriented to the understanding of the brain impaired individual from a holistic stance. As we look toward evaluation and treatment, the reader needs to be cognizant of the following guiding principles:

1. The person with brain impairment is best understood as a whole, integrated being — not as set of discrete systems that function independently. It is of paramount importance to us as occupational therapists to understand that purposeful activity, i.e., baking a cake, creating a collage, hammering nails, or enjoying a concert or a walk cannot be localized in any portion of the brain.
2. An assault on any part of the person will result in a reorganization and effort to accommodate to that change from the microscopic to the macroscopic level.
3. The individual impacts and is influenced by his environment. The environment may be structured to facilitate his learning and optimum function; or, it may unwittingly respond to make his readjustment more difficult.
4. The attitude of the therapist and significant others will have a significant influence on the ultimate outcome of the therapeutic effort.

Evaluation

Orienting to the Evaluation Process

It is not within the scope of this text to describe extensive sensory, motor, or cognitive neurological assessment; nor would such assessment typically be pursued by the occupational therapist in a psychosocial setting. However, the therapist needs to be knowledgeable about the scope of evaluation that occurs in working with a brain injured individual, and she needs to be able to contribute to the continued assessment of functional changes.

In the broadest terms, the therapist needs to gather data and monitor change in the following:

1. Sensory perception, analysis, and integration;
2. Motor function;
3. Higher cognitive function;
4. Problem solving, especially as relates to self-care, activities of daily living, work, and avocational interests;
5. Social facility;
6. Emotional and affective parameters;

The goal of gathering and evaluating information in these areas will be to:

1. Aid in differential diagnosis, when necessary;

2. Identify specific strengths and limitations;
3. Target areas that best can be remediated or where function can be improved;
4. Clarify the conditions under which success is most likely to occur;
5. Establish specific goals; and
6. Aid in gauging progress.

Before addressing each area, the authors underscore that each system to be assessed functions in relation to a unified whole. What is especially important is ascertaining the effectiveness of all "systems" in contributing to successful problem solving and meaningful activity. While the assessment areas are the same as those typically approached by occupational therapists in a diversity of treatment problems, the discussion in this test will highlight functional aspects especially common to brain injury.

Sensory Perception and Sensory Synthesis

The reader was oriented to perception in Chapter 5, "The Overview of the Cognitive Process." Here we will add to that information. *Perception* consists of the ability of the CNS to detect or discern sensation; the faculty to discriminate or "know" what that sensation is and to distinguish it from other sensation; and to retain in memory the impression of that sensation long enough to respond to it purposefully (Mosey, 1970 p. 151). Once accurately perceived, the organism must then be able to simultaneously relate or integrate sensory data coming from a variety of sources and through a variety of sensory modes through a process frequently called *synthesis* or *integration*. This synthesis occurs at all levels of the brain cortex, cerebellum, and brainstem. Separate from perception and synthesis but complementary to them, the organism must be able to screen out or ignore irrelevant sensory information.

Owing much to the work of Luria, researchers and clinicians have become more aware of the important and integral role played by language in mainstreaming sensory data. By language or speech, one refers to the ability to think in words rather than images. Speech production is itself a motor act, but the comprehension of language and verbal reasoning do not require motorization. When sensory information comes into the individual, upon recognizing it he tends to categorize the data by assigning it a "name" or quality. Thus, an individual does not see random lines, rather he sees shapes, or identifiable objects; or he feels textures that he calls "rough," or "smooth," or "cool," or "wet." Because of the functional relationship of speech to all modes of perception, it often follows that when a sensory system is assaulted, speech may be impaired; or, when a speech center is adversely affected, aspects of sense perception or sense synthesis are disturbed. It is because of the integration of vast amounts of sensory data, at both the conscious (cortical) level and at subcortical levels, that the individual is able to know where he is in space, to develop a meaningful body scheme, and to derive meaning from the objects and events he encounters in his environment.

The rehabilitation literature (see Najenson, et al., and Toglia and Abreu for discussions particular to occupational therapy) conceptualizes a developmental hierarchy of increasing complexity in perception and synthesis.

For example:

Simple Visual Perception Tasks:
1. Focus the eyes on an object; and
2. Recognize shapes, colors, and objects.

Intermediate Visual Perception Task:
1. Distinguish a shape from within a field of distracting shapes (figure-ground perception); and
2. Recognize that foreground objects are closer, and background is farther in a photograph (depth perception).

Complex Visual-Auditory Synthesis:
1. Derive meaning from a television program.

With each sense modality, vision, touch, kinesthetic input from joints and muscles, vestibular input, smell, taste, and hearing, the individual learns, as he develops, first the simplest, then increasingly complex ability to perceive, analyze, synthesize, and make meaningful sensory data. When there is brain insult it is frequently (though not always) the more complex sensory perceptual and sensory synthesis skills that show impairment. For example, stimuli received via one sense at a time may be interpretable, but the ability to understand multidimensional data may be interpreted; or, subtle differences in or changes in sensation may not be perceived. However, because of the ability to call upon other intact sensory-perceptive constellations to function for those that cannot, the individual may not give evidence of the dysfunction until his skills are pressed. To cite a deficit discussed by Luria (1963):

When there is a temporal lobe compromise and a problem with phonemic hearing, the patient may be able to "hear" (sound registers in the CNS), but have difficulty synthesizing sound. He might be able to reproduce a rhythm only if it is slow enough to be counted; or, he may have difficulty comprehending speech when sounds are similar, but not when sounds are distinctly different.

Agnosia. The inability to comprehend sensory information due to CNS damage is termed agnosia. The agnosias most commonly tested and discussed in the literature are: visual agnosias, tactile agnosias, and auditory agnosias. Actually, all sense perceptions (including taste, smell, and kinesthetic) may be disturbed. The agnosias are further categorized to best describe the exact nature of the perceptual problem (Appendix J). In an attempt to compensate for milder sensory dysfunction, the individual may do one or more of the following:
1. Restrict his sphere of attention;
2. Respond to only the obvious or unambiguous aspects of a sensory message;
3. Create barriers or isolate himself to cut down on the amount of auditory or visual stimuli coming into the CNS;
4. Avoid touch or being touched;
5. Demonstrate a slowed, more deliberate response; and
6. Demonstrate a quickened or more irritable response.

The therapist in the psychosocial setting would be unlikely to do an extensive sensory evaluation; however, she needs to be aware of the presence of sensory-perceptive deficits. It is virtually impossible in the clinic setting to ascertain the existence of sensory-perceptual problems without including an aspect of motor function — that is, the individual must "do" something to indicate that he understands a sensory message. Thus, sensory perception and synthesis are typically assessed, formally or informally, within an individual's sensory-motor performance. Tasks typically cited as representative of sensory function are listed in Appendix I, with suggestions for formal assessment later in the chapter.

Also, note the performance of so-called "sensory" or "motor" tasks cannot be separated from the ability to concentrate, to process intellectually, or any number of other cognitive variables. The therapist needs to be aware always of the holism of function.

Body Awareness Synthesis

An important aspect of sensory-motor and cognitive synthesis relates to the ability of the individual to interpret sensory data in order to ascertain his own position in space. Included in this is the ability to know where each body part is in relation to the others, to understand concepts of directionality (right-left; or up-down) to synthesize information received from all environmental and body planes and in relation to gravity; and to coordinate activity in a three-dimensional way. For the sake of clarity in this discussion, the authors would conceive spatial relationship and vestibular-kinesthetic synthesis as directly influenced by and influencing each other as well as body awareness.

Spatial relationship synthesis, or *spatial awareness*, includes the ability to orient oneself in space, and to visualize what an object looks like from all angles; to know where sounds are coming from; and to know where body parts are in space. It is easily disturbed by visual and tactile agnosias, as the individual has impaired ability to localize and synthesize sensory data. What may not be as obvious to the neurologically naive is that with a disturbance of spatial relationship comes also a disturbance in understanding all directional and comparative relationships. For example, the individual may be unable to tell time, or to place an object "to the right of, or left of another." Or, he may be unable to understand the comparison, "Tom is lighter than Harry, but heavier than Marge." Further, mathematic computations involving multicolumn numbers (i.e., 192 + 468) cannot be conceptualized as representing "one hundred, nine tens, and two ones" (Luria, 1966, pp. 150-160).

Vestibular Kinesthetic Synthesis

Vestibular kinesthetic synthesis refers to the ability to discriminate and evaluate data received about the pull of gravity and position in space through the vestibular apparatus within the ears and from the kinesthetic receptors in joints, tendons, and muscles. The work of Ayres, Moore, and King has contributed significantly to the knowledge of how vestibular-kinesthetic synthesis is achieved and maintains smooth body movement. Vestibular-kinesthetic synthesis relates directly to the ability to maintain balance (eyes open and closed) and the ability to orient and potentially "right" oneself in three-dimensional space.

Much vestibular-kinesthetic synthesis occurs in the CNS at the subcortical level, when information is assessed and corresponding muscle tone mediated without the necessity of the individual to think about coordinated and balanced movement. When brain assault interferes with automatic, subcortical regulation of movement, tone, timing, and balance, the individual may try to compensate by thinking consciously about movement. The result is a loss of stability and fluidity in movement, a loss in coordination, or a reduction in movement in order that the individual might eliminate or lessen the amount of sensory input that needs to be synthesized.

Interference with vestibular-kinesthetic pathways at any level of the central nervous system may result in one or more of the following:

1. Loss of "smoothness" and fluidity in motor function;
2. Loss of timing;
3. Loss of stability and balance; and
4. Lessened movement or rigidity, which will ultimately impact general motor performance (gross and fine). This will be discussed later.

Motor Synthesis

Purposeful activity requires the ability to perceive and synthesize sensory data, use higher cortical function (typically in a language-related process) to analyze the aspects of a motor problem, plan action, and synthesize movement into a meaningful whole.

Disturbances of voluntary or purposeful movement at the CNS level is termed *apraxia*. Apraxias are further labeled to describe more exactly the specific nature of the deficit (Appendix J). Frequently, as with deficits in sensory perception, simpler or more familiar motor schemes may be intact, while more complex or unfamiliar schemes show the deficit. The deficit may be exhibited as a slowed or jerky response; or there may be a loss of ability to stop one movement pattern and go onto the next; i.e., a person asked to clap might be unable (without outside intervention) to stop clapping. The inability to interrupt a motor pattern is called *perseveration*. It is frequently seen when patients are asked to copy a visual pattern, and may appear as "scribbling," when an individual gets "stuck" on one portion of a given scheme (Fig. 9-1), or as an obvious continuation of a visual pattern (Fig. 9-2). Perseveration is also often evidenced in speech, with an affected individual unable to change topics. There may be an inability to sustain a motor action, termed *motor impersistence*.

When the intention for cortically planned movement is intact, but the ability to mobilize (or organize) in action is assailed, the individual may describe vocally what he wishes (but is unable) to execute.

Although all aspects of the CNS are ultimately involved in the smooth execution of intentional activity, the reticular activating system has been cited as especially significant in the ability to select from a large range of learned behavior patterns the appropriate motor response, while suppressing inappropriate response (Mosey, 1970, p.153).

The attempt to compensate or reorganize in adjustment to assaults on motor performance links lead to a constellation of:

1. Avoiding novelty;
2. Staying rigidly with familiar schemes;

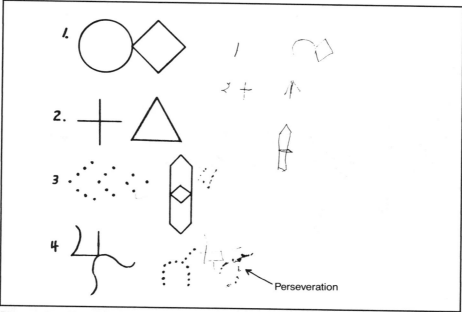

Figure 9-1. Preservation due to organic brain syndrome.

3. Slowed response;
4. Tendency to home in on one aspect of a motor task, with resultant failure to respond to the whole; and
5. Fatigue, due to the extra effort needed to synthesize movement. The tasks typifying motor function are listed in Appendix I.

Speech Synthesis

The ability to think effectively via private speech, to communicate through language, and to comprehend language is a complex function dependent, as with all the performance components discussed, on the ability to attend and synthesize sensory data, organize thoughts through use of cognitive process, and utilize speech-motor pathways. Adult language involves five basic processes: (1) understanding spoken language, (2) verbal reasoning, (3) speech production, (4) decoding written language, and (5) writing (Strub and Black, 1981, p. 30). An impairment in the CNS aspect of speech is called *aphasia*. Specific categories of aphasia are outlined in Appendix J.

Although damage to the left hemisphere in the right-handed person is often found in individuals with aphasia, due to its complex representation throughout the brain, speech is derailed by insult in diverse brain areas. Thus, even though she is not primarily concerned

297

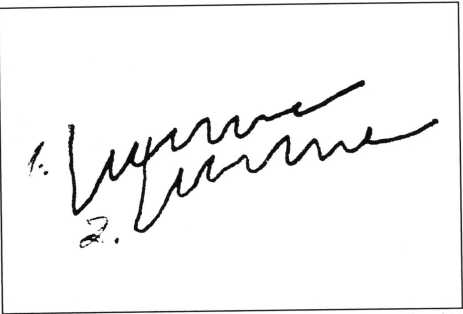

Figure 9-2. Preservation of pattern done by man who twice attempted to write his name.

with the evaluation of speech, the occupational therapist needs to be aware of the potential impact of language difficulties on all aspects of activity. In a response pattern similar to that seen with sensory and motor synthesis, interference with language pathways may, in milder interruptions, be exhibited as a slowing of language comprehension or language response; i.e., the individual may falter; be unable to "find the right word" without much deliberation; may need to have the speaker talk more slowly, or use shorter phrases, or repeat; may seem to have a limited vocabulary; or may have increased pausing.

The occupational therapist is concerned with not just speech, per se, but with the ability for what Kent-Udolf calls *functional communication*. That is, the ability to participate in casual everyday conversation. This includes the ability to understand implied meaning and to enjoy humor (Kent-Udolf, 1984, p. 23). Limitations in the ability for functional communication will seriously interrupt socialization, and may result in social isolation by the patient: isolation noted by his withdrawal, or the withdrawal of others who find social discourse with him to be cumbersome.

When language reception or communication is impaired, the individual may respond to open-ended conversation with irrelevance, confabulation, or with very abbreviated replies

(Kent-Udolf, 1984, p. 32). It should be recognized that the patient's ability to comprehend speech is not necessarily best evaluated by asking complex or open-ended questions. Such questions require much more than verbal comprehension. It may be more useful, when language comprehension is a concern, to ask patients to follow simple commands or to ask questions that can be answered "yes" or "no" or with a nod (Strub and Black, 1981, p. 53).

It needs to be remembered that the ability for language is at its heart the ability to think in words, not images. When this is impaired, the ability to read, write, and mathematically compute is also interrupted. Further, because the ability to use higher cognitive functions (to be addressed later) is generally judged by speech facility, when there is an impairment of language, the individual may be inaccurately perceived as having limited intelligence. The result may be a further tendency by others to "talk around" the individual, as if he were not there.

When there is a language impairment, the occupational therapist may wish to consult with a speech or language specialist to help ascertain the strategies that could help the patient better communicate. Without effective communication, the individual is in an intolerable position of frustration and isolation.

In summary, speech and language impairment may result from or lead to deficits in sensory synthesis, motor performance, or cognition. It can easily impede social process and the ability for meaningful activity. Attempts to compensate and reorganize may be demonstrated in the individual as follows:

1. Restricted use of language; limited vocabulary;
2. Requests to others to speak more slowly or to repeat;
3. Focus on only one aspect of a verbal request;
4. Avoidance of reading, writing, or calculation;
5. Avoidance of social situations; and
6. Slowness to respond to a verbal request.

Cognition

The most complex cortical function is that referred to as cognition. Cognition includes the ability to assimilate and assess sensory data, retain this information over time in memory, and to consciously manipulate it in problem solving. Higher cognitive function is made possible by the extensive association of multifaceted information at the brain's cortex. Such function is also predicated on vast subcortical activity charged with handling background stimuli, keeping irrelevant detail from awareness, and maintaining a normalized (unconscious) homeostasis that frees conscious, cortical function from a devotion to survival concerns. As discussed in Chapter 5, "Overview of the Cognitive Process," the higher cognitive processes are frequently perceived as those that enable the individual to proceed past the concrete or tangible aspect of stimuli and problems, to deal symbolically (or ideationally), to imagine, to create, and generate multiple alternative or hypothetical conscious structures.

The following are frequently cited in psychiatry as elements basic to cognition. The reader will note they differ in emphasis from the aspects of cognition discussed in Chapter 5 of this text. They are summarized here in this manner since it is in this following general format that most psychoscial assessments are oriented. However, the reader needs to be aware that these represent rather arbitrary structures, always interrelating, both in the theoretical and functional sense.

Attention

Attention refers to the ability of the central nervous system to focus on relevant stimuli or information while screening out or keeping from conscious awareness irrelevant information. Further, the CNS must be able to sustain attention over a period of time. Attention occurs at both the cortical and sucortical level. At the subcortical level, the CNS must be able to maintain necessary arousal or alertness while dampening any overarousal. In practice, the ability to attend is often assessed by the individual's motor performance: Does the individual display an ability to focus on the salient features of a task, conversation, or problem? Further, is the individual able to maintain attention to these salient features? Attentional difficulties might be described clinically as "irritability," "distractibility," "overarousal," and "hyperactivity," or "apathy," "dullness," or "underarousal." The therapist might note significant differences in the ability of the individual to attend in various environmental settings; i.e., in a dyadic conversation; in a small group interaction; in a familiar setting; in an unfamiliar setting — as well as differences in the ability to attend to varying modes or intensities of sensory input; and to input coming from varying positions in the environment (i.e., from the patient's right side, or from the patient's left).

The patient attempting to compensate for his own attentional difficulties might do the following:

1. Describe noises, lights, and other environmental stimuli as "annoying" or "confusing";
2. Seek to isolate himself in his environment, or seek to reduce stimulation;
3. Limit the task to which he attends;
4. Employ strategies to help himself maintain attention, i.e., talk aloud to himself, follow along with his finger as he reads; and
5. Employ self-stimulation.

When attentional dysfunction is excessive, the individual may be barraged with what has become meaningless stimuli and he understandably responds with anxious, confused, or nongoal directed behavior. He may be so underaroused that relevant information goes unnoticed, or the ability to sustain attention may be sporadic, yielding unpredictable, inconsistent cognitive and motor behavior.

Concentration

Closely related to attention, *concentration* refers to the ability of the individual to maintain attention for longer periods of time in order that he can keep his thoughts directed toward completing a given task or bringing closure to a given cognitive scheme. It too necessitates a homeostatic balance of sufficient arousal, while avoiding overarousal. Individuals unable to concentrate refer to "loosing my train of thought." Others may perceive these individuals as daydreaming, switching from one subject to another, rambling, or being unable to finish tasks once started. There may be a strong affective component to the ability for concentration as is demonstrated by our everyday difficulty with "keeping our thoughts" on a task when we are especially worried about or looking forward to a meaningful encounter. Concentration problems result in a lack of goal directed behavior.

Orientation

Orientation refers to a specific aspect of personal attention, knowledge, and memory — the knowledge one has about his own relationship to the environment. Frequently referred to as orientation to *time*, *place*, and *person* (sometimes written as "orientation × 3"), it includes the awareness of one's own name, roles, likes, dislikes; the names and roles of significant others; the awareness of one's own physical location; and the awareness of time parameters. In an initial assessment, the individual is frequently asked to give his name (orientation to person), the name of the interviewer (orientation to person), to indicate his whereabouts in the treatment setting (orientation to place), and to state the day, time, or month and year (orientation to time). Orientation is an ongoing reassessment of one's own relationship within the environment. Loss of orientation is most often evidenced with mild to extreme confusion.

Knowledge

Incoming data becomes knowledge when it has meaning to the individual. Guidano and Liotti (1983) speak of the acquisition of both preverbal (tacit) knowledge and verbal (explicit) knowledge. *Tacit knowledge* includes the incorporation of images, affect, and instruction in early childhood, and ultimately permits the internal representation of objects, events, and persons. *Explicit knowledge* allows for the conscious manipulation of ideas over time, and includes the symbolic-representational knowledge that is language encoded (Chapter 5). It is explicit knowledge that is most frequently assessed when working with brain impaired individuals. Frequently, when explicit knowledge becomes less available to a severely impaired individual, his behavior appears to reflect a reliance on tacit knowledge. That is, the individual responds nonverbally to familiar tastes, touch, and smells, and behavior takes on a primitive quality.

The ability to acquire explicit knowledge may be understood developmentally, as discussed by Piaget and cited by Flavell (1977). Essential is the ability to experience objects and events as separate from oneself; name objects and events and recognize their essential properties; categorize objects and events according to similarities and differences; infer cause and effect in the observance of action; arrange events seriately; infer logical relationships in terms of concrete (observable) events; read signs and symbols; and infer logical relationships in abstract or hypothetical events.

In clinical practice, knowledge has often been assessed in terms of a *fund of knowledge*. For example, the individual is asked to name the current governor, or to discuss current events. This is viewed by the authors as a restricted use of the term knowledge, and a more functional understanding, as follows, is suggested.

One cannot separate the evaluation of knowledge and the assessment of memory (a discussion on memory follows). Permanent knowledge may be conceived of as including three kinds of information: sensory-perceptual, procedural-motoric, and propositional beliefs (Bower and Hilgard, 1981, p. 422). *Sensory-perceptual knowledge* includes knowledge of images and internal maps for finding one's way around. *Procedural-motoric knowledge* is knowledge of how to do things, including motor, speech, and intellectual function (for example, knowing how to ride a bike, solve a math problem, or bake a cake). *Propositional beliefs* include our beliefs about ourselves and others, our knowledge and concept of word meanings, our knowledge of objects and events over time, and our knowledge regarding values (Bower and Hilgard, 1981, p. 423).

The therapist assessing knowledge may find it useful to have an individual demonstrate knowledge representative of learning in each of the preceding areas (Appendix I). The person with knowledge deficits may appear immature or unskilled if his behavior does not appear grounded in prior experience. He may be described as impulsive when his actions do not appear to anticipate probable outcome. He may be described as intellectually deficient when his fund of common information appears limited, or when his command of language is compromised. Mild deficits in knowledge synthesis are often difficult to separate from misperception and memory deficits. Globally, knowledge insufficiency may be exhibited by the individual through the following:

1. Ineffective or inappropriate task and social behavior;
2. Withdrawal from former work-related tasks;
3. Avoidance of new tasks;
4. Rigidity in problem solving;
5. Expressions of frustration over one's own inability to "think" or function;
6. Denial or confabulation or both to cover deficits; and
7. Obvious inaccurate recitation of or manipulation of data (including verbal, written, and mathematical).

Memory

Memory is a complex function, but it is only partially understood. It involves the ability of the central nervous system to take in information (*input*); code, categorize, and store information (*maintenance*); as well as the ability of the individual to willfully retrieve or remember that information (*retrieval*). As discussed by Guidano and Liotti (1983), and Flavell (1977), memory is an exquisitely personalized process by which the individual actively selects data and interprets it or gives it meaning in the context of his own experience. Memory is not static maintenance, but it is a process in which "old" information may be constantly re-evaluated and remembered differently as new experiences are integrated. (Think for example of how you remember your first bicycle, or first date. First you may have remembered the bicycle as being huge. Then later the bicycle may have been remembered as smaller and less significant. Your first date may also be remembered quite differently now than it was 10 years ago.

Memory includes both the explicit holding of information as verbal knowledge, as well as the more primitive preverbal (tacit) experiencing of the infant (see end note 1). Tacit or unconscious memory may be viewed as providing a contextual background without which explicit information cannot be sought and maintained in memory.

Mental health clinicians have frequently referred to and assessed three temporal aspects of memory: *immediate recall*, *short term memory*, and *long term memory*. These divisions apply to the ability to recall newly given information, information frequently as given by the practitioner in assessment:

Immediate recall:The ability to recall information within one minute of its inception;

Short term memory: The ability to recall information within one minute to one hour after its inception;

Long term memory: The ability to recall information after one hour (including over weeks, months, and years).

The recent cognitive literature speaks more to two major temporal divisions: the separation of short term memory (STM) from long term memory (LTM), conceptualizing the two as "stored" differently (Atkinson and Shiffinn, 1968). *Long term memory* is the repository of permanent knowledge and skills (sensory-perceptual, procedural-motoric, and proposi-tional). *Short term memory*, or "working memory," is of a limited capacity, as it constantly provides a context for current activity and deals with new information (Bower and Hilgard, 1981, p. 427). Think for a moment about what has happened in your experience over the last hour. While fairly easily recalled at his moment, a year from now very little (perhaps none) of the information in this short time span will have been established into long term memory. Short term memory is prone to disruption by attentional difficulties or by distraction. (Think, for example, of how quickly you "forget" to turn off the stove, if something distracts you, or how quickly you forget the name of a newly introduced acquaintance if you are not really paying attention.) The ability for information to transfer from STM to LTM appears related to its repetition or rehearsal during the short span, and also is facilitated by the ability of the individual to make *meaningful* or *personal* associations between the new information and knowledge already contained in long tem memory (Bower and Hilgard, 1981, p. 433; Luria, 1966). Bower and Hilgard refer the interested reader to Craik and Lockhart (1972) for a more extensive discussion of the role of association in memory.

Modern theorists are beginning to believe that the ability to draw upon or retrieve memory is akin to "opening a locked treasure chest," requiring just the right "key" or retrieval cue

(Bower and Hilgard, 1981, pp. 446-447). *Cues* are words, images, sounds, or perceptions that are associated with and elicit the memory. For example, the smell of baking bread may act as a cue for remembering days spent at Grandma's house; or the word "wrinkled" may be for an individual the cue to the memory of ironing.

The therapist assessing memory both formally and informally would note effective memory as related to the following:

1. Short term memory/ long term memory;
2. Meaningful (personal) memory/ nonmeaningful (impersonal) memory; and
3. Sensory-perceptual/procedural-motoric/propositional memory.

The therapist would also assess the role played by cueing (the patient's own cueing, or cues provided by the therapist); and by noting the role played by attentional function or dysfunction in short term memory.

It is quite common with brain impairment to see daily fluctuations in memory: that is, the patient who appeared quite clear one day or one hour may have less functional memory at another time. Memory is also influenced by affective components. We all, for example, are often less able to remember when we are very anxious or depressed.

Individuals experiencing mild memory problems may describe themselves as "forgetful"; i.e., unable to remember appointments, annniversaries, or the names of acquaintances. They may find themselves in the midst of an errand, and forget what they had gone for; or in the midst of a conversation, and lose track of its content. They may "misplace" household items put away for safekeeping.

Efforts to compensate for mild memory loss include:

1. Making Lists;
2. Writing notes to oneself;
3. Asking others to remind oneself;
4. Confabulation;
5. Rambling or "talking around" an event not remembered;
6. Perseveration; and
7. Avoiding tasks requiring good memory.

Severe memory loss is frightening, disorienting, and immobilizing. The individual loses a sense of continuity over time and with events. He becomes incapable of deriving meaning from everyday events and from negotiating the tasks of daily living.

Judgment and Insight

Sometimes addressed separately, judgment and insight are conceptualized here as being closely related. *Insight* refers to he ability to "see into" a situation and imagine "what would happen if" or "what has happened because." In applying *judgment*, the individual anticipates the likely consequences of his actions — including their likely social acceptance — and plans his behavior accordingly. The individual with insight is freed from the necessity of trying out a series of actions to ascertain their appropriateness or likely outcome. He can, rather, hypothesize based on past learning. Further, when an event has occurred and he looks at it in retrospect, he generates a reasonable hypothesis regarding why it happened. For example, the individual with insight can state why he is in the treatment setting; hypothesize why another patient is angry about missing the bus; or describe what would happen if he does not pay a parking fine.

In the psychoscial setting, much of the ability to engage in meaningful process-oriented group interaction depends on the ability of the individual to understand insightfully the actions and interactions of others.

Frequently with mildly lessened insight, the behavior of the individual is described as indicative of poor judgment. This would be exemplified by mismanagement of finances; loss of social polish; failure to observe safety precautions (i.e., while driving, or when using tools), or by lack of apparent concern regarding dress, hygiene, or eating.

Judgment and insight can be addressed by asking questions about why events occur or what behavior would be considered appropriate in a given situation (Appendix I). However, judgment and insight are most accurately assessed through the observation, over time, of an individual's task and social behavior.

Abstraction

Abstract thinking is the ability to derive meaning from an event or experience beyond the tangible aspects of the event itself. It involves being able to perceive the symbolic or conceptual nature of an object and event, and to extrapolate the similar and unique features of objects and events beyond the concrete. For example, when he reads the book *Moby Dick*, he can understand that in addition to it being a story about a man hunting a whale, it is also a depiction of the struggle between good and evil. Abstraction includes the ability to de-center and imagine the feelings of others. It includes the ability to use Piaget's formal operational thinking (Flavell, 1977), and complex (hypothetical) problem solving.

Einstein's ability to hypothesize about the (unseen) actions of the particles within an atom represents the ultimate in abstract thinking.

Some individuals seem naturally more (or less) comfortable with and able to deal in the abstract domain. The individual with limited ability for abstraction has special difficulty imagining "what would happen if" in a hypothetical problem. The ability to have insight becomes in a practical sense closely related to the ability for abstraction.

Frequently, with milder impairment, the patient may be able to describe one appropriate (and, most likely, familiar) strategy for solving a problem — but remains stimulus bound and cannot generate any other alternative approach. He cannot discern the "moral of the story" when others speak and cannot, therefore, derive the most significant meaning in social discourse. The classic test in psychiatry for the ability to abstract is when the patient is requested to interpret proverbs; i.e., "What is meant by 'people in glass houses shouldn't throw stones?' "

A reduction in the ability for abstract thinking frequently leads to behavior that is described by others as rigid, egocentric, opinionated, or missing the point. Because of its relatedness to insight and judgment, limited ability for abstraction is frequently associated with behavior described as inappropriate, narrow, thoughtless, or careless.

A functional assessment approach is for the therapist to observe the patient's ability to function with flexibility in a diversity of problem solving tasks, and to appreciate subtlety, humor, hypotheses, and implied meaning in social discourse.

In summary, cognition is a complex, internally mediated process by which the individual attends to internal and external information, analyzes the meaning of objects and events, and retains and manipulates data toward the ultimate end of engaging successfully with his environment. A breakdown in any aspect of cognitive function is detrimental to the entire thinking process. Compromise in cognitive function is a frequent result of brain assault, and is often the most distressing residual dysfunction for individuals and their families. While treatment strategies can assist in the regaining of cognitive ability or assist in building compensatory behaviors by the individual, most often the premorbid level of cognitive function is not expected.

Problem Solving

As discussed in Chapter 5, "Overview of Cognition," the traditional approach in assessing problem solving has been for the therapist to identify the existence and efficacy of the following seven general steps: (1) identify that a problem exists, (2) analyze the problem and identify its salient features, (3) identify alternative solutions for solving the problem, (4) select one of the alternatives, (5) make a list of action, (6) implement the plan, and (7) evaluate the outcome.

In assessing problem solving, the therapist attempts to determine how all the "threads" of function come together in handling both the practical and more esoteric events of living. Keeping the above sequence in mind, Bara's broad categories are useful in pinpointing specific kinds of problems that a patient can or cannot handle effectively. Bara (1984) identified six classifications of problems: (1) formal, (2) mundane, (3) physical, (4) interactive, (5) personal, and (6) self-problems. These were discussed further in Chapter 5, "Overview of Cognition." (These categories should not be construed as related to any specific area of brain function.) In actual assessment, one cannot separate the assessment of problem solving from the assessment of knowledge (i.e., the existence of knowledge needed to solve the problem), memory, sensation, motor ability, and other components of function. Indeed, for a person with limited function, any daily task can present a difficult problem. Typically, however, in assessing problem solving, occupational therapists have selected problems that, in their resolution, allow opportuniy for the use of such higher cognitive processes as those involved in insight and hypothesis. The therapist is also interested in ascertaining the patient's ability for conjecture, or his ability to act upon more than one solution to a problem. Therefore, she frequently selects problems in assessment that have two or more reasonable means of resolution, and then asks the patient to identify these alternative means. The reader may find the Table, "Analysis of Activity Complexity," in Appendix I to be helpful in judging the relative complexity of a range of problem solving tasks.

Affective States

As discussed previously, brain dysfunction frequently results in significant personality or emotional changes. These may be as a result of brain trauma to a specific arousal or control center, or a combined result of increased physiological and psychological stress.

With mild brain dysfunction, the personality may be described as similar to the premorbid personality, but personality traits or affective reaction may be more exaggerated. In some instances, the individual is described by others as having a marked personality change. With diminished sensory-motor function, and lessened or slowed cognitive synthesis, there results a frequent constellation of two or more of the following affective reactions:

1. Increased frustration or lessened ability to deal with frustration;
2. Poor impulse control;
3. Dimunition or alteration in body image;
4. Affective change related to under or overarousal;
5. Loss of self-esteem;
6. Anxiety or irritability;
7. Worry regarding the future;
8. Feelings of hopelessness;
9. Feelings of helplessness;
10. Feelings of depersonalization;
11. Depression or euphoria; and
12. Suspiciousness and distrust.

The assessment will attempt to establish the relationship of premorbid personality variables with current affective states, as well as to note affective changes influenced by the task demands, and social and environmental setting.

Social Parameters

The impairment of brain function frequently jeopardizes the individual's ability to function successfully in a social context. This may be due to lessened social astuteness, loss of judgment, lessened affective and behavioral control, diminished ability to perceive and respond to verbal and nonverbal messages, and attentional or arousal difficulties. Additionally, there may be withdrawal by the individual who has a diminished self-esteem, or social isolation by others who find his behavior discomforting.

The therapist will assess the individual's ability for appropriate social discourse in the dyadic relationship. Additionally, the individual should, if possible, be observed in one or more group settings. The therapist will make observations regarding the following:

1. What skills facilitate the individual's interaction with others?

2. What behaviors interfere with successful interaction?
3. Does he approach others? How?
4. Do others approach him? Do others isolate him?
5. Does he seem able to comprehend what is said to him? (Concrete meaning? Implied or subtle meaning?)
6. Does he seem to comprehend when others are speaking but not directing their discourse to him?
7. Does he maintain appropriate eye contact?
8. Is he able to share materials or to share space?
9. Is he able to cooperate in a task?
10. Does his behavior suggest that he values himself within the setting?
11. Does his behavior suggest that he values others in the setting?
12. What role does he take in the setting? Is he able to appropriately assume more than one role?
13. In what kind of social setting does he appear most successful?

Given her observations, the occupational therapist can use her knowledge of group structure and group dynamics, and select social and therapeutic experiences in which the patient can experience success or regain social skill and confidence.

Assessment Process

The occupational therapist working in the psychosocial setting will most likely not have a formalized assessment battery on hand for use with brain impairment since patients with organically induced deficits are not the primary population in such settings. She will need to be able to adapt the assessments with which she is familiar, whether these are standardized or idiosyncratic to the setting, or she may wish to select from one or more of the testing procedures highlighted in this chapter. As she considers what approach she wishes to take in evaluation, the therapist should consider the ability of a given assessment or procedure to give the kind of information about which she is most concerned. For example, if she is primarily concerned about an individual's ability to function independently at home, she needs to select an assessment that provides information about the patient's ability to do practical tasks of daily living and to approach problems in an organized fashion. If the patient's referral describes a presenting problem with socialization, she may wish to use an evaluation that speaks primarily to social skills (and skill components). If she is in a position to do more extensive sensory-perceptual, sensory-motor, or cognitive testing, she needs to select an assessment tool that will provide baseline data with which later comparisons can be made. Unless the therapist has been requested to do extensive sensory or sensory-motor testing and is prepared to do this, the authors would suggest that a broadly based assessment, designed to gain information about a patient's ability to function in a variety of task, social, and environmental situations would be most appropriate.

Before beginning her assessment, the occupational therapist needs to consider two factors:

a brain impaired individual frequently has difficulty with maintaining attention for any extended period of time, and performance tends to be irregular; that is, tends be good on a given task on one day, and poorer on another, without predictability. With these two factors in mind, the therapist usually gains more reliable information by extending the evaluation process over two or more brief evaluation sessions.

Before a final decision is made regarding what testing will be done, it is suggested that the therapist acquaint herself with all available medical history, including any input from other professionals who have worked with the patient. This will assist the therapist in her selection of evaluation procedures that are most likely to accommodate the patient's limitation and skills. Finally, it is suggested that she spend time in an initial interview with the patient. Such an interview, in addition to helping to establish rapport, helps the therapist gain insight into the patient's mode of communication, strengths and limitations, and in his ability to sustain attention. Fatigue and loss of attention are suggested by an increase in perseverative behaviors, signs of irritability, and signs of drowsiness. During the initial interview, the therapist may use some of the questions or avenues of exploration suggested in Appendix I to gain information about the patient's cognitive abilities (including orientation, memory, general awareness of events, and ability for abstract as well as concrete thinking). From this interview, she can also learn more about his moods, his attitude toward treatment, and his concerns and expectations for himself and others. From this, she may gear the assessment to his special needs. It must be stressed that no one evaluation battery can be expected to deal best with all patients, or all types of difficulty. If the therapist does this preliminary preassessment groundwork, she may be able to avoid a plethora of initial testing, which is testing that can overwhelm a patient. If, in the course of treatment she finds that more specific information is needed, she may choose to employ additional test batteries.

While there is a variety of assessment material available in occupational therapy (as described in previous chapters of this text), the authors are not aware of any standardized occupational therapy assessment batteries specific for brain impairment. If the therapist is concerned primarily with gaining baseline information about an individual's ability to function on given tasks, this may not present a problem. If, however, the therapist is unclear regarding what is "normal" adult function, what is subnormal, and what is directly indicative of brain dysfunction, she may need to select a battery outside of the usual occupational therapy domain.

Assessment Tools

The following are representative of assessments used in the preliminary evaluation of brain impaired individuals:

Bay Area Functional Performance Evaluation (BaFPE)

This evaluation is described with behavioral and occupational behavioral assessment tools in Chapters 4 and 8. Although it is not designed for the assessment of organic brain dysfunction, it does provide the opportunity to assess a broad range of functional, language, social, and cognitive skills. It requires the therapist to have knowledge about brain dysfunction if it is used diagnostically. The test manual and materials are available from Consulting Psychologists Press.

The "Magazine Method of Testing"

This is a method (cited by Holden and Woods, 1982, p. 124) which is a nonthreatening, nontestlike task that can be easily done in a clinic or home setting. A magazine is opened to a two page advertisement with pictures. The individual is asked to read the text aloud, name the objects, and describe the purpose or "message" in the advertisement. The therapist can note the patient's ability to read (large and small print), name objects, to attend to a full visual field, to visually scan, and to discern abstract as well as concrete meaning. It is not a standardized test and requires the therapist to be an astute observer.

The Person Drawing

The person drawing may be conceived of as an assessment tool in itself, or as a part of a larger assessment battery. The request for a person drawing is, for example, a part of the Schroeder-Block-Campbell, BaFPE, and other evaluations which have been described in this text.

King supports the use of a person drawing as a means to help ascertain dysfunction in the central nervous system, noting that the ability to depict a person in a visual symbol depends on the ability to abstract, successfully integrate body awareness and spatial orientation, and to integrate visual and motor planning. In the authors' experience, loss of integration or loss of wholeness in the person drawing is a very frequent adjunct to brain dysfunction, and they recommend the person drawing as a screening tool. The interested reader is referred to Cohn's *The Person Symbol in Clinical Medicine* (1960) for a thorough discussion of how brain impairment may manifest in figure drawings.

Bender-Gestalt Test

A standardized assessment tool. The individual is shown figures one at a time, then is asked to copy each. Upon completion, the individual is asked to duplicate from memory those figures he can recall. This test has been used by occupational therapists as a screening tool for visual-perceptual and motor function, and has been used by psychologists as a projective test. The assessment is discussed in the literature (Hutt and Briskin, 1961, pp. 126-138) as a screening tool for organic impairment. It is available from the American Orthopsychiatric Association, 1790 Broadway, New York, New York 10019.

Schroeder-Block-Campbell Sensory-Integration Evaluation

This is an evaluation designed to assess sensory integrative function in the adult psychiatric population, and is not specifically designed for assessment of brain dysfunction. However, it provides many opportunities for the therapist to test perceptual sybthesis and body awareness synthesis. For more information and a test manual, write to SBC Research Association, La Jolla, California. (The SBC is also discussed in Chapter 7.)

Benton Neuropsychological Assessment

This is a test designed by Benton, a neuropsychologist. It includes a series of 12 separate neuropsychological tests designed specifically for screening for and specifying the nature of CNS deficit. The manual (Benton, 1983) gives a description of each test, and provides sample forms, administration and scoring procedures, and normative data for "normal" as well as dysfunctional adults. Of the 12 tests, some can be replicated from reading in the manual; others require special materials available from the author. The 12 tests described are for the assessment of the following:

1. Temporal orientation;
2. Right-left orientation;
3. Serial-digit learning;
4. Facial recognition;
5. Judgment of line orientation;
6. Visual form discrimination;
7. Pantomime recognition;
8. Tactile form perception;
9. Finger localization;
10. Phoneme discrimination;
11. Three-dimensional block construction; and
12. Motor impersistence.

Although the primary author is a neuropsychologist, the tests are very similar to those that have long been used by occupational therapists. For the interested reader, this assessment as described in Benton, A, et al., *Contributions to Neuropsychological Assessment: A Clinical Manual* (1983) is recommended because of its clarity and because normative data is given for many groups including: normal children, older adults, normal adults, and brain injured adults.

Regardless of the assessment chosen, there are important variables that need to be noted by the occupational therapist. These include the following:

1. The ability to maintain attention and persist on a task;
2. The method of dealing with frustration;
3. The ability to deal with distracting stimuli;
4. The ability to recognize error;
5. The ability to correct error;
6. The ability to recognize alternate means of problem solving;
7. The predominant sensory, motor, or cognitive approach taken during task

performance;

8. The consistency of performance over time;
9. The changes in affect and emotional tone;
10. Comments made about self and one's performance; and
11. The ability to ask for clarification or assistance as needed.

Assessment of the Environment

As part of the evaluation process, the therapist should gather information about the patient's academic or work history, including the current status of his schooling or employment; his interests (premorbid as well as those skills presently enjoyed); the nature of his family roles and interactions; and the nature and demands of the environment in which he will be expected to function. The patient may be able to give this information, or the therapist may need to gather some information from medical records, family members, or other professionals. When possible, the authors favor gathering this information from dialogue with the patient. It is not just the history, per se, but the patient's current attitudes and interests in activities and roles that are especially important. Also, it is through discussion that the therapist and patient can often begin to understand the complex interplay of function and dysfunction in all areas of the individual's everyday world.

The therapist should attempt to ascertain the degree to which social activities have been maintained or curtailed. Frequently, the brain impaired individual, even when highly functional, regards himself as "different" or "handicapped," and will tend to be isolated within the community. The therapist may be aware, in some communities, of support groups created especially to meet the needs of the brain impaired.

One should look at activities of daily living in the broadest sense. Even when dressing, eating, and hygiene are easily accomplished, the individual may be restricted in other activities of special importance to him. For example, he may be restricted from strenuous physical activities, and may no longer be able to participate in the sports he so enjoyed. Or, he may not be allowed to drive an automobile or use other machinery. These restrictions may dramatically alter his life style, academic, and vocational plans and his sense of purpose.

In many instances, the therapist's assessment at the conclusion of treatment will be utilized to aid in determining whether or not the individual can return home, or whether he will need some degree of partial or full care. The scope and focus of the assessment will need to be individualized to accommodate this issue.

Final Assessment Comments

While the preceding discussion might suggest a high demand in the area of assessment, the occupational therapist need not let her assessment get in the way of knowing the patient. Learning about a patient is an ongoing, unfolding process. Some information may be gained quickly in formal testing; some will emerge gradually in the process of treatment. The treatment or therapy process really begins from the moment the therapist and patient meet. Get to know the individual, and interact with him. You can learn a wealth of information that no assessment would reveal. Also, in coming out from behind your tests, you are giving him an added opportunity to know and interact with you, and to experience himself in a meaningful way.

Treatment Process

Establishing Treatment Goals

Having identified specific areas of function and dysfunction, treatment goals will be established with the individual. Lynch suggests making a problem list, from which problems can be prioritized in accordance to their urgency for the patient and feasibility within the treatment setting (Lynch, 1984, pp. 292-294). This is especially important since the extent of problems may be broad, while the duration of treatment is often shorter than what the therapist would wish for. When possible, the treatment goals will be established in the areas and toward the end that the individual has communicated his desire for improvement. Treatment success will be measured in relation to changes in the individual's own function, not in relation to his ability to meet the norm.

The individual may be able to make only global statements about his treatment hopes; i.e., he may state his wishes to "remember better," or "get around town more," or "learn some games to help pass time." It is the therapist's responsibility to break down global goals or problems into manageable, accomplishable smaller units that will ultimately lead to goal attainment. With brain impaired individuals, this involves looking carefully at the complexity of sensory and motor synthesis involved, the complexity of cognitive organization and processing, and the environmental demands. When activities are to be done stepwise, the individual needs to be made aware of how each step ultimately leads to the accomplishment of desired goals. When there is an impairment of cognitive function, this relationship of steps to the final outcome may not be obvious to the patient, and the therapist needs to pay special attention that the relationship is understood. Once goals are established, they will be communicated to family and other involved staff.

In addition to the pursuit of formalized treatment goals, the therapist is often, along with other staff, in the position to engage in more casual, everyday encounters that can serve to increase the individual's awareness of everyday events and social expectations, and to increase his ease in social encounters. These are discussed further as "reality orientation."

No one technique or strategy or combination is appropriate or best for all patients; further, a variety of treatment tasks may be individualized to meet an individual's specific strengths and limitations. The literature describes strategies that are primarily reality oriented, behavioral, cognitive, cognitive-behavioral, or sensory-integrative in basis. Though emerging from diverse treatment frameworks, most of the strategies suggested are quite similar, and are summarized here. It will be noted, however, that some principles basic to sensory-integration are in contradiction to those primarily cognitive strategies. The reader will find also that many strategies involve the direct manipulation of the environment and activity; others speak to the therapist-patient interaction.

Making Treatment Meaningful

As has been stated, the activity(s) selected for avenues of treatment need to be activities that the patient has indicated have relevance for him. This is understandable and essential if he is to be motivated and sustain interest in the therapy process.

An activity or task has meaning on a sensory level when sensory data is received and understood by the nervous system. The therapist must be certain that the sensory stimuli integral to an activity are clear enough, slow enough, and given through sensory modes able to be integrated by the individual.

On a task level, the individual must perceive how a given task is designed to lead to the goal of treatment. If, for example, he desires to gain skills that will enhance his ability to return to his job, the therapist may begin with simple, repetitive tasks designed to increase his ability for sustained attention, or to rebuild familiar motor schemes. These initial tasks may be in the form of a game, or as part of a craft. Some individuals do not, without explanation, see the relationship of play to work.

In the psychosocial setting, the brain impaired individual may perceive himself and his problems as far different from those other individuals with whom he shares his treatment environment. This can serve to make ward meetings and group activities appear initially less relevant, from his perspective. The therapist can assist by highlighting for him the parallel or common problems shared with him by many of the patients. She can also highlight for him the manner in which hospital or clinic situations parallel the social, work, or ADL demands that he has or will encounter at home.

Simplification

In simplification, the requirements of a task (be it work, play, ADL, or social) are reduced to a level at which the patient can successfully function. Gradually, the complexity of the task is increased as each step or task is successfully accomplished. Simplification may be conceived of in two ways: some activities are inherently more simple than others; and the therapist may, for example, select a simpler method of attaining a desired outcome; i.e., weaving on a handheld or cardboard loom is simpler than weaving on a floor loom.

A therapist may be able to simplify a complex task, making it ultimately attainable, by breaking it into its component parts, and reteaching one part at a time. To illustrate, a patient may indicate a desire to be able to play a card game. The occupational therapist might begin by seeing if the patient can recognize and sort the playing cards according to color. If he can do this, she might see if he can sort them according to suit. If he exhibits confusion with this, she could demonstrate how this was done, then have the patient imitate and practice until sorting by suit is easily accomplished. She will continue to break the activity into its integral parts, having the patient practice each new skill until it is "overlearned" (done without hesitation or automatically).

Simple Retraining Through Repetition

This is a principle taken from physical rehabilitation. This approach, as it implies, is relearning through practice. The therapist determines the specific skill level a patient has, and then sets small goals to keep just ahead of the patient. As was described in reference to learning a card game, each step is practiced until it comes easily, before a new skill is attempted. The therapist should strive to add only one new behavior or skill at a time. A patient learning to dress himself might, for example, practice putting his arms into the sleeves of his shirt and repeat this many times until this was easily accomplished. Then he would practice getting buttons properly aligned, and finally, approach the task of buttoning the shirt.

The principle behind such repetition is the recognition of the brain's ability to establish alternate pathways for function. Further, it has been demonstrated that repetition enhances the likelihood that short term memory will be translated into long term memory. Integral to the development of these new pathways is consistent feedback to the CNS regarding its own success. The therapist will, for example, draw the patient's attention to his success with each attempt.

While repetition and practice are recognized as essential in relearning there is an important caution. When an activity becomes too repetitive, it begins to lose its meaning (Moore, 1980, p. 74; Bower and Hilgard, 1981, p. 492). On a sensory level, the individual may begin to ignore sensory stimuli. This is termed *CNS habituation*. On an attentional level, the individual may lose his attention. We can pause to consider our own reactions to repetitive music; we may habituate to it and stop "hearing" it. Or, consider our reaction to piano or typing drills; they become boring. The therapist may be able to assist by providing simple variation through her interacting with the patient; enthusiastic comments, and a slight touch to the hand can serve to bring back the patient's attention. Drills, per se, would seem less desirable than repetition in the context of a meaningful whole.

Feedback

A patient attempting to relearn a skill needs frequent and immediate reinforcement regarding his success. When sensory-perception, synthesis, or cognitive processing is impaired, this will be especially important because he may not be otherwise aware that he has succeeded. If, for example, an individual is sorting cards in preparation for a game of cards, very clear statements, such as, "Good, you put the RED HEART (verbal emphasis) with the RED HEARTS" give him clear information that he has succeeded and reaffirms to his reintegrating nervous system the accuracy of what it has perceived. Feedback includes also correction of error: "Oops! You put a BLACK HEART with the RED HEARTS".

Feedback is equally important in the social setting. An individual may have difficulty perceiving the theme or meaning of a group interaction. Not only does the therapist attempt to place the individual in a smaller, less demanding group setting, she will pay close attention to and encourage the individual's appropriate response in the group. This may involve responding to his affect and not just his verbalization; i.e., "I see the smile on your face, Tom, and I can tell you enjoyed Mr. Barr's story as much as I did."

The therapist is engaged in a constant process of giving the patient feedback. She does this through her verbal and nonverbal responses to him, by her praise, her smiles, and frowns, and by the enthusiasm in her voice. The communication of genuine caring cannot be over-emphasized for its importance. Because of the possible loss by a brain impaired individual of the ability to perceive subtle messages, the therapist would be advised to "err" in the direction of paying special attention to the clarity and frequency of demonstrations of concern, regard, and approval.

Amplification

(Also called *highlighting*, Kent-Udolf, 1984.)

The therapist cognizant of this strategy will help an individual compensate for sensory losses, attentional, arousal, or cognitive problems by making stimuli louder or bolder, and by making the salient features of a problem more obvious. For example, a patient experiencing visual perception problems might be better able to attend to data by means of larger, thicker lettering or outlining. A patient with attentional difficulties may be assisted by the therapist's talking louder, or using more intonation in her voice. A patient with tactile perception problems may be able to dress himself more easily through the use of larger buttons or zippers.

The individual may become more aware of the important aspects of a living or social problem by the therapist's highlighting its significant features. For example, an individual might not understand why another patient has responded abruptly or angrily to him, or why his neighbors regard his dress as "odd." The therapist can assist by drawing his attention to the key aspects of his own behavior, and the key features of appropriate behavior.

One additional way that a given message is made more obvious is by the elimination or dampening of distracting messages. It is often appropriate for a therapist to select an environment (or create a place in the environment) that is especially quiet, or visually nonstimulating, and that is without the usual traffic of patients and staff, if the individual is to perceive the essential sensory messages in his activity.

Substitution

In substitution, one intact perceptual or motor system, or one intact behavior is substituted for another that is impaired. For example, an individual with visual agnosia may be able to enjoy the "talking books" available at libraries and on cassettes. An individual who can no longer wash and iron his own clothes may be taught to use the local cleaners. The successful use of substitution requires the therapist to be knowledgeable regarding the exact nature of a patient's deficient and intact processing system.

Substitution is also at the heart of many memory strategies (to be discussed) when visual or auditory messages take the place of memory.

Modeling and Physical Guidance

Especially in reteaching functional motor skills, the therapist may use modeling and physical guidance. If teaching a patient to tie a simple macrame knot, for example, the therapist would give directions, model, and if necessary, guide the patient's hands by placing her own on his and taking them through the scheme. She would do this hands-on guidance many times. She would then gradually provide less and less guidance until the patient could complete the procedure on his own.

As another illustration, an individual having difficulty finding his way around the treatment center might be guided by the therapist through a specific path many times until it was familiar. No new or alternate paths would be shown until the first one was clearly established. (The path might be made more obvious or highlighted by the addition of visual cues, i.e., red tape along corridors; once established, the cues might be removed.)

Brainstorming and Guided Search

Malec (1984, pp. 138-140) suggests brainstorming and guided search as a means to generate more potential solutions in problem solving. Frequently, patients with impaired brain function are stimulus bound in problem solving. That is, they can not get beyond the obvious aspects of a problem, or they cannot generate more than one possible solution to a problem. One patient, for example, verbalized concern regarding what she would do if Meals on Wheels would "forget" to bring her meal. The only solution she could come up with was "I'd call my daughter," but she then persisted with the fact that her daughter is "never home."

Through brainstorming, and with some prompting from the occupational therapist, she was able to develop two other possibilities: notify Meals on Wheels, or ask a neighbor for assistance. It should be emphasized these solutions were not obvious to the patient, as they might be to the reader, and by being able to essentially draw from her own information and come up with these alternatives, she was able to re-establish a significant cognitive link.

In *brainstorming,* there are three basic steps:

1. The individual is asked to generate as many solutions to a problem as possible. Any ideas, even the most ridiculous "off the top of the head" are encouraged. The therapist may have to pick up on words or gestures to bring the idea to fruition.
2. The therapist lists the ideas and reviews them with the patient. The most appropriate are either discussed or, if appropriate, may be attempted.
3. A decision is made to select the most effective one or two solutions. These may then be practiced (Malec, 1984, p.138).

A *guided search* may be used as a part of the brainstorming procedure. Through a guided search the patient is cued to help identify relevant information needed for problem solving (Malec, 1984, p. 140). For example, a patient unsure of who to call to ask for help might be asked "Who are your friends?" or "Who lives next door?"; or an individual uncertain of the day of the week might be asked "What activity did you do this morning? Bowling? Then is must be Monday, since Monday is the day on which the group goes bowling."

Generalization

Whether seeking to build work related, leisure, ADL, or social skills, it is essential that any skill learned in the context of therapy be able to be carried over into a wide variety of settings and contexts. The therapist conducting home care is in the best position to assure this occurs, but even she must be aware that her approval may be serving as a significant reward for behavior, and that once she discontinues treatment, other naturally occurring or intrinsic rewards must now be sustaining the behavior.

The therapist working in a hospital or clinical setting would frequently profit from a home visit in order to assist in ascertaining for herself the key features of the home environment so that these might be more closely approximated in the therapy setting. This concern regarding generalization is especially important because with cognitive loss there is frequently a reduction in the individual's ability to see the similarities in given situations. One way that generalization can be facilitated is to have a new skill practiced in a variety of similar settings. For example, a patient who has relearned to use a telephone might be initially taught on the clinic phone. He might then practice with a pay phone, or a touch tone phone. A patient regaining social confidence might begin with one primary social group, and then be encouraged to try out his skills in several group situations. The therapist might assist by pointing out the similar features and expectations across groups. Role playing and rehearsal in a therapeutic setting might begin with one primary social group, and then the patient might be encouraged to try out his skills in several group situations. The therapist could assist by pointing out the similar features and expectations across groups. Role playing and rehearsal in a therapeutic setting might also facilitate generalization.

Reality Orientation

Reality orientation is a term applied to an ongoing process, used especially with confused patients. While most often discussed in relation to nursing home care, it is appropriate for use with any individual experiencing cognitive dysfunction. Confused individuals are continuously reminded by the therapist of names, places, events, and temporal relationships (Holden and Woods, 1982, p. 156). Upon greeting the individual, the therapist says, "Hello, Mr. Barnes. I'm Mary and it's 10 o'clock, time for occupational therapy." During the therapy session, the patient might be reminded, "Let's look out the window. . . . It's snowing very hard today. . . what a cold Tuesday we're having, Mr. Barnes." The occupational therapist speaks slowly, clearly, and supplements her speech with nonambiguous nonverbal messages.

In order to assist in establishing orientation, calenders and clocks will be conspicuous in the clinic. Where at all possible, the schedule and routine will be rigidly adhered to.

In order to facilitate appropriate response, the therapist frequently encourages conversation around specific tasks or events. For example, rather than asking "What's new?" she might say, "I saw your daughter and you visiting in the day room today. Did you enjoy your visit?" In order to help the patient succeed, she may use prompting so a patient can give a correct answer; i.e., if another patient asks, "Did you watch that musical special on T.V. last night?" the patient might be prompted by the therapist who says, "Yes, Mr. Barnes, wasn't that Perry . . . " (allowing the patient time to complete his response).

An important aspect of reality-orientation is the interruption of confabulation and confused talk. To readdress a previous example, if a patient states incorrectly, "I had pancakes, eggs, and bacon for breakfast," the therapist might gently disagree, without diminishing the individual's esteem. She might say, "Well, I believe I saw oatmeal and fruit, but I can understand how one day might seem like the next." Another way of interrupting confabulation and perseverative talk is to interrupt the discourse and direct the patient to a specific subject in the here and now, and require a response: "Oh, Mr. Barnes, I see you have a haircut. Did you go to the barbershop today?" In some cases, the therapist may be able to ascertain an underlying feeling or concern that is in part generating the individual's discourse. She might then be able to respond to the feeling she discerns.

The reader wishing to know more about the use of reality orientation with individuals and in a group context is referred to Holden and Woods, *Reality Orientation: Psychological Approaches to the Confused Elderly* (1982).

Memory Strategies

Memory strategies are designed to (a) increase the likelihood a given message is perceived, (b) help in storing information in an easily retrievable form, (c) provide cues for retrieval, and (d) rebuild long term memory through repetition and association. The environment needs to be arranged in order to decrease distraction while maintaining necessary arousal. In some instances, memory of stimuli or of an event will be enhanced by the attempt to incorporate all (or many) senses. Thus, a patient will be instructed to not only see an object, but to touch, and even to smell it. Further, he may be asked to incorporate speech pathways, being directed to describe aloud what he sees and what he is doing. This multisensory approach is capable of providing extra sensory cues and extra associations for memory.

Repetition of a task many times during a short span (as in practicing a tennis swing) may serve to increase the likelihood of storage as long term memory. Events being remembered are more likely to be retained when the individual can make a meaningful association. Thus, the therapist may attempt to draw out these associations, i.e., assisting the patient to state aloud his memories or images which are being triggered by a task.

An individual may be taught to use substitutions for memory; he may be taught to make lists, put visual or written reminders to himself in conspicious places (or others may be asked to do this for him), and he may be taught to tape record or log important information for easier retrieval (Kent-Udolf, 1984, p. 56).

It has been found that memory losses with brain impairment are not usually recoverable. It is most often helpful to assist the individual in re-establishing associative links for functional information; i.e., the patient may be reintroduced to familiar objects with a multisensory approach in an effort to trigger intact memory pathways or rebuild memory associations. Further, the individual may be taught compensatory memory strategies, such as those cited regarding substitution, in order that he can function in his everyday world. It will not, however, be likely that he will again have what is called a good memory. This needs to be considered as he looks ahead to employment objectives.

Sensory-Integration

The sensory-integrative approach to the treatment of brain dysfunction is, in some respects, quite different than some of the preceding strategies described. The reader is referred to Moore (1980) for a more thorough discussion.

Recognizing the developmental progression of central nervous system control over activity, Moore emphasizes that subcortical integration precedes cortical. Many activities are done most smoothly when an individual does not "think" about them too much. The authors are reminded of attempts at skiing and learning to play tennis. It often appears that skiing (or tennis, or any number of sports) is accomplished quite easily until one tries, consciously, to think about what she is doing, perhaps in an effort to correct an error or improve her style. Moore uses the term "cortical overdrive" to describe this conscious interference with skill (Moore, 1980, p. 81). This same effect may be demonstrated in speech activity, when for example, one may be able to speak easily and comfortably until she consciously attempts to improve her delivery. This principle depends on the ability of subcortical brain centers to direct and automatize skilled movement without conscious (cortical) brain direction.

While most of the references previously cited have emphasized the corticalization of function, Moore suggests an opposite approach. Instead of giving a patient a verbal direction to do (or imitate) a specific activity, the patient is taken through the motor aspects of the task by hands-on assistance by the therapist. Rather than asking the patient to verbalize aloud regarding what he is doing, his conscious attention will be taken away from the task, perhaps by means of distracting stimuli or comments. This will be repeated until the action is "automatic."

While addressing the re-establishment of motor function, the sensory-integrative approach has powerful implication for the systematic retraining of all function. The therapist who expects to work extensively with organic impairment is advised to gain a further understanding of sensory-integrative theory and principles, as well as those professed by cognitive therapies, in order that she might compare them most judiciously.

Responding to Affective Changes

In working with the patient, the therapist needs to be aware of affective changes as influenced by the activity, environmental setting, and social process that provides parameters in which the individual functions. The therapist must be especially attuned to the necessity of providing an emotionally and physically safe, consistent, and trustworthy interactive and environmental framework for treatment. Essential in establishing this trust is the therapist's verbal and nonverbal congruence, genuineness, and regard for the individual. One must remember that simply stating "I want to help you or I care about you" may be quite insufficient when cognitive impairment has interceded. Consistent, caring behavior must be communicated through all means. While in-depth psychotherapy may be inappropriate, the brain impaired individual is always viewed as a person whose feelings and emotions are as important as anyone else's.

At times, the individual may wish to talk about his own emotional concerns. The therapist may be able to assist him by the following:

1. Helping him to clarify what he is feeling;
2. Validating his feelings and emotions as having worth;
3. Being perceptive of and responsive to nonverbal as well as verbal messages;
4. Providing alternate means of communication when verbalization is ineffective; and
5. Being patient in allowing the individual to gather and make concrete his own thoughts.

Many times the less medical, more functional aspects of the occupational therapy setting provide a naturally facilitating atmosphere in which, given the opportunity and encouragement, the individual will draw upon experiences, develop associations, and ultimately integrate important feelings.

The individual who is suspicious, angry, or uncooperative in treatment presents special difficulties. It is sometimes helpful for the therapist to:

1. Help the patient with reality orientation when perceptual distortions are at play;
2. Understand that some of this affect may be due to fright as the individual seeks to retain a sense of dignity;
3. Avoid touching the patient unless he indicates a desire for touch;
4. Approach the patient from a position and in a manner that will not surprise him;
5. Speak slowly, clearly, and be certain communication is understood;
6. Support the individual's efforts to realistically and reasonably exert influence over his own treatment;
7. Assure (and be sure) that the patient will not be allowed to be in a position to harm others;
8. Give maximal information to the patient about what you, the therapist, are doing and why; and
9. Provide the patient with opportunities for "time-out" from interaction or therapy.

The individual who is experiencing feelings of depression, loss, and grief is encouraged to communicate these feelings while being kept cognizant of the progress he has made or can reasonably expect to make.

The therapist may consider the following:

1. Avoid the oversoliticous "Everything will be all right";
2. Provide realistic information about function, dysfunction, treatment, and goals;
3. Provide the individual an opportunity for expression of sadness (this may need to occur many times, and in ways and in duration the patient can tolerate);
4. Validate the individual's right to his sadness;
5. Assist the individual to put words (or thoughts) to affective states and to actions when affect seems random;
6. Assist the patient in realistically assessing his losses (in order that these may be grieved) and in assessing his strengths (in order that these may be maximized);
7. Assist the individual in making memory associations with persons, objects, and events to facilitate the expression of grief;

8. Assist in values clarification when values need to be reassessed;
9. Provide avenues for closure (saying "goodbye" to a relationship, role, or skill) as needed; and
10. Listen carefully for suicide indicators.

When lability of affect, or under or overemotionality presents a problem, the therapist might be able to assist the individual by doing the following:

1. Moderating the environment to increase or decrease stimuli, as needed;
2. Assessing the (possible) calming effects of soft music, rocking in a chair, and other sensory-integrative variables;
3. Helping the patient become sensitive to his body's own cues regarding arousal;
4. Encouraging the patient to take time out from activity or interaction as needed (providing a place where he can do this); and
5. Breaking activity into smaller temporal units.

Whatever the affective state of the individual, it may be helpful for him to understand how the physical assault to his nervous system, as well as the psychological assault to his sense of self, has helped lead to the feelings he now experiences. In so understanding, he will hopefully be freed from the burden of believing his emotional states are due to his being a "bad person," a "selfish person," or a "crazy" person. When the individual has some context in which to understand his own emotions, he gains some ability to more successfully manage these feelings and incorporate them in a meaningful way. Without such a context, the individual may feel at the mercy of feelings that seem outside of himself; he may experience a loss of personalization as he views thoughts, actions, and feelings as without apparent cause, aim, or connection.

Chapter Summary

One can reflect here, that the "Founding Father of Psychiatry," Sigmund Freud, never gave up his belief that the secrets of the human psyche would someday be uncovered in the matter of the brain itself. To some extent, he may have been proved correct, with the stacks of any medical library attesting to the vast amount of information that has been gathered about the brain and its function. However, even with the information now available about discrete centers of mood and need, and chemical constituents of learning and memory, a great deal yet remains a mystery. In supporting a holistic framework as a basis for understanding brain function and response to dysfunction, we have encouraged the reader to consider a framework capable of integrating not only what is known about the brain, but also one that can flexibly accommodate what is unknown. At its heart, holism proposes that the "sum is more than the total of the parts." In terms of the brain, this means that what we call "consciousness," "purposeful behavior," and "personality" are not fully understood by dissecting the brain. Rather, they can best be appreciated as changing or fluid in their representation throughout a nervous system that is constant itself only in its vigilance toward the aim of making meaningful human experience.

Using holism also as a basis for rehabilitation, we cited examples of the brain's plasticity and ability to reorganize in response to trauma. We are not so naive as to believe that all patients with organic brain syndrome have deficits that are easily remediated or compensative (if at all), especially given the limitations of accepted parameters for length of care.

However, in our practice and that of our colleagues we have seen many organically impaired individuals whose quality of life was enhanced as a result of therapeutic intervention within the arena of psychosocial practice.

End Notes

1. Jung's hypotheses regarding the integration of a collective unconscious could be postulated as the acquisition of tacit knowledge by the celluar matter of the individual before his birth.

References

American Psychiatric Association: Diagnostic and Statistical Manual of Mental Disorders (DSM III) Ed 3. Washington, DC, American Psychiatric Association, 1980.

Atkinson R, Shiffrin R: Human Memory: A Proposed System and Its Control Processes. In Spence K, Spence J (Eds): The Psychology of Learning and Motivation. Vol. 2. New York, Academic Press, Incorporated, 1968.

Bara B: Modifications of Knowledge by Memory Processes. In Reda M, Mahoney M: Cognitive Psychotherapies. Cambridge, MA, Ballinger Publishing Company, 1984.

Benton A, Hamsher K, Varney N, et al.: Contributions to Neuropsychological Assessment: A Clinical Manual. New York, Oxford University Press, Incorporated, 1983.

Bower G, Hilgard E: Theories of Learning. Ed 5. Englewood Cliffs, NJ, Prentice-Hall, Incorporated, 1981.

Cohn R: The Person Symbol in Clinical Medicine. Springfield, IL, Charles C Thomas Publisher, 1960.

Craik R, Lockhart R: Levels of processing: A framework for memory research. J Verb Learn Verb Behav 11: 671-684, 1972.

Franco L, Sperry R: Hemispheric lateralization for cognitive processing of geometry. Neuropsychologia 15: 107, 1977.

Flavell J: Cognitive Development Ed 2. Englewood Cliffs, NJ, Prentice-Hall, Incorporated, 1977.

Flavell J: Cognitive Development. Englewood Cliffs, NJ, Prentice-Hall, Incorporated, 1985.

Gazzangia M: The split brain in man. Sci Am (August): 24-29, 1967.

Gazzangia M: The Bisected Brain. New York, Appleton-Century-Crofts, 1970.

Glees P: Functional cerebral reorganization following hemispherectomy in men and after small experimental lesions in primates. In Bach-y-Rita P (Ed): Recovery of Function: Theoretical Considerations for Brain Injury Rehabilitation. Bern, Switzerland, Hans Huber, Publishers, 1980, pp 106-126.

Golden C: Rehabilitation and Luria-Nebraska Neuropsychologial Battery. In Edelstein B, Couture E (Eds): Behavioral Assessment and Rehabilitation of the Traumatically Brain Damaged. New York, Plenum Press, 1984, pp 83-120.

Guidano V, Liotti G: Cognitive Processes and Emotional Disorders. New York, The Guilford Press, 1983.

Harris D: Children's Drawings as a Measure of Mental Maturity. New York, Harcourt Brace Jovanovich, Incorporated, 1963.

Holden U, Woods R: Reality Orientation: Psychological Appraoches to the Confused Elderly. Edinburgh, Churchill Livingstone, Incorporated 1982.

Horenstein S: Effects of cerebrovascular disease on personality and emotionality. In Benton A (Ed): Behavior Change in Cerebrovascular Disease. New York, Harper & Row Publishers, Incorporated, 1970.

Hutt M, Briskin G: The Clinical Use of the Revised Bender-Gestalt Test. New York, Grune & Stratton, 1961.

Kent-Udolf L: Functional appraisal and therapy for communication disorders of traumatically brain injured persons. In Edelstein B, Couture E (Eds): Behavioral Assessment and Rehabilitation of the Traumatically Brain Damaged. New York, Plenum Press, 1984.

King L: The person symbol as an assessment tool. In Hemphill B (Ed): The Evaluation Process in Psychiatric Occupational Therapy. Thorofare, NJ, Slack Incorporated, 1982.

Luria A: Restoration of Function After Brain Injury. New York, Macmillian Publishing Company, Incorporated, 1963.

Luria A: Higher Cortical Function in Man. New York, Basic Books, Incorporated (Consultants Bureau), 1966.

Luria A: The Working Brain. New York, Basic Books, Incorporated, 1973.

Lynch W: A rehabilitation program for brain-injured adults. In Edelstein B, Couture E: Behavior Assessment and Rehabilitation of the Traumatically Brain Damaged. New York, Plenum Press, 1984, pp. 273-312.

Malec J: Training the brain injured client. In Edelstein B, Couture E (Eds): Behavioral Assessment and Rehabilitation of the Traumatically Brain Damaged. New York, Plenum Press, 1984, pp. 121-150.

Miller R: Meaning and Purpose in the Intact Brain. Oxford, England, Clarendon Press, 1981.

Moore J: Neuroanatomical consideration relating to recovery of function following brain lesions. In Bach-y-Rita P (Ed): Recovery of Function: Theoretical Considerations for Brain Injury Rehabilitation. Bern, Hans Huber Publishers, 1980.

Najenson R, Rahmani L, Elazer B, et al: An elementary cognitive assessment and treatment of the craniocerebrally injured patient. In Edelstein B, Couture E (Eds): Behavioral Assessment and Rehabilitation of the Traumatically Brain Damaged. New York, Plenum Press, 1984, pp. 313-338.

Ornstein R: The Psychology of Consciousness. New York, W. H. Freeman and Co., 1972.

Rosenthal M: Strategies for intervention with families of brain injured patients. In Edelstein B, Couture E (Eds): Behavioral Assessment and Rehabilitation of Traumatically Brain Damaged. New York, Plenum Press, 1984, pp. 23-81.

Sperry R: The Great Cerebral Commissure. Sci Am (January): 142-152, 1964.

Strub R, Black F: Organic Brain Syndromes: An Introduction to Neurobehavioral Disorders. Philadelphia, F. A. Davis Company, 1981.

Sufrin E: Physical rehabilitation of brain damaged elderly. In Edelstein B, Coutrue E (Eds): Behavioral Assessment and Rehabilitation of the Traumatically Brain Damaged. New York, Plenum Press, 1984, pp. 191-226.

Toglia J, Abreu B: Cognitive Rehabilitation, unpublished manual in preparation for publication.

Walsh K: Neurophychological aspects of rehabilitation following brain injury. In Garret J (Ed): Australian Approaches to Rehabilitation in Neurotrauma and Spinal Cord Injury. New York, International Exchange of Information in Rehabilitation, World Rehabilitation Fund, Incorporated, 1982 (monograph #19).

Williams M: Brain Damage, Behavior and the Mind. New York, John Wiley and Sons, 1979.

Wolanin M, Phillips L: Confusion: Prevention and Care St. Louis: C. V. Mosby Company, 1981.

Chapter 10

The Suicidal Patient

The problem of suicide cannot be understood apart from the theoretical frameworks that have been summarized for the reader in this text. Depending upon one's theoretical orientation, suicide will be understood in terms of given compatible assumptions regarding the etiology of dysfunction, the general nature of man, and activity and remediation. However, the additional information in the following chapter is provided to help the reader become better acquainted with some of the general knowldege that has been gained across the social sciences in regard to suicide as a "special" problem.

Here, we treat suicide as a "special problem" because we have, in our work with students, found the suicidal patient to be one the new (and seasoned) therapist often responds to with trepidation. The information provided here may help the reader to use and appraise her own treatment assumptions, and may assist her in understanding and responding to the needs of the suicidal patient. We hope this information will be useful, regardless of the theoretical framework favored. We recognize that not every treatment guideline proposed in the ensuing discussion is equally compatible with all treatment frameworks. Where we create disagreement, we encourage the reader to engage in dialogue with colleagues.

At some point, the occupational therapist is likely to become involved with a person who is considering suicide. Professionally, this may occur not only with psychiatric patients, but also with individuals who are dealng with physical loss or limitations, as well as with family concerns. The therapist may be the first to recognize the suicide wish, or the patient may be in treatment because his suicidal depression is well known. It was the recommendation of the Center for Studies of Suicide Prevention, National Institute of Mental Health (Resnik and Hathorne, 1973, p. 3), and the belief of the authors that all individuals in health fields need to have "core" information regarding suicide: information that includes suicide theory, suicide predictors, and basic concepts of suicide prevention. Even if health professionals are not directly providing treatment to suicidal individuals, they need information regarding the resources available in their own communities — resources that can respond to the needs of the individual during the "crisis" phase, as well as afterward as a vehicle for support. The student who has not already done so is encouraged to participate in courses or seminars designed to enhance her understanding and skills in the area of suicide prevention.

Current Understanding of Suicide

Suicide is the deliberate self-inflicted termination of one's life. In contemporary literature, it is regarded as existing on one end of a broad continuum of what are termed self-destructive or life-threatening behaviors (Weisman, et al., 1973; Worden, 1976; Farberow, 1980; Maris, 1981; de Catanzaro, 1981; and Victoroff, 1983). Thus, while taking a gun to one's head is clearly self-destructive, one can discern also the self-destructive potential of forgetting to take one's insulin, if diabetic, or of drinking alcohol to excess. Many (but not all) patients who eventually make a clear suicide attempt have a prior history of self-destructive behavior (see end note 1). Many individuals who ultimately die of "disease" may, in retrospect, be viewed as having taken quite active steps to hasten their own death. While the discussion of suicide theory and prevention in this text focuses on the more obvious suicide behaviors and expressed "plans" to kill oneself, the therapist will undoubtedly encounter equally troubling instances of less clear, yet very self-destructive patterns in the patients for whom she cares. While it was once generally believed that no one tried to take their own life unless they were "mentally ill," that theme is no longer evident in contemporary suicide literature. Rather, the wish to die, even if it is a transient desire that is not well-developed, is conceived or experienced by most persons at some time in their lives. A suicide wish, even if well-developed, is not perceived as a sign of mental "illness" as such. However, when there are physical or emotional problems, the risk of suicide becomes much greater.

Suicide has been related to many emotional states: depression, anger, guilt, hopelessness, and apathy. Suicide and suicide attempts have been conceived as a wish to "sleep"; a wish for psychological "rebirth" (see end note 2); a way to become immortal; and a way to escape the unbearable. For a long time, the traditional Freudian psychoanalytical posture regarding suicide dominated the literature and generally dictated the treatment response. Briefly stated, Freud postulated that depression is a response to the loss of a significant love object. Loss of the object (loss may be actual separation from the object, or at lesser level, inability to be as dependent on the loved person as one wishes) elicits conscious or unconscious rage. This anger is turned inward against the self in an act of self-destruction (Shneidman, 1976, p. 10; Hendin, 1961, p. 183; Freud, 1949). Currently, less emphasis is placed on the role of hostility, while hopelessness and loss of self-esteem are given more focus. Further, as behavioral theory, existential-humanism, and social and cognitive psychology continue to impact suicide theory as well as general psychosocial treatment, they have significantly modified the view of health, stress, distress, and helping in response to suicide. Overall, there has been more emphasis given to the relationship of the suicidal individual within the whole social milieu; the patterns of coping by the individual in all areas of his life; and the conscious and cognitive components of the individual's actions (Weisman, et al., 1973, p. 18). Further, while not conclusive, information is being gathered about the biochemical changes in the human body that are related to states of depression and stress. Those substances of special interest include the neurotransmitter substance of the central nervous system, especially the catecholamines (norepinephrine and dopamine) and the indoleamine serotonin. The reader is referred to de Catanzaro (pp. 125-138, 1981), and Maris (pp. 180-188, 1981) for literature reviews in this area.

Above and beyond the personality aspects of suicide, which will be discussed, there are three psychosocial characteristics of suicide that bear directly on the understanding and prevention of suicide (Shneidman, 1976, pp. 10-12):

1. Suicide crisis is an acute, and not a chronic state, which is usually measured in hours or days, not months or years. While many individuals have a life history of self-destructive behavior, or make many suicide threats or attempts during a life time, the actual crisis that occurs when one seriously contemplates decisive action is either alleviated or else the person makes his attempt in a short period of time. This perspective on suicide as a "crisis" problem has significantly impacted the current approach to suicide across a variety of theoretical treatment frameworks. This is not to say that all suicidal individuals receive only brief, crisis treatment, for many suicidal individuals experience a suicide crisis in the context of general stress (physical or psychological) that involves them in long term treatment. Treatment which usually undergoes change in response to the crisis will focus definitely on the individual's present experiencing. The alleviation of intense symptoms is sought, success is nurtured, and frequently the therapist becomes more directive and parental (see end note 3).

2. The death wish is viewed by virtually all students of human nature as one of ambivalence. The paradigm of suicide is not merely a matter of "wanting to die or not wanting to," but rather one in which there often appears to be both a desire to die and a wish to live, or be rescued.

3. Most suicidal events are dyadic: that is, there is often a significant other person about whom the individual is thinking when he considers his own demise. This significant other may be someone whom the person wishes to make "take notice," or "punish," or someone whose burden he wishes to lessen. The significant other may be someone already dead whom the individual wishes to join.

Demography of Suicide

There have been innumerable attempts by suicidologists to correlate statistical or demographic data in an attempt to identify high risk individuals. All authors in this field emphasize that such demographic data may be accurate or misleading because (1) this data does not accurately reflect suicide attempts that have failed, and (2) many deaths that were in fact suicide are not identified as such. Suicide deaths are sometimes covered up by family members or members of the community because of the stigma attached to suicide, and because of the punitive laws (and insurance disclaimers) pertaining to suicide. The following data are frequently cited:

Sex: The most statistically significant and consistent differential in suicide rates is between men and women. The rate for men ranges from two to seven times greater than for women (Linden and Breed, 1976, p. 82).

Age: The second most significant, relatively consistent factor relates to that of age. The suicide rate of white males tends to increase consistently with age; the highest rate of suicide is among the eldest males. The suicide rate for white females increases until the age of 64, then decreases slightly thereafter (Linden and Breed, 1976, pp. 85-86). It should be noted that while still very low in comparison to other previously mentioned groups, the suicide rate of young people (ages 15 to 24, and 25 to 35 years) is increasing rapidly (Linden and Breed, 1976, p. 87).

Race: The suicide rate of Blacks is significantly less (less than half) that of Caucasians. While suicide rates for whites increase with age, the Black rate increases through ages 25 to 29, and then declines (Swanson and Breed, 1976, p. 107).

Social Involvement: Any factors that lessen social contact tend to increase suicide risk. These include death of spouse, living alone, emotional isolation within a marriage (Worden, 1976, p. 157), downward economic mobility, unemployment, and low participation in social groups.

Separation: A history of early (childhood) loss or recent loss of a significant other has been consistently correlated with suicide.

Health Factors: Poor physical or emotional health is correlated to an increased rate of suicide. This includes chronic or acute health problems, a history of emotional or mental disorder, and substance abuse. Alcoholism and cyclothymic (also called manic depressive) episodes have been especially implicated (Maris, Dorpat, Hawthorne, et al., 1973, p. 33; Robins, Gassner, Keyes, et al., 1959; Dorpat and Ripley, 1960; Worden, 1976).

Judgment: Anything known to decrease the ability of an individual to exert sound judgment increases the risk of suicide. Judgment may be diminished by high emotionality, loss of ego in the state determined as psychosis, cognitive dysfuncton, organic mental disorder, intoxication, and sleep or food deprivation.

Other factors known to correlate statistically with suicide include a family history of suicide and a history of previous attempts.

While the preceding may be of special significance to those attempting to identify high risk individuals, these findings should not be construed as a means of deciding whether or not an individual is going to succeed at suicide. When dealing with individuals in one's own practice, statistics may not bear out. Certainly, the emotional character of the individual to be discussed is of additional and critical importance. However, there are no "pat" profiles or statistics that can assure us that our patient will be safe from his own self-destruction. When his hopelessness is great enough by his own measures, suicide looms as a possibility.

Characteristic Emotion and Cognition of Suicide

Depression is very frequently referred to as the key emotion of suicide, but depression, as such, may be a misleading indicator. Severe depression, as exemplified by both physical and emotional lassitude, and associated with biochemical findings, may render an individual too lethargic to carry out a suicide wish. It may be with the lifting of depression and with renewed energy that suicide is attempted. There are other emotional and cognitive factors that emerge frequently (but not always) and should be highlighted. (Except where otherwise noted, these factors originate from Weisman, et al., 1973; Swanson and Breed, 1976, pp. 115-116; Shneidman, 1976, pp. 1-22; Beck, 1979; James, 1984; and Richman, 1986, pp. 49-68.)

1. Hopelessness: It is most often a diminished self-esteem that leads to hopelessness. Not only is the individual in a situation that seems unredeemable, as may occur with chronic illness, but he also frequently feels shame, disgrace, and "impoverishment of life itself" (Shneidman, 1976, p. 20). Especially significant is the impact of loss — loss of a loved one, or a part of the self, or self-esteem. A person who loses the ability to walk and holds no hope that this function will return may see suicide as a way out of a hopeless situation. When a loved one will not come back, suicide may be a means to escape that reality, or to try to force the other to realize how much pain he has caused.

Closely related to hopelessness is a disturbance in motivation. While the dynamics of motivation are subject to interpretation according to theoretical framework, it is evident that many suicidal patients are not unable to produce actions on their own behalf, but they no longer experience the desire to do so. Suicide preoccupation thus serves to be an immobilizing influence.

2. Rigidity: Frequently the individual committing suicide is regarded by others as relatively inflexible and unable to shift roles. He is unable to perceive alternatives, keeping himself in a mold that he blames others for creating. James (in Hatton and Valente (Eds), 1984) refers to this as "tunnel vision" (p. 48) and suggests that this rigidity may be a way for the patient to prevent being flooded with too many choices, and to keep from feeling fragmented and out of control.

Rigidity is often demonstrated in the thinking of the suicidal individual. There is a tendency toward polar or "dichotomous thinking" (Neuringer, 1976, p. 238); that is, the individual tends to think in terms of right or wrong, moral or immoral, always or never. When involved in activity, he may be able to see only task involvement as resulting in "success" or "failure," and not in terms of enjoying the process, or the opportunities for socialization it affords. Such thinking reduces the ability for effective problem solving, and especially for compromise.

3. Commitment: Many suicidal individuals have high goals or aspirations, be they occupational or relational. These expectations cannot be moderated, and when not met, lead to a sense of failure, which will be discussed later in this book.

4. Failure: The individual feels he has failed to live up to his own (often high) expectations,

and he can perceive no other standards as viable. Failure may be task related, i.e., being unable to hold down the "right" kind of job, or get into the college of one's choice. Failure in a simple task, for example, being unable to complete an occupational therapy project, may be viewed as a blow to the esteem as much as failure in a life task (i.e., gaining employment) when the individual employs idiosyncratic logic. Failure may also be relationship oriented, i.e., failure to be a "good" mother, inability to sustain the interest and attention of a spouse, or inability to engage with friends comfortably. Guilt is a frequent adjunct to failure. For example, the individual feels guilty because he feels he has disappointed others, or perceives himself as a burden to them.

5. Shame: The individual experiences shame when his failures are brought into the public arena. When one loses a job, or fails school, the failure is no longer private. This leads to a loss of self-esteem and a loss of pride. This sense of shame may be a distorted response in that the individual may assume that others have a negative opinion of him when they may not.

6. Isolation: Isolation may precede or become an integral part of the suicide picture. The person with few significant others in his life is already at greater risk. Additionally, with the loss of self-esteem and hope, the individual emphasizes to himself the relative "strength" and success of others and his own lack of significance. There exists also a kind of cognitive isolation in which the individual, even if with others, feels increasingly that "no one can know how I really feel" and "I am really different from everyone else."

What follows is increased withdrawal from others, which serves only to lessen the potential support others might give, and to reduce the opportunity for positive experiencing.

7. Anger: While anger does not necessarily "cause" suicide, there is often a great deal of anger experienced by the person who attempts suicide. This may appear as overt, acting out behavior, or may seem to be hidden. Anger may relate to shame, as when an individual makes the supposition, "Because I am angry, I am not worthy of being cared about."

8. Perception of time: Brockopp and Lester (1970), Greaves (1971), Binswanger (1958), and Neuringer (1976) have all studied the perception of time as it is experienced by the suicidal individual. They all concluded that suicidal individuals are more present oriented. These individuals find it difficult to project themselves into the future, and imagine "what would happen if." Also, Neuringer found evidence that time, in the present, is perceived by them as moving very quickly. The self-destructive person feels that his present condition is "changeless" over "endless" time, while the future is too far away to offer any hope (Neuringer, 1976, p. 244).

9. Idiosyncratic logic: The lack of logic or what might be better conceived as idiosyncratic logic has been frequently noted (see especially Tripodes, 1976, pp. 212-221; Neuringer, 1976; Alvarez, 1970; Beck, 1979, pp. 208-224; and James, in Hatton and Valente (Eds), 1984). What seems to occur often is that the decision to act out is made, and then the individual interprets all subsequent events as pointing to the validity of the decision. Tripodes looks at suicide notes as a means to better understand this logic. He emphasizes that frequently suicide notes dwell on issues or incidents, or cite as obvious concerns events which would be

regarded as irrelevent by others (Tripodes, 1976, p. 221). The individual writing the note describes himself as "different" from others and, therefore, feels that he should not to be evaluated according to common beliefs (Tripodes, 1976, p. 216). The individual inaccurately perceives a cause and effect relationship in which two events occur together (Tripodes, 1976, p. 218). The individual can not "de-center," or see how his perceptions and opinions are different from others, and tends to think in terms of absolutes, or else the individual tends to perceive all circumstances as having equal importance (Tripodes, 1976, pp. 220-222).

Alvarez also speaks about the "private logic" of suicide. As he discusses, suicide may become to the self an act of "success" where indecisiveness and powerlessness had before prevailed. It may seem to be an act of great power and control, despite the fact that it leads to an extinction of power. Perhaps where suicide is most difficult to accept by those left behind is when it is the choice of an individual whose life, by external measures, seems to be very successful. The person may have an internal belief that he does not deserve success or happiness, or success, as culturally defined, may seem empty and pointless to him. When there is no major obvious loss, yet there is a diminution of self and purpose in the eyes of the self, to the outsider the reason for suicide is beyond reason.

Crisis Model Within a Broader Treatment Scope

In general, suicidal intent or the act of suicide is seen as a response to a crisis in which the individual's perceptions about what is wrong with himself and his life are not countered by a belief that he can somehow change what he experiences as intolerable, or change his feelings.

We might think of living as something of a balancing act. On the one hand are life's demands as exemplified by personal and role expectation, losses and disappointments. On the other are life's rewards or "pluses" as provided by social contact and interpersonal sharing, personal satisfaction, accomplishments at work and play, increases in status, and joys. Balancing these is the individual's coping capacity. This includes, but is not limited to, his capacity for self-observation, insight, and judgment; his ability for perseverance; his beliefs about purpose; his values; and his repertoire of life skills (Fig. 10-1).

In a time of exceptional stress, coping capacity may be diminished, or may be perceived as inadequate to deal with all that life is demanding. When there is a loss of a loved one, or of wage earning capability, or of self-esteem, then not only do demands become greater, but personal resources may dwindle. How often and unfortunate it is that when we experience the loss of someone we love, it is they we identify as "the one person" who could help us. Added to this is a loss of coping capacity — perhaps due to fatigue, or emotional "burnout"; or perhaps due to a recent questioning of values and purpose. Also, the mediator — the part of the person that normally restores equilibrium — is ineffective.

It should be emphasized that the suicidal person is frequently an individual who has had or is currently identified as having psychiatric problems (see end note 4). Thus, many suicidal crises occur in the context of a broader treatment approach or preventative stance with the

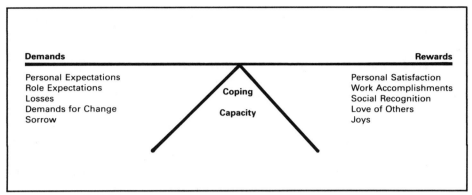

Figure 10-1. Suicide.

psycho-emotionally disturbed individual. Such an individual is one whose coping capacity has already been shown to be less effective, and often one whose demands and rewards are in a precarious balance.

It is becoming increasingly clear to health professionals that the now familiar crisis model is not sufficient to deal with suicide. Much more attention is being given to less intensive but longer term follow-up within the community to assist the individual to improve his quality of life, to increase his awareness regarding avenues of support, and hopefully to help the individual avert future crises.

Intervention

The occupational therapist may become involved in intervention at several levels. When the suicide crisis occurs with an individual who is already in a treatment program (for example, in an inpatient or community mental health setting), the occupational therapist would likely be involved as a member of the treatment team. This would also occur when the individual is brought into a short or longer term treatment program at a mental health facility, as a response not only to the crisis, but what is envisioned as a broader dysfunction. When the individual is a patient of the occupational therapist, but not within a psychosocial setting (as with home health care or physical-dysfunction treatment settings), the therapist's primary role in intervention would be to be alert to suicidal messages, to assist in clarifying that a suicide intent exists, and to guide the individual to appropriate treatment. (This will be covered in more detail later in this chapter.) When the individual receives crisis treatment only, as might occur through a crisis mental health program, the occupational therapist would less likely become involved. Many crisis centers, for example, conceive of crisis treatment as from one to six individual psychotherapeutic sessions with a staff counselor. More recently, attention has been given to the usefulness of providing community support groups and activities for the individual after the crisis has abated. Although the authors could find no discussion specific to occupational therapy in this regard, such community follow-up would seem to be a viable avenue for occupational therapy involvement.

Attempts to prevent suicide are aimed at picking up suicide messages; providing protection, when necessary; helping the individual more realistically assess his demands and alternatives; rebuilding self-esteem through successful experiences; rebuilding a supportive social network; increasing the individual's self-reliance; and increasing the individual's ability to identify and respond effectively to stress situations that trigger suicidal thoughts.

Ambivalence

One key ingredient in suicide prevention is the existence of ambivalence. Almost always, an individual will be personally ambivalent, even when the wish for death or relief is strong. There appears in most suicide wishes a strong contrasting instinct for survival. Suicide is not conceived of as an easy act to accomplish. Perhaps that is why many individuals contemplating suicide will talk about it, or drop hints, knowing that this increases the likelihood of rescue. While it is generally believed that most persons who commmit suicide wanted to die, the study of attempted suicides does not support this premise (Stengal, 1964; as cited by Worden, 1976, p. 135). Many suicide attempts and actual suicides are carried out with the thought "I don't care whether I live or die." Often, the emotional stress of the suicide attempt adds to the mental muddling that may well have existed before the attempt (Stengel, 1964; as cited by Worden, 1976, p. 135). Thus, ambivalence is compounded by confusion. This ambivalence "buys time" for would-be helpers. How much time is obtained is not always clear. The helping community must, however, make contact during this period, establish some trust and rapport, and impact on the individual enough that the decision is made by him to postpone any definitive self-destructive action and wait and see what happens.

It is not possible, at this writing, to know how many occupational therapists treat suicidal individuals, since treatment statistics tend to be gathered using other kinds of diagnostic and problem categories. In the authors' experience, suicidal individuals are encountered frequently by therapists working in psychosocial settings.

Psychoeducational Model of Treatment

Although not describing an occupational therapy program, Kiev (1976) offers a model of therapy for suicidal individuals that is compatible with the authors' and consonant with principles of occupational therapy across a variety of treatment settings and frameworks. As Kiev writes, "Personality changes do not come about in therapy sessions but in real life situations when patients are able to experiment with new ways of being and behaving. This is particularly true for those individuals with chronic difficulties in adjustment and getting along. For this reason, treatment moves most rapidly when patients can focus on concrete problems in work, at home or in interpersonal relationships" (Kiev, 1976, p. 471).

The authors are not suggesting that occupational therapy is a panacea for suicide, but in being offered an opportunity for active involvement, the individual has a chance to experience

335

himself more successfully and renegotiate some of his cognitive distortions. It must be reiterated that many patients who are suicidally depressed have an apparent problem with motivation. These are often individuals who avoid occupational therapy (and other forms of active engagement) because, as they say, they are "too tired" or "no longer interested" in accomplishing anything. Presuming the individual is in attendance within the occupational therapy setting, Kiev's guidelines (which he termed a "psychoeducational" frame) may be useful. In Kiev's model the individual is helped to:

1. Concretize goals;
2. Ascertain what is standing in the way of goal attainment;
3. Look realistically at the feasibility of goals. This includes a realistic evaluation of his own skills and abilities, and the availability of others;
4. Assess what can and cannot be changed;
5. Determine which of his own assumptions and patterns of behaving are standing in the way of positive change;
6. Establish feasible strategies for achieving goals, based on his own strengths;
7. Check to be certain that goals are ones that suit himself and are not tailored to imitate others; and
8. Check to be certain that goals are kept to a reasonable number.

Once treatment goals have been established, the individual is encouraged in pursuing these goals to:

1. Focus on present and daily events;
2. Look to himself, not others, for approval;
3. Avoid preoccupation with detail and overattention to mistakes. Such preoccupation tends to create tension or tedium;
4. Avoid comparing his performance to that of those around him;
5. Become increasingly self-reliant: self-reliance is seen as essential to self-esteem;
6. Look realistically at failure and "rejection." Tolerance for mistakes will be sought; and both success and failure will be judged by his own standards, not by the expectations of others. Relatedness to others will be encouraged, but the individual must realize that others have needs and demands that do not include him (Kiev, 1976, pp. 472-475).

As therapy proceeds and the crisis passes, the patient needs help in identifying and monitoring those visceral changes and situational events that tend to signal he is in a situation that feels overwhelming. For example, he might be assisted in identifying:

1. Bodily changes that signify stress, i.e., muscles feel tight, and the individual feels tired;
2. Problem situations that make him feel especially vulnerable, i.e., arguments with a spouse, loss of employment, and frustration during tasks;
3. Personal responses that indicate he feels overwhelmed, i.e., he starts to avoid normal social discourse, avoids calling friends, starts skipping classes, or calls in "sick" to work.

Maintaining the Therapeutic Relationship

An important aspect of the treatment process concerns the therapeutic relationship. There has been much written about the therapeutic relationship, and some discussion has ensued in this text. The therapeutic relationship is not different when working with the suicidal individual. However, there may be extra demands placed on the therapist.

The suicidal individual is often one who wishes to have a dependent relationship on another. He frequently looks to others for approval and nurturance; he sees them as having high expectations for him; and is frequently angry when others do not allow him the closeness and dependency he seeks. (With severe depression, this may at first not be apparent as the person may withdraw from others; however, the dynamics will often emerge later on in the therapy process.) It may be quite natural to encourage dependency when an individual is in great distress. In fact, when the individual is in severe crisis, appears out of control, or with limited ability for sound judgment, many professionals, across disciplines, take a parental, protective stance. However, such dependency, over any extended period, does not serve the best interests of the patient and tends to "wear out" the treatment staff. Being overly dependent keeps an individual from realizing his own strengths, keeps him from accepting responsibility for his own well-being, and keeps him in a very vulnerable position. The helping staff tend to become drained and frustrated, feeling that they have given all that they can. The therapist needs to realize that in fostering dependency, the ultimate message is not, as we might believe, "I care for you" (though well we may); but rather, "I don't believe that you can take care of yourself."

The individual wishing to be taken care of may intentionally (or unintentionally) use his suicide as a way to mobilize others around him. He can further keep them there by suggesting "If you don't take care of me as I have asked, I will kill myself," with the implied "And it will be your fault." At times, the staff will become angry, feeling controlled or manipulated. In response, they may push away an individual who has a genuine need for contact. It is for this reason that the therapist needs to work with the person to help increase his own sense of strength and resourcefulness; that she communicate her belief in his abilities; and that she help him to look more realistically at the extent to which she can meet his needs. This is written with the authors' full understanding of the excess demands that a suicidal individual may place on the helping staff, and with the realization that many suicidal individuals will choose to continue a needy and helpless posture in regard to others. It can be an advantage to work along with other staff in a team approach in order that the staff have the chance to gain support and a broadened perspective through their interaction with each other.

Another impediment to the therapeutic relationship may arise when the therapist is particularly uncomfortable with thinking or talking about death. She may, for example, tend to cut off any dialogue in this area. While there are particular instances of therapists refusing to talk about suicide with their patients (see end note 5), it is often held that the suicidal individual needs to be allowed to consider the ramifications of taking his own life, as he would consider any important decision (see end note 6). What is essential is that he look realistically at the decision, and not with a lot of distortions and fantasies about what would be accomplished. When the therapist's response to the individual's suicide talk is "Oh, let's not dwell on this; let's think about the positive" she may unwittingly increase his sense of isolation and further the cognitive distortion he has. The extent to which the therapist believes the patient should be allowed or encouraged to talk about his feelings will depend in part also on the theoretical treatment of her choice.

Most therapists agree that in order for an individual to experience himself in a more positive way, he needs to experience himself through active engagement. Further, most realize that the patient may well profit from a "break" from thinking about dilemmas that are not going to be quickly resolved. However, the therapist will need to balance this recognition with the realization that the exhortation to participate in activity may be misinterpreted as a demand to perform, and not entirely unlike the demands the individual already puts upon himself, or perceives that others put on him. Also, many suicidal individuals are not those who wish to talk about feelings, be they feelings about suicide, or any other kind of feeling. Rather, the suicidal individual may, as part of his increasing disengagement and isolation, be very uncommunicative. It is with this noncommunicative patient that the therapist will be particularly sensitive so as not to inadvertently "shut him off" and "shut him out" in her striving to involve him in therapeutic activity.

A third difficulty can arise in the therapeutic relationship that is often quite particular to occupational therapy. When the therapist fears the patient's suicide potential, she may be reluctant to allow him to participate in occupational therapy, the "domain" in which she has primary responsibility. Fearing that he might use occupational therapy materials to harm himself, or feeling that she is (in some settings) off by herself with a patient that she cannot effectively watch, she suggests that he not be allowed to come with the other patients to the clinic. She might offer instead to "bring some materials to the ward," or indicate that he can participate in occupational therapy after he has "stopped feeling suicidal." The result can be that the patient is more isolated, and has less opportunity to experience himself in a positive way. Also, the therapist has communicated her belief, "I believe you are out of control" or "I am frightened of being with you."

Certainly, occupational therapy settings tend to offer a myriad of potentially lethal materials. They range from machinery to toxic glues, and from kitchen knives to potential ropes. The material is there. If one resticts material, the list can become endless. It can be very frightening to think that a patient might use something acquired in occupational therapy to take his own life, and the instinct might be to restrict or prohibit his participation. However, it is hoped that the decision will be considered carefully. Occupational therapy offers an opportunity for the individual to begin to regain a sense of worth and mastery that he has lost. Monitoring media by making certain that all materials are accounted for before the person leaves the occupational therapy setting may be preferred. It often makes sense to ask a staff member to stay with the individual while he is in the occupational therapy setting — not just

The following may be useful

to watch him, but to provide support and encouragement during this stressful time. One may see this as a way of communicating, "I know you are having difficulty with self-control. I respect this, and I will help you with setting limits." In allowing the patient to participate in occupational therapy, the message is given that the therapist sees coping skills and positive potential that the individual may not see in himself; also, the individual is given the chance to re-establish social contact and useful re-engagement when the tendency may have been toward disengagement. While a severe suicide crisis may in some instances be judged as necessitating strong protective measures by treatment staff, when such "protection" lasts for weeks and months, the situation may need reappraisal.

Other Therapeutic Guidelines

The following may be useful as further general guidelines in dealing with the suicidal individual across a variety of treatment settings:

1. A patient may select indirect ways to tell you about his suicidal intent. It is difficult for many individuals to admit, even to themselves, that they are contemplating suicide. They may fear that if they tell you, you will judge them harshly, or reject them; or that you will try to stop them. However, as discussed earlier, there is often an ambivalence that also comes into play. This ambivalence may be acted out as hints; i.e., the individual communicates that he is finishing up family business or he will not start any new occupational therapy projects. Or, he may tell you "good-by" when you are unaware that treatment was to be terminated. A person drawing may show him fading into nonexistence, or engaged in a self-destructive act (see end note 7). A direct question, such as "Are you thinking about taking your own life?" is considered better than beating around the bush, and may help alleviate the person's anxiety as he wrestles with keeping his thoughts a secret (MacKinnon and Michels, 1971, p. 208). We do not give the person the idea of committing suicide by asking such a question. Certainly, he may answer "no" and may have other explanations for his behavior. But, we have communicated our willingness to continue to work with him in therapy, or to assist him in gaining access to the other avenues of treatment he might require.

2. If a patient tells you, even offhandedly, that he is considering suicide, take the remark seriously. The information needs to be shared with all involved health professionals. Again, the indirect or casual mentioning of the suicidal wish may be a reflection of his ambivalence. Do not assume that the individual has told everyone his thoughts; he may have selected you and only you to share this information with.

3. Know your community resources well and know the steps to make a referral. For referrals outside of your own agency:

(a) Be familiar with community mental health resources identified as specific to crisis intervention. These may include public facilities, private care therapists, and physicians. Have telephone numbers close at hand. If a patient is in distress and wants to walk out of a treatment session, this is not the time to be fumbling through the Yellow Pages of your telephone directory.

(b) Discuss with your patient what agency or individual you are referring him to and why you have selected this referral.

(c) Determine if the patient is able to follow through with the referral. If not, contact the agency or individual and set up an appointment. Identify yourself, your relationship to the patient, the patient, and his needs.

(d) Make sure the patient and the agency "connect." This may mean you or a designated other will accompany the patient to the agency.

(e) Follow up on the referral as is appropriate to the patient's needs and the policies of your setting.

(Summarized from Valente and Hatton, in Hatton and Valente (Eds), 1984, p. 110).

4. Play for time. Recognizing his ambivalence, try to arouse the patient's curiosity and interest, in order that he continues to postpone any definitive action while he sees where therapy might take him. Make provocative references to the next session, or the next person he will be seeing, references designed not to be coy, but to stimulate his curiosity and to concretize his image of himself as projected into the future (Beck, 1979, p.214).

5. Facilitate the expression and clarification of concerns. A patient who is very depressed often lacks the energy to talk about his feelings and concerns, and he may need much support and encouragement from all concerned to help him identify these. It is not just feelings about suicide that may need to be expressed, but concerns about all areas of the individual's functioning. If for example, he can talk about his fears of failure, his confusion about values, his concerns regarding losses of role, or esteem, there is more opportunity for him to clarify his own needs, and to renegotiate his own distortions. In occupational therapy, as the patient re-enters into active participation, the therapist may find it helpful to assist the patient to recognize his own feelings about himself "doing." This does not suggest that the individual must examine every one of his own actions, but that he have the opportunity to talk about and learn from his experiences. Expressing feelings may help to alleviate stress and may provide an opportunity for the following:

(a) Reduce his feelings of isolation;

(b) Allow you and others to provide emotional support and physical limits if needed; and

(c) Begin the process by which he can start becoming aware of alternatives for coping that may have been out of his awareness.

6. Ascertain the degree to which the following lethal "danger signals" are in play. These factors are considered indicative of increased suicide danger, for they serve to either (a) decrease the ability of the self to judge a situation accurately; (b) lessen the internal constraints that stop destructive action; or (c) indicate that a choice to act has been made and accepted by the individual:

(1) Distrust and withdrawal from significant others;

(2) Mental confusion;

(3) Use of drugs or alcohol (including overuse of medication);

(4) Extreme hopelessness;

(5) A history of impulsiveness, or current impulsive behavior;

(6) Family history of suicide;

(7) Paradoxic calm or sudden uplift in mood, indicating the decision to act has been made; and

(8) The existence of a specific plan (see 7 following).

7. Ascertain whether the patient has a specific plan to accomplish the suicide. It is believed that the person who has a specific plan is more likely to commit the act. However, there is twice as much at stake here. If the patient tells you his plans, at some future time this information may help you or others intervene on his behalf. For example, if he suddenly disappears from the treatment setting, you may have information about where he would go. If he tells you that he plans to drive his car into oncoming traffic, the treatment team may act to prevent his access to driving.

8. Let the patient know what you intend to do. While confidentiality is respected, the individual needs to know that you will not keep anything secret that he has told you if it is toward the end of aiding his suicide. He may get angry with you for this, but you must emphasize that his welfare is the most important issue. If you intend to limit his access to tools or materials, you need to let him know your reasons and under what conditions those restrictions will be lifted.

9. Help the treatment team and the individual assess his strengths and resources. Although this may not occur immediately in the treatment process, occupational therapy provides the patient a chance to get a tangible as well as intellectual understanding of his own situation — of his limits, coping skills, and resources. Given this, a patient may start to feel less confused and overwhelmed by his own difficulties. He may at least feel that he "has a place to start."

10. Communicate your belief that there is hope. This is not to suggest you be a Pollyanna; rather, that you communicate you see the patient as worthwhile, and you believe viable options exist that can prove useful to him.

11. Be aware that the suicidally depressed patient may be acutely sensitive to any perceived criticisms from you, or any perceived task failures. Try to keep the channels of communication and expression of feeling very open. This would be a time that structuring for success would be appropriate. Learning to deal with failure may need to be saved for the time when at least some equilibrium has been restored.

12. As the patient becomes able, help him explore alternative coping methods. As therapy progresses and the patient is more amenable to trying new behaviors, role playing may be useful. Help the patient identify personal and community resources, provide opportunities for task accomplishment, and eventually, for new ways to judge task "failure." Help identify how coping skills gained in occupational therapy are the same skills which will assist him to function in the everyday world. Be aware that the patient's pessimism and low esteem tend to block any easy access to perceiving alternatives. Do not allow yourself to be put off by this.

13. Be aware of the influence and interrelatedness of other patients. There are two main aspects of concern. A misguided patient or patients may be talked into "helping" the suicidal

patient gain access to restricted materials, or into helping him "cover his tracks." The other patients' dynamics and personal needs come into play, also. When one patient becomes suicidal, it may stir the suicidal thoughts of other patients and provide a type of permission for them to pursue their wishes. When there is a community approach to treatment, the issue of suicide becomes everyone's issue. Priorities may rearrange themselves in order to allow everyone a chance to explore their own feelings around this issue.

14. Be aware of your own boundaries, and communicate them clearly to the patient. Let him know when you will see him, and when you cannot. If an individual or individuals are designated as contact persons to be called on (i.e., by phone) after hours, encourage the patient to use the appropriate channels.

If a patient seems reluctant to end his therapy sessions with you, it may be helpful for you to alert him 10 to 15 minutes before time is up and ask if he has any issues he wishes to raise. It may also be helpful in establishing a sense of completion if you talk with the patient at the end of each session and summarize what he has accomplished.

Termination of Treatment

While the manner of termination and extent of follow-up will depend on the type of treatment program in which the individual has been involved, there have been significant findings that may influence programming.

In a study of clients at the Los Angeles Suicide Prevention Center, it was determined that approximately one half of those who commit suicide were "chronically suicidal," tending to be "needy," dependent, chronically depressed, and often chronic abusers of drugs and alcohol (Litman and Wold, 1976, pp. 530-533). These individuals tended to make frequent demands on the treatment staff, and eventually "wore out" staff who found them to be incessantly demanding. In response, the center developed a reach-out service that they called "Continuing Relationship Maintainance." This program was not considered therapy, per se, and was conducted by volunteers, who were supervised by paraprofessionals and professional staff. The individuals, post-crisis, were taught to use community resources, and met both individually and in groups to engage in supportive activities. Activities included both social activities and "active listening" by an attentive volunteer. This experimental program, in a manner consistent with the recommendation of the Center for Studies of Suicide Prevention, National Institute of Mental Health, emphasized the importance of the gradual "amelioration of self-destructive lifestyles" (Litman and Wold, 1976, p. 530) with less emphasis on the "active intervention to ensure temporary safety of the patients (Litman and Wold, 1976, p. 530). Follow-up studies of this program revealed that misuse of alcohol was very high in those who used this program, and that volunteers tended to "wear out" when dealing with these chronic alcohol abusers, thus suggesting some problems that would require further inquiry and possible program adjustments (Wold, in Hatton and Valente (Eds), 1984, p. 234).

While occupational therapy services were not discussed in this preventative program (no specifics regarding ancillary services were given), it would seem that the role in such a preventative program would be very viable for occupational therapy and consistent with the beliefs and aims of the profession.

Endnotes

1. "Self-destructive" refers here to behaviors that may lead to death and not to self-mutilating behaviors such as superficial cutting and burning oneself with cigarettes. These behaviors are viewed as having a different psychological purpose.

2. Klopfer (1961) discusses the Jungian perspective as one in which attempted suicide is viewed as a move by the ego to "start over" in a symbolic rebirth. This is not to be confused with a literal interpretation of rebirth through reincarnation. Although not cognizant of Jungian theory, some individuals known by the authors have, after a brush with death, described the feeling that they had been given a "second chance" and felt "reborn."

3. Therapists who follow a Rogerian, "nondirective" approach do not necessarily make the shift to a directive approach. They continue to believe in the essential health of the individual and to base their therapeutic actions accordingly.

4. In two often cited studies, Robins, et al. (1959) and Dorpat and Ripley (1960) investigated large groups of "successful" (completed) suicides. Using hospital records and talking to family members, associates, and physicians the investigators concluded that 95 percent to 100 percent of the individuals were "psychiatrically ill." Both studies especially implicated alcoholism and manic-depression (bipolar depression). More recent descriptions of practice have also cited schizophrenic process as a primary psychiatric problem correlated with suicide.

5. Some behaviorally oriented therapists might, for example, refuse to discuss the individual's suicide plans because they would perceive themselves as thereby giving attention to or rewarding suicidal thinking. As an alternative, they would give attention to any verbalization or other behavior in which the individual pursued matters pertaining to his own well-being and productivity.

6. Although this text will not delve into the ethics of suicide, there are differing views regarding the morality of suicide, views that are likely to surface and influence the response of the occupational therapist as well as other helping personnel. Whether or not the therapist sees suicide to ever be a reasonable solution will undoubtedly color the response she makes to an individual. The reader might consider the following:

(1) Can the decision to commit suicide ever be a healthy decision?

(2) Should an individual ever be allowed to take his own life, if the decision seems well thought out?

(3) How far should one go to protect a person from himself — to the point of depriving him of his rights?

(4) What if the individual is terminally ill? or chronically miserable?

(5) If the individual does not have the final word about his own life, who should?

(6) Who and what determines competence? Incompetence?

The interested reader is referred to Brandt (1976); Kastenbaum (1976); and Pretzel and Heilig, in Hatton and Valente (Eds), (1984) for provocative discussions of these issues.

7. The use of the Machover Figure Drawing Test as a screening device for suicide is described by Richman, 1986.

References

Alvarez A: The Savage God: A Study of Suicide. New York, Bantam Books, Incorporated, Random House, Incorporated, 1970.

Beck A: Cognitive Therapy of Depression. New York, The Guilford Press, 1979.

Binswanger L: The case of Ellen West. In May R, Angel E, Ellenberger H (Eds): Existence. New York, Basic Books, Incorporated, 1958.

Brandt R: The morality and rationality of suicide. In Shneidman E (Ed): Suicidology: Contemporary Developments. New York, Grune & Stratton, 1976.

Brockopp G, Lester D: Time Perception in Suicidal and Nonsuicidal Individuals in Crisis Intervention. Vol. 2, 1970, pp 98-100.

de Catanzaro D: Suicide and Self-damaging Behavior. New York, Academic Press, Incorporated, 1986.

Diggory J: United States suicide rates, 1933-1968: An analysis of some trends. In Shneidman E (Ed): Suicidology: Contemporary Developments. New York, Grune & Stratton, 1976.

Dorpat T, Ripley H: A Study of Suicide in the Seattle Area, Comprehensive Psychiatry. Vol.1, 1960, pp 349-359.

Farberow N (Ed): The Many Faces of Suicide. New York, McGraw-Hill Book Company, 1980.

Farberow N, Shneidman E (Eds): The Cry for Help. New York, McGraw-Hill Book Company, 1961.

Farberow N, Breed W, Bunney W, et al: Research in suicide. In Resnik H, Hathorne B (Eds): Suicide Prevention in the 70's. Rockville, MD, National Institute of Mental Health Center for Studies of Suicide Prevention. US Dept of Health, Education, and Welfare publication (HSM0) 72-9054, 1973, pp 45-80.

Fawcett J, Comstock E, Hendin H, et al: Priorities for improved treatment approaches. In Resnik H, Hathorne B (Eds): Suicide Prevention in the 70's. Rockville, MD, US Dept of Health, Education, and Welfare publication (HSM) 72-9054. National Institute of Mental Health Center for Studies of Suicide Prevention, 1973.

Freud S: Mourning and Melancholia. (1917) Vol. 4. In collected papers. London, Hogarth Press, Limited, 1949.

Greaves G: Temporal orientation in suicidal patients, Perceptual Motor Skills. Vol. 33. 1971, p 1020.

Helig S: A personal statement. In Hatton CL, Valente SM (Eds): Suicide: Assessment and Intervention. Ed 2. Norwalk, CT, Appleton-Century-Crofts, 1984, pp. 256-261.

Hendin H: Suicide: Psychoanalytic point of view. In Farberow N, Shneidman E (Eds): The Cry for Help. New York, McGraw-Hill Book Company, Incorporated, 1961, pp 181-192.

James N: Psychology of suicide. In Hatton CL, Valente SM (Eds): Suicide: Assessment and Intervention. Ed 2. Norwalk, CT, Appleton-Century-Crofts, 1984, pp. 33-53.

Kastenbaum R: Suicide as the preferred way of death. In Shneidman E (Ed): Suicidology: Contemporary Developments. New York, Grune & Stratton, 1976, p 421-441.

Kiev A: Crisis intervention and suicide prevention. In Shneidman E (Ed): Suicidology: Contemporary Developments. New York, Grune & Stratton, 1976, pp 445-478.

Klopfer B: Suicide: The Jungian point of view. In Farberow N, Shneidman E (Eds): The Cry for Help. New York, McGraw-Hill Book Company, Incorporated, 1961, pp 193-203.

Linden L, Breed W: The demographic epidemiology of suicide. In Shneidman W (Ed): Suicidology: Contemporary Developments. New York, Grune & Stratton, 1976, pp 71-98.

Litman R, Wold C: Beyond crisis intervention. In Shneidman E (Ed): Suicidology: Contemporary Developments. New York, Grune & Stratton, 1976, pp 525-546.

MacKinnon R, Michels R: The Psychiatric Interview in Clinical Practice. Philadelphia, W. B. Saunders Company, 1971.

Maris RW: Pathways to Suicide: A Survey of Self-destructive Behaviors. Baltimore, Johns Hopkins University Press, 1981.

Maris R, Dorpat T, Hathorne B, et al: Education and training in suicidology for the Seventies. In Resnik H, Hathorne B (Eds): Suicide Prevention in the Seventies. Bethesda, MD, National Institute of Mental Health, 1973.

Neuringer C: Current developments in the study of suicidal thinking In Shneidman E (Ed): Suicidology: Contemporary Developments. New York, Grune & Stratton, 1976, pp 229-252.

Pretzel P: A personal statement. In Hatton CL, Valente SM (Eds): Suicide: Assessment and Intervention. Ed 2. Norwalk, CT, Appleton-Century-Crofts, 1984, pp 249-255.

Resnik H, Hathorne B (Eds): Suicide Prevention in the 70's. Rockville, MD, National Institute of Mental Health Center for Studies of Suicide Prevention. US Dept of Health, Education, and Welfare publication No. (HMS) 72-9054, 1973.

Resnik H, Hathorne B: The challenge of the Seventies. In Resnik H, Hathorne B (Eds): Suicide Prevention in the 70's. Rockville, MD, National Institute of Mental Health Center for Studies of Suicide Prevention. US Dept of Health, Education, and Welfare publication No. (HMS) 72-9054. 1973.

Richman J: Family Therapy for Suicidal People. New York, Springer Publishing Company, Incorporated, 1986.

Robins E, Gassner S, Kayes J, et al: The Communication of Suicidal Intent: A Study of 134 Consecutive Cases of Successful (Completed) Suicides. Am J Psychiatry 115: 724-733, 1959.

Shneidman E: Current overview of suicide In Shneidman E (Ed): Suicidology: Contemporary Developments. New York, Grune & Stratton, 1976, pp 1-22.

Swanson W, Breed W: Black suicide in New Orleans. In Shneidman E (Ed): Suicidology: Contemporary Developments. New York, Grune & Stratton, 1976, pp 99-128.

Stengel E: Suicide and Attempted Suicide. Baltimore, Penguin Books, Incorporated, 1964.

Tripodes P: Reasoning patterns in suicide notes. In Shneidman E (Ed): Suicidology: Contemporary Developments. New York, Grune & Stratton, 1976, pp 203-233.

Valente SM, Hatton CL: Intervention. In Hatton CL, Valente SM (Eds): Suicide: Assessment and Intervention. Ed 2. Norwalk, CT, Appleton-Century-Crofts, 1984, pp 83-148.

Victoroff V: The Suicidal Patient: Recognition, Intervention, Management. Oradell, NJ, Medical Economics Company, Incorporated, 1983.

Weisman A, Feifel H, Henley C, et al: Death and self-destructive behaviors. In Resnik H, Hathorne B (Eds): Suicide Prevention in the 70's. Rockville, MD, National Institute of Mental Health Center for Studies of Suicide Prevention. US Dept of Health, Education, and Welfare publication No. (HMS) 72-9054, 1973, pp 13-22.

Wold C: The chronically suicidal person. In Hatton CL, Valente SM (Eds): Suicide: Assessment and Intervention. Ed 2. Norwalk, CT, Appleton-Century-Crofts, 1984, pp 230-237.

Worden J: Lethality factors and the suicide attempt. In Shneidman E (Ed): Suicidology: Contemporay Developments. New York, Grune & Stratton, 1976, pp 131-162.

Additional Readings

Bellak L: Intensive brief and emergency psychotherapy. In Grinspoon L (Ed): Psychiatry Update. Vol.III. Washington, DC, American Psychiatric Press, Incorporated, 1984.

Gaylin W (Ed): The Meaning of Despair. New York, Science House, 1968.

Chapter 11

Conclusion

As we come to the end of our journey, we are aware of the wealth of information that exists, the alternative frames of reference that are applied in practice, and the concerns and questions posed by educators, clinicians, and students as they look toward their future practice in psychosocial occupational therapy.

When one completes a journey, he reflects on his travels, and within the context of the entire journey may highlight what he has seen and learned; reflect on meaningful sights, events and personal encounters; and often becomes aware of how he has changed since his journey began. Thus we will take this opportunity to reflect on our journey, to respond to some of the criticisms leveled at multiframework approaches to education and practice, and to suggest from our own perspective what is gained from a broadly based development of knowledge. We will summarize the psychosocial occupational therapy process that exists regardless of the framework applied, and note the potential value of activity as therapy, as well as the limitations of occupational therapy as a profession contributing to contemporary mental health care.

Multiframeworks for Education and Practice

Occupational therapy resides in the realm of applied science, and each of the frames of reference included in this text have had a dual task. First, each must select and organize information and provide logical and internally related assumptions judged to be essential in understanding how man engages with persons, objects, and events to achieve meaning, identity, and purpose in his life. Second, each frame of reference must state how this understanding of the man-activity relationship can be applied in the context of therapy to promote an individual's well-being. These frames of reference often (but not always) include statements about:

1. Criteria for selecting information into the framework;
2. The nature of man — including the relative relationship of biological, psychological, and social-cultural forces;
3. The person's relationship to his environment;
4. The nature, purpose, and organization of activity as it enables persons to achieve meaning;
5. The nature of motivation — including the relative importance of internal and external determinants;
6. What constitutes optimum function;
7. What constitutes dysfunction;
8. The conditions (internal or external) believed to promote and sustain optimum function;
9. The means, tools, and criteria for assessing function/dysfunction;
10. What constitutes therapy — including areas identified for remediation, goals, and expectations for therapist and patient;
11. Therapeutic principles for implementing treatment;
12. The suitability of the framework to designated patients or clients; and
13. Recommendations and parameters for research.

Each frame of reference described in this text places a different emphasis in addressing these issues, and not all issues are treated by each with the same clarity, or conceived as having equivalent importance. That each of the frameworks is far from complete is evidenced by the relatively vague development of and lack of empirical support for many of the theoretical assumptions upon which the individual frameworks lie, and on the very limited research regarding the efficacy of treatment.

However, each frame of reference does serve an important function, as it acts as a "pair of glasses," providing a unique perspective on man, activity, and therapy. Recognizing that no therapist, indeed no individual, can at any given time attend equally to every aspect of the human condition, the frame of reference helps the therapist determine what is most important as she plans, implements, and evaluates treatment. Towards this end, each of the frameworks in this text can act as a basis for further, and much needed, exploration and study; and each, we believe, adds to the knowledge occupational therapy has as a profession about how man achieves purpose through his investment in activity, and how activity can best be utilized as therapy.

If, as we contend, all of the frameworks in this text are useful, we need to pause and clarify, "Useful to whom?" As authors, our supposition throughout this text has been that adult psychosocial occupational therapy is concerned with serving a broad spectrum of adults. This supposition is challenged, by Allen, in her elucidation of cognitive therapy and by some proponents of the occupational behavior frame of reference. While coming to some very different conclusions, these theorists propose in common three general beliefs:

(1) Occupational therapy has too much knowledge or irrelevant knowledge. The knowledge needs to be confined to a more manageable amount;

(2) Theoretical development in and the practice of occupational therapy should be restricted to one frame of reference; and

(3) Occupational therapists treat primarily the "chronically" disabled, and should be most concerned as a profession with meeting the needs of the "chronic" patient.

Here we can respond to these three assumptions but briefly, on the hope that we stimulate critical thinking.

(1) In response to the contention that occupational therapy has too much knowledge, we would only wish to reiterate that it is the role of a frame of reference to select and organize information to keep it from being unwieldy. No one person is expected to be expert in all frameworks, or to have a depth of information in all frames. If one looks at the relative lack of research, the only limited availability of program descriptions and case studies in the literature, and the as yet vague development of many theoretical and practice oriented premises, one could argue that occupational therapy has many areas of knowledge deficit.

(2) Should occupational therapy then limit itself to development and practice within the confines of a single frame of reference? We believe that no one frame of reference has proven more legitimate for understanding the man-activity relationship, or has been more helpful when applied within the context of patient care. It is not just the lack of rigorous and broad empirical evidence, but it is also the denial of individual difference and the limitation of individual preference and option that is a concern. Stated simply, in looking about in everyday practice, we see that given patients seek and profit from different emphases in practice as a result of their own unique needs and preferences. Some patients are concerned strictly with tangible results, and find stringently applied behavioral programs a helpful vehicle for monitoring their own success. Others desire by their own account to "know themselves better." These are the patients who engage the therapist in "how" and "why" questions, who endeavor to clarify their own motives, or who find self-expression in media to be a legitimate and helpful endeavor. The individual who needs to learn more self-control may be contrasted with the individual whose over-control renders him ineffective and anxious. Some individuals can learn from activity without any need to verbalize about it; others learn more readily when they can talk about the activities in which they have participated. Some individuals lack physical ease, and move about in a manner that appears stiff and overprotective; others display physical ease, but disregard social mores. Not surprisingly, therapists also bring to therapy their own strengths, limitations, interests, values, and needs; and as a result, they are often much more at home within one frame of reference than another.

Thus far, no one frame of reference has been able to attend to all treatment challenges with comparable effectiveness, and it seems unlikely any will in the forseeable future.

If, as some suggest, we put all our professional "eggs in one basket" and attempt to develop one framework to the extent that it addresses "all" the needs of all our patients, will we unwittingly move away from our commitment to the individualization of care? Is individualization of treatment a priority? If, in fact, one frame of reference could be developed to the status of a paradigm, is it so evident which would best serve this function?

We have in this text indicated both contributions and limitations of all the frameworks discussed. But, beyond this, we have tried to present the frameworks in a positive light. It does not appear to us that occupational therapy is so well grounded in psychosocial practice to suggest that now is the time to close our doors on avenues of learning. Where theoretical frameworks are presented with an emphasis only on what they fail to do, then they are unlikely to generate interest or development. Further, the notion is often promulgated that one can learn only from those things which fit nicely with his own biases; and often, critical thinking suffers. We believe that any student of occupational therapy, as well as the seasoned professional, profits from being cognizant of the key premises of all the frames of reference that exist in psychosocial practice. Given this, the individual has a means to compare and critique theoretical assumptions, and a basis to choose for herself the framework in which she will go beyond the general and seek expertise.

(3) Finally, we address the proposal that occupational therapy should be primarily concerned with meeting the needs of the "chronic" patient. What constitutes criteria for chronicity, and perhaps more important, why and in what way the preparation to meet the needs of the chronic patient should be different than that preparation needed to serve the needs of the more general population is not clear. If, however, in their education we prepare our new therapists to deal only with a select population, then obviously, their skills will only be in this area of treatment, and our statistics will show that these are the patients occupational therapy serves. Given the uncertain and ever-changing nature of public health needs, is this the preparedness we want in order to meet the health needs of the 1980s, 1990s, and beyond? If indeed, the profession determines that it will henceforth specialize in the treatment of a select patient population, then we all must recognize that at that point occupational therapy has defined itself in a new way.

While we propose that all frameworks offer a legitimate girder for therapy, we all are well aware of the need for occupational therapists in psychosocial practice to better clarify and document their contribution in patient care. This is parallel to the need within the broader mental health community to better determine what it can and cannot offer the populace.

For all the theories and alternatives in mental health practice, many patients make no demonstrable progress — neither in our nor their estimation. The treatment of psychosocial problems is by no means the exact science anyone might hope it to be. Even where we can predict likelihood, or trends in macrostructures of behavior, we cannot make any one patient profit from his participation in therapy. However, we have seen in the work of our colleagues, in clinics, and research endeavors, and have found in the literature, treatment programs representative of all the frameworks discussed in this text, and professionals who are committed to further development of theoretical and practice principles within their area of expertise. While we as a profession will assuredly wish to encourage therapists to venture out and look creatively at what may prove to be new, as yet unconceived ways for conceptualizing therapeutic activity, we must not cease to support and encourage all those individuals who continue to learn within their chosen domain. Rather, we must enhance the opportunity for all these individuals to develop knowledge, assess it critically, and communicate their learning.

Psychosocial Occupational Therapy

Whatever the frame of reference chosen, the occupational therapy process in psychosocial practice has consistent boundaries which identify and define psychosocial occupational therapy. These boundaries are: (1) purposeful activities; (2) an occupational therapist who is knowledgeable of psychosocial theories, activity analysis, and occupational therapy theory; effectively uses her interpersonal skills to work with patients and colleagues; and implements occupational therapy services within the guides of an ethical code; (3) a patient who seeks to change what he knows, what he does, how he does it, the satisfaction he gains, his participation and control within his environment or the quality of life that he experiences; and (4) an environment that has available given (but not unlimited) resources which support the patient in his quest for change, and an environment that sanctions certain behaviors. Using these boundaries, the authors define psychosocial occupational therapy as follows:

Psychosocial occupational therapy is a major rehabilitation service, based in theoretical principles that emphasize the role that activity has in the development of personhood and the achievement and maintenance of optimum well-being. Psychosocial occupational therapy principles are compatible with many theories within psychology, sociology, education, and rehabilitation. Within the theoretical framework, the occupational therapist and patient work together to assess the patient's level of function (physical and psychosocial) within the environment, to target areas needing change, and to implement intervention which will utilize the patient's abilities and promote competent function in his environment. *Competent function* indicates that the patient has adequate knowledge, skills, and attitudes to function in his environment, to communicate effectively, to meet his daily needs, to contribute to his community, to participate in recreation and be renewed for work and maintain health, and to use his time meaningfully, efficiently, and effectively. Change in function is brought about through the dynamic interaction between the therapeutic activity, the patient, and the therapist within his environment.

We can look further at the components of this definition as we summarize what has been posited by the frameworks for therapy discussed in this text.

Activity as Therapy

The choice of activity and the manner in which activities are used by the occupational therapist to promote growth and to facilitate change in function is determined by the frame of reference chosen. Regardless of the theoretical framework, the authors feel that the effectiveness of an activity is determined by the context in which it occurs. That is, activity becomes meaningful because of the interaction between patient, therapist, activity, and the environment.

In this text, therapeutic activities are identified as being capable of serving one or more of the following functions:

    1. As a bridge to the community;

2. As a catalyst for social, vocational, recreational, or task related interaction;
3. As a means for expression;
4. As enabling the creation of an end-product by the patient;
5. As a desired behavioral outcome;
6. As a reinforcer of behavior;
7. As a tangible indicator of progress;
8. As a means to master developmental tasks;
9. As a means to assess the individual's knowledge, skills, beliefs, and values;
10. As a way to achieve meaning or purpose;
11. As a vehicle for trying out or practicing roles or different facets of selfhood;
12. As a means to increase competent function and help the individual to achieve a realistic sense of control within his environment;
13. As the tools and outcome of the education process;
14. As occupation;
15. As corrective learning experiences;
16. As a focus for dialogue; and
17. As a means to engage the "whole" person in a way that is satisfying for him, optimizes his physical and emotional well-being, and helps to prevent "dis-ease" and disability.

Roles of the Occupational Therapist

The role of the occupational therapist also depends upon the frame of reference within which she operates, the environment in which she works, the focus of the treatment/health setting, the needs of the patient, the purpose (function) of the activity, and the desired treatment outcome.

As identified in this text, the occupational therapist has multiple role choices: educator-facilitator, motivator, teacher, trainer, role model, participant-observer, observer, resource, or supporting agent. Regardless of the role she assumes, the therapist establishes and maintains a therapeutic relationship based upon understanding, open communication, and a valuing of change. In this relationship, the therapist facilitates an interactive process between the patient, the activity, and the environment and assures the patient that she offers a safe, and caring environment which will assist the patient to "risk" change.

The Patient in Occupational Therapy

The frame of reference chosen influences the therapist's view of the patient's level of function as well as determines what will be conceived as the optimum or desired level of function for each patient. In this text, the view of the person and his behavior is described within the context of particular theories, and guides are provided to determine function or dysfunction.

The patient in occupational therapy need not be labeled or categorized by a diagnosis in order for the determination to be made that occupational therapy services are needed. The patient's knowledge, skills, and attitudes, and how these influence his function in his environment are the focus of occupational therapy evaluation and treatment. The therapist asks: Does the patient have knowledge and skills needed to function competently in his environment? Does he use his knowledge and skills toward an effective outcome? Can he make use of available resources when his level of skill or information base is inadequate? What are his beliefs about himself and others? Does he feel in control and competent?

Dynamic Interaction in Occupational Therapy

The term "dynamic interaction" connotes change in the relationship between patient, therapist, activity, and the environment as each of these four elements constantly influences the other.

This interaction will influence the assessment and treatment services that the occupational therapist provides. The interaction in assessment promotes "purposeful inquiry" to gather data that identifies the patient's physical or psychosocial level of function in his environment. This data is used to determine short term and long term goals, to identify expected functional outcomes, and to evaluate the efficacy of treatment. The data may be used to compare the patient's performance to a norm, or may identify and measure the individual's function according to particular performance criteria. Aware of this dynamism, the therapist frequently reassesses treatment goals and is open to making treatment changes that are responsive to her patient's changing needs.

During treatment, the interaction between patient activity and therapist can occur in individual or group situations, and it provides experiences through which the patient can (1) gain knowledge and skills, (2) practice skills and problem solving, (3) develop coping patterns, (4) learn more about his abilities and limitations, (5) better learn the rules for social interaction and role performance, and (6) become more independent.

Theoretical Principles

In this text, the frames of reference provide the guidelines for understanding patients and determining how to use activities to assess function and produce the desired treatment outcome. Thus, the theoretical principles or assumptions of each frame of reference are capable of guiding or of influencing the dynamic interaction that exists in the occupational therapy process.

The theoretical assumptions listed with each frame of reference in this text are compatible with or within the guides of the broader principles that underlie psychosocial occupational therapy. Those emphasized in this text include:

1. The patient is an individual who needs and is capable of change.
2. The therapist's primary and guiding concern is the well-being of her patient and the needs he experiences within his milieu.
3. Occupational therapy practice is based within identified theoretical and practice frameworks.
4. Occupational therapy is a dynamic process in which therapist, patient, and activity

interact within and with the environment, and none of these can adequately be understood in isolation.

5. Occupational therapy uses a combination of tasks and dialogue to facilitate change.
6. Occupational therapy experiences are designed to promote the maintenance or improvement of function.
7. The occupational therapist is concerned not only with remediation of function, but also the maintenance of health and the prevention of further (or future) disability.
8. The individual is understood as an integrated biopsychosocial "whole" whose health care needs must be addressed accordingly.
9. In practice, occupational therapy activities are graded to adapt to the developmental and functional needs of the patient and the resources and demands of the environment.
10. Participation in activity provides a means by which the individual can improve his skills, broaden his knowledge base, perceive himself in a more positive way, and become better prepared to meet the expectations of his tomorrow.

The Promise: The Reality

This book has been about the potential of therapeutic activity in bringing about positive change for the individuals whom we serve. This potential may in a sense be thought of as the "promise" of occupational therapy. In actual practice, the promise has not always come to fruition, and occupational therapy, as well as the mental health care of which it is a part, must be accountable. The following are some of the concerns and problems confronting occupational therapy in psychosocial practice:

1. The concept of "activity as therapy" is a tremendously broad and inclusive one. Therapists engaged in practice, education, and research must grapple with determining which human "activities" are the legitimate vehicles for occupational therapy intervention, and which are the primary concern of other helping disciplines.
2. Occupational therapy is conceived of as both an "art" and a science. The profession as a whole and the individual in practice, education, or research must find a way to respect and integrate both aspects of the therapy process.
3. The theory and practice of occupational therapy is poorly understood by the health community, by the public, and by third-party payers. Ask even the enthusiastic occupational therapy student to describe her chosen field, and the lack of clarity quickly becomes evident. One result is that occupational therapy has varying and often limited support within the mental health care community, and there exists reluctance on the part of third-party payers to reimburse occupational therapy services. Contributing to this dilemma, and at the same time resulting from it, there exists only limited research in support of the practice of occupational therapy.
4. As evidenced in the literature, there are multiple assessment instruments. However, very few of them have reliability and validity standards. This compounds the problem

experienced by the professional in her need to clarify and document what occupational therapy can reasonably be expected to accomplish.

5. The desire to clarify and better manage the parameters of therapy have led some educators, clinicians, and students to limit the theoretical assumptions and practices subsumed within occupational therapy. Lacking a sound research base, it becomes very difficult (perhaps impossible at this point) to assess which theoretical assumptions and practices should be excluded.

It has been our perception that in its desire to be responsive to changes in the health care system, occupational therapy has had a tendency to move quickly from one "bandwagon" to another. We must, we feel, strike a balance between the need to be both responsive and also pro-active in our service to the public, with the need to be diligent and patient in developing and testing the assumptions we purport. We must educate ourselves before we can educate others in what is not only the promise but the benefit of occupational therapy.

Appendices

Appendix A
Principles of Occupational Therapy Ethics

Adopted April 1977; Adopted, Revised, April 1979

PREAMBLE:

The American Occupational Therapy Association (AOTA) and its component members are committed to furthering man's ability to function fully within his total environment. To this end the occupational therapist renders service to clients in all stages of health and illness, to institutions, other professionals, colleagues, students and to the general public.

In furthering this commitment the American Occupational Therapy Association has established the Principles of Occupational Therapy Ethics. The Principles are intended for use by all occupational therapy personnel, including practitioners in all settings, administrators, educators, and students. Licensure laws and regulations should reflect and support these Principles which are intended to be action oriented, guiding and preventive rather than negative or merely disciplinary. The Principles, likewise, should influence the consulting, planning, and teaching of occupational therapists.

It should be noted that these Principles are intended only for internal use by the American Occupational Therapy Association as a guide to appropriate conduct of its members. The Principles are not intended to define a standard of care for patients or clients of a particular community.

Professional maturity will be demonstrated in applying these basic Principles while exercising the large measure of freedom which they provide and which is essential to responsible and creative occupational therapy service.

For the purpose of continuity the following definitions will support information in this document: Occupational therapist includes registered occupational therapists, certified occupational therapy assistants, occupational therapy students; clients include patients, students, and those to whom occupational therapy services are delivered.

I. Related to the Recipient of Service

The occupational therapist demonstrates a beneficent concern for the recipient of services and maintains a goal-directed relationship with the recipient which furthers the objectives for which it is established. Services are evaluated against objectives and accountability is maintained therefore. Respect shall be shown for the recipients' rights and the occupational therapist will preserve the confidence of the client relationship.

Guidelines: Recipients of occupational therapy services refer to clients, patients, students and the employers of occupational therapists, i.e., agencies, facilities, institutions, etc.

It is the professional responsibility of occupational therapists to provide services for clients without regard to race, creed, national origin, sex, handicap or religious affiliation. Occupational therapists recognize each client's individuality and worth as a unique person.

Services provided should be planned in concert with clients' involvement in goal-directed activities, in accordance with the overall habilitation or rehabilitation plan. Treatment objectives and the therapeutic process must be measurable to insure professional accountability.

Clients' and students' rights are to be protected as stipulated in the Federal Privacy Act of 1974, in addition to any specified rules, regulations or procedures as may be required by the employer.

The financial gain of occupational therapists should never be paramount to the delivery of services. Those occupational therapists who are compensated by virtue of being a direct service provider or vendor have the right to assess reasonable fees for profit.

Occupational therapists are obligated to provide the highest quality of service to the recipient. If further services would be beneficial to the client, the referring practitioner should be informed. It is also incumbent upon occupational therapists to recommend termination of services when established goals have been met, or when further services would not produce improved recipient performance.

Occupational therapy educators are obligated to provide the highest quality educational services supporting the AOTA "Essentials" and the current theory that supports service delivery.

II. Related to Competence

The occupational therapist shall actively maintain and improve one's professional competence, represent it accurately, and function within its parameters.

Guidelines: Occupational therapists recognize the need for continuing education and where relevent, they obtain training, experience, self-study or counsel to assure competent occupational therapy services.

Occupational therapists accurately represent their competence, education, training, and experience. Occupational therapists must accurately represent their skills and should not provide services or instructions, either for pay or in a voluntary capacity, that are not within their demonstrated competencies.

Occupational therapists must recognize the skills necessary to manage a client or a position. If client needs exist that the therapist cannot effectively manage, the therapist should seek consultation or refer the client to an occupational therapist or another professional who can provide the required service.

III. Related to Records, Reports, Grades and Recommendations

The occupational therapist shall conform to local, state and federal laws and regulations, and regulations applicable to records and reports. The occupational therapist abides by the employing institution's rules. Objective data shall govern subjective data in evaluations, grades, recommendations, records and reports.

Guidelines: Occupational therapists realize that reports are a required function of any position. Occupational therapists accurately record information and report information as required by AOTA standards, facility standards and state and national laws.

Occupational therapists fulfilling a teaching role utilize objective data in determining student grades.

All data recorded in permanent files or records should be supported by the occupational therapist's observations or by objective measures of data collection.

Students' records can only be divulged as authorized by law or the students' consent for release of information.

IV. Related to Intra-Professional Colleagues

The occupational therapist shall function with discretion and integrity in relations with other members of the profession and shall be concerned with the quality of their services. Upon becoming aware of objective evidence of a breach of ethics or substandard service, the occupational therapist shall take action according to established procedure.

Guidelines: Information gained or data gathered on a client shall only be divulged as expedient to other professional colleagues, students, referring practitioner, and employers. This includes data used in the course of in-service programs, professional meetings, prepared papers for presentation or publication, and educational materials. Undue invasion of privacy should be of utmost concern. Any reference to quality or service rendered by, or the integrity of a professional colleague will be expressed with due care to protect the reputation of that person.

It is the obligation of occupational therapists with first-hand knowledge of a breach of the ethical principles of this Association, by a colleague or student, to attempt to rectify the situation. If informal attempts fail, such activities or incidents against the ethical principles of this Association, should immediately be brought to the attention of the appropriate local, regional or national Association committee/commission on ethical standards. Designated procedures should be followed and at all times the confidentiality of the information must be respected to protect the alleged party.

Practices by an employer which are in conflict with the ethical principles of this Association, should also be brought to the immediate attention of the appropriate body(ies).

Information gained in peer review procedures should be held within the realm of confidentiality and be dealt with according to established procedures.

Publication credit for material developed by colleagues must be given. Also, credit for materials used in the classroom, manuals, in-service training, and oral or written reports, for example, should acknowledge the name of the individual or group who developed the material.

V. Related to Other Personnel

The occupational therapist shall function with discretion and integrity in relations with personnel and cooperate with them as may be appropriate. Similarly, the occupational therapist expects others to demonstrate a high level of competence. Upon becoming aware of objective evidence of a breach of ethics or substandard service, the occupational therapist shall take action according to established procedure.

Guidelines: Occupational therapists understand the scope of education and practice of related professions, and make full use of all the professional, technical and administrative resources that best serve the interests of consumers.

Occupational therapists do not delegate to other personnel those client related services where the clinical skills and expertise of an occupational therapist is required. Other personnel or students may support treatment or educational goals, but must have demonstrated competency in each aspect of service to the occupational therapist before the responsibility can be delegated.

Occupational therapists who employ or supervise other professionals or technicians, or professionals or technicians in training, accept the obligation to facilitate their further development by providing suitable working conditions, consultation and experience opportunities.

Occupational therapists protect the privacy of all persons with whom professional collaboration occurs. If, however, an occupational therapist has first-hand knowledge of a colleague's performance which is in conflict with ethical standards, the therapist shall attempt to rectify the situation. Failing an informal solution, the occupational therapist shall utilize procedures established within the facility or agency, or to call the behavior to the attention of management, or utilize procedures established by the profession to handle such situations. Under no circumstances should the occupational therapist remain silent when a client, student or facility's status is in jeopardy.

VI. Related to Employers and Payers

The occupational therapist shall render service with discretion and integrity and shall protect the property and property rights of the employers and payers.

Guidelines: Occupational therapists function within the parameter of the job description or the goals established mutually between the employer or agency, and the occupational therapist. Occupational therapists use the utmost integrity in all dealings with the facility, university/college or contracting agency. Established procedures are followed regarding purchasing and bids.

Occupational therapists recommend appropriate fees for services and gain necessary acceptance for fees from the facility, agency and payers. Fees must be based upon cost analysis or a factor that can be justified upon request.

Occupational therapists shall not use the property, such as supplies and equipment, of the employer for their own personal use and aggrandizement.

VII. Related to Education

The occupational therapist implements a commitment to the education of society and the consumer of health services as well as to the education of health personnel on matters of health which are within the purview of occupational therapy.

Guidelines: Occupational therapists do not only provide direct service to alleviate specific problems with clients, programs or a community, but in addition, include education of all phases of services which can be provided to the public. This should include education of situations and conditions for which the competency of occupational therapists is recognized to assist in alleviating barriers limiting a person's ability to function socially, emotionally, cognitively or physically.

The public includes not only individuals concerned with the well-being of a member of their family, but also federal, state and local governmental agencies, educational systems and social agencies dealing with the health and well-being of the public.

VIII. Related to Evaluation and Research

Occupational therapists shall accept responsibility for evaluating, developing and refining service and the body of knowledge and skills which underlie the education and practice of occupational therapy and at all times protects the rights of subjects, clients, institutions and collaborators. The work of others shall be acknowledged.

Guidelines: Clients' families have the right to have, and occupational therapists have the responsibility to provide explanations of the nature, the purposes, and results of the occupational therapy services unless, as in some employment or treatment settings, there is an explicit exception to this right agreed upon in advance.

In reporting test results, occupational therapists indicate any reservations regarding validity or reliability resulting from testing circumstances or inappropriateness of the test norms for the person tested.

In performing research and reporting research results, occupational therapists must use accepted scientific methodology.

IX. Related to the Profession

The occupational therapist shall be responsible for gaining information and understanding of the principles, policies and standards of the profession. The occupational therapist functions as a representative of the profession.

Guidelines: Occupational therapists should provide accurate information to the public about the profession and the services that can be provided. Occupational therapists should remain informed about changes in the profession and represent the profession accurately to the consumer.

Occupational therapists should conduct themselves in a manner befitting professionals. The profession is judged in part by the conduct of its members as they carry out their functions.

Occupational therapists should show support and loyalty to the Association by cooperating with the Representatives in collecting information regarding proposed Association policy, replying to official requests for information and supporting the policies of the Association. It is the member's duty if he disagrees with an Association policy to work through existing channels to effect change.

Occupational therapists who engage in work or volunteer activities in addition to professional occupational therapy responsibilities, shall not violate the ethical principles of the Association in such activities.

X. Related to Advertising

Advertising by therapists under their professional title shall be in accordance with propriety and precedent in health professions.

Guidelines: Occupational therapists may provide information to the public about available services through procedures established by the employing facility or contracting agency. If an occupational therapist provides an independent service, it is appropriate to advertise those services.

The occupational therapist shall not use, or participate in the use of, any form of communication containing a false, fraudulent, misleading, deceptive, self-laudatory or unfair statement or claim. Testimonials or statements which promise a favorable result shall be avoided.

XI. Related to Law and Regulations

The occupational therapist shall seek to acquire information about applicable local, state, federal and institutional rules and shall function accordingly thereto.

Guidelines: Occupational therapists are obligated to function professionally as a practitioner within the limits of all laws related to the delivery of health services, and applicable to the practice of occupational therapy. Occupational therapists will not engage in any cruel, inhumane or degrading practices in the treatment of clients or in the education of students, or in supervision of others or in peer relationships with other individuals.

It is the responsibility of occupational therapists to make known to their employers, employees and colleagues, those laws applicable to the practice of occupational therapy and education of occupational therapists.

XII. Related to Misconduct

The occupational therapist shall not appear to act with impropriety nor engage in illegal conduct involving moral turpitude and will not circumvent the principles of occupational therapy ethics through actions of another.

Guidelines: As employees, occupational therapists refuse to participate in practices inconsistent with legal, moral and ethical standards regarding the treatment of employees or the public. For example, occupational therapists will not condone practices that are inhumane, or that result in illegal or otherwise unjustifiable discrimination on the basis of race, age, sex, religion, handicap or national origin in hiring, promotion or training.

In providing occupational therapy services, occupational therapists avoid any action that will violate or diminish the legal and civil rights of clients or of others who may be affected.

As practitioners and educations, occupational therapists keep abreast of relevant federal, state, local and agency regulations and American Occupational Therapy Association Standards of Practice and education essentials concerning the conduct of their practice. They are concerned with developing such legal and quasi-legal regulations that support the interests of the public, students and the profession.

XIII. Related to Bioethical Issues and Problems of Society

The occupational therapist seeks information about the major health problems and issues to learn their implications for occupational therapy and for one's own services.

Guidelines: The principle is a philosophical statement that encourages occupational therapists to be global in their views of health in relationship to society.

Reproduced with permission. *American Journal of Occupational Therapy,* Vol. 38, No. 12, 1984 pp. 799-802.

Enforcement Procedures are available from The Division of Practice, 1383 Piccard Drive, Rockville, MD 20850. Complaints should be addressed to the Standards and Ethics Chair, 1383 Piccard Drive, Rockville, MD 20850.

Appendix B

Standards in Practice for Occupational Therapy Services in a Mental Health Program

Preface

These standards are intended for internal use by the AOTA as guidelines to assist members in the practice of their profession. These standards by themselves cannot be interpreted to constitute a standard of care in any particular locality.

Standard I

A Referral for Occupational Therapy Must Be Based Upon the Provisions as Outlined in the Statement on Occupational Therapy Referral.

1. When a referral is received, the therapist shall:
    a. document the date of receipt and referral source
    b. document the occupational therapy services requested in the referral

Standard II

The Occupational Therapist Shall Evaluate the Client's Performance.

1. The therapist shall evaluate and document the client's goals, functional abilities and deficits in occupational performance (activities of daily living):
    a. self-care skills
    b. work skills
    c. play/leisure skills
2. The therapist shall evaluate and document the client's goals, functional abilities and deficits in the following performance component areas:
    a. psychological/intrapersonal skills
    b. social/interpersonal skills
    c. cognitive skills
3. If the results of the occupational performance evaluation indicate possible deficits in the client's motor and/or sensory-integrative skills, the therapist should evaluate these areas and document any functional deficits; or should refer the client to another practitioner for evaluation.
4. If any of the above evaluation results indicate the client's need for referral to community services or programs, the therapist should determine the availability of such community resources; or should refer the evaluation to another.

Standard III

The Therapist Shall Prepare and Document a Program Plan Based Upon an Analysis of the Occupational Therapy Evaluation Data and the Client's Expected Prognosis.

1. The documented program plan shall consist of a statement of achievable program goals and the methods to achieve the goals.

2. The program plan goals and methods shall be consistent with the evaluation data on the client's goals, functional abilities and deficits, community resources, and expected prognosis.

3. The program plan goals and methods shall be compatible with the program plans of the other health practitioners.

Standard IV

The Therapist Shall Implement the Occupational Therapy Program According to the Program Plan.

1. The therapist shall periodically document the occupational therapy services provided and the frequency of the services.

2. The therapist shall periodically re-evaluate and document the changes in the client's occupational performance and performance component skills.

3. The therapist shall formulate, document and implement program changes consistent with changes in the client's occupation, performance and performance component skills.

Standard V

The Therapist Shall Prepare and Document the Occupational Therapy Discharge Plan

1. The discharge plan shall be consistent with the client's goals, functional abilities and deficits, community resources, and expected prognosis.

2. The discharge plan shall be consistent with the discharge plans of the other health care practitioners.

3. Sufficient time should be allowed for coordination, acceptance and effective implementation of the discharge plan.

4. The therapist shall document the client's functional abilities and deficits in occupational performance and performance component skills at time of discharge.

5. The therapist shall terminate occupational therapy services when the client has achieved the goals, or when the client has achieved maximum benefit from occupational therapy.

Standard VI

The Therapist Should Re-evaluate the Client with Chronic Conditions at an Appropriate Time Interval Following Discharge.

1. The re-evaluation results shall be documented.

2. If the client needs further service, the therapist shall refer the client to the services needed.

Standard VII

The Occupational Therapist Shall Systematically Review the Quality, Including Outcomes, of Services Delivered, Using Predetermined Criteria Reflecting Professional Consensus and Recent Developments in Research and Theory.

1. If actual care does not meet the criteria, it may be justified by peer review.

2. If justification by peer review fails, a program to improve care shall be planned and implemented.

3. Patient care review will be repeated to assess the success of the corrective action.

Approved by Representative Assembly May 1978
Reproduced with permission from the American Occupational Therapy Association.

Appendix C
Developmental Groups

Parallel Group

A group composed of patients who have the ability to trust others enough to tolerate being with more than one person at a time. They can acknowledge the presence of other group members through eye contact or casual conversation. The occupational therapist is the leader of the group, and thus provides the group boundaries, explains the purpose of the group, the expectations for behavior in the group, and is responsible for giving feedback to the patients regarding their performance during the group. She provides an occupational therapy environment which is a safe place to work and where the patient can feel accepted and valued. The goal of the group is to have each patient work on his own chosen task while sharing space with other patients. For example, a craft group may be started in which each patient is working on a craft project of his choice.

Project Group

A group experience in which the patients are expected to come together to interact with each other in casual conversation and in order to complete a short term task (about one half hour work period). Patients are expected to work together cooperatively, share space, materials and tools, and be able to cope with limited competition. The occupational therapist is a leader who plans and presents the short term task to the patients and is available during the work period to support, assist, and guide patients as needed. The goal of the group is to provide the patients with an opportunity for trial and error learning, for group interaction around a task, and for a balance of cooperative and competitive experiences. These experiences may be, for example, team sports and games, making holiday decorations, or planning and preparing a patient party.

Egocentric-Cooperative Group

A group in which the patients come together to work on a task that is completed in one or two work sessions (one hour per session). During the task, the patients learn to express their needs, acknowledge the needs of other patients, ask for feedback, and give feedback to the other patients. The occupational therapist is a democratic leader that makes suggestions and allows the patients to choose and carry out the task and group plan. She is a resource for facilitating task completion and a support that promotes an atmosphere of acceptance and safety. The goal of the group is to have a task experience in which the patients will learn to (1) identify group norms and goals, (2) use their own knowledge and skills to respond in the group, (3) experiment with different group roles, (4) identify themselves as a group member with rights, (5) respect the rights of other group members, (6) respond empathetically to group members' needs, and (7) gain satisfaction from participating in the group experience. Examples may include structured learning experiences such as assertiveness, communications skills, or stress management.

Cooperative Group

A cohesive group in which patients come together to express and share their needs, thoughts, and feelings, and in which they listen to each other. The task of this group is used to promote sharing and listening, and does not seek to produce an end product. The occupational therapist serves as an advisor rather than as a leader. She helps form the group and initiate the task experience, and then becomes a participant who freely shares her thoughts and feelings. The goal of the group is to provide an experience for the patients that helps them to share their thoughts, feelings, values, and common interests, and to gain pleasure and satisfaction from this shared experience. Behavior change is not the focus of the group. Examples are art, music, poetry, or other creative experiences which facilitate the discussion of thoughts and feelings; another example is a values clarification group.

Mature Group

A group experience in which patients independently select, plan, and complete a group task which is time limited and produces a specific end product. The occupational therapist is a group member, and not the identified leader. During the task, the function of the group and group needs have priority over the needs of the individual. The task experience is processed in order to help the patients learn the social-emotional and task roles of the group. The goal of the group is to provide an activity that will allow the individual patient to put aside his needs for the betterment of the group, and to help the group accomplish its goal. During the task, from the group "process" discussion each patient will identify the social-emotional and task roles that they assume. Examples of this are a community transition group or group in the community.

Note: Material used for these descriptions is taken from Mosey A: *Three Frames of Reference for Mental Health*, (pp. 201-206), and from Mosey A: *Activities Therapy* (pp. 120-136).

Appendix D
Activity Groups

Evaluation Group

During an evaluation group, the occupational therapist uses a short term activity to observe the patient's interpersonal skills and response to the activity. The specific areas of function which are evaluated are determined by the frame of reference that is applied. Intervention strategies are not planned during this evaluation experience.

Task Oriented Group

A task group is a group which has a tangible outcome (end product or service). During the group, the patient learns from his interactions with others and the activity. He increases his awareness and understanding of himself and other patients. He learns interpersonal skills, practices new behaviors, and explores the interaction of thoughts, feelings, and behaviors that occur. The occupational therapist helps the patient process the activity experience and actively seeks to change the patient's behavior through the group interaction that occurs.

Developmental Groups

This is a group in which the patient learns group interaction skills through sequential, stage specific activities. The therapist uses activities, which are graded from simple to complex and short term to long term, in order to provide progressive challenges which require collaborative effort, the ability to compete, and increased independence in problem solving and task completion.

Thematic Groups

A thematic group is one in which the therapist uses purposeful activities to help the patients gain knowledge, skills, and attitudes necessary for function in a protective environment. The patient learns activities of daily living, work, and leisure skills through didactic, directive, and supportive experiences.

Topical Groups

Topical groups are ones in which the patient learns to independently use in the community the knowledge, skills, and attitudes gained in a protective environment. The two types of topical groups are (1) anticipatory groups in which patients focus on the future and the performance expectations needed in their future environment; and (2) concurrent groups in which patients focus on the knowledge, skills, and attitudes needed to function in the present roles that the patient has in his community. During these groups, the occupational therapist may prescribe activities and facilitate discussion of role expectations, identify the knowledge and skills needed to identify problems, and promote brainstorming and skill practice for solving problems.

Instrumental Groups

An instrumental group is one in which the occupational therapist uses activities to maintain the patient's present level of function and to promote an optimum level of health.

Note: Material for these descriptions is taken from Mosey A: *Occupational Therapy — Configuration of a Profession*, pp. 110-112.

Appendix E
Defense Mechanisms

Defense mechanisms are unconscious intrapsychic processes by which anxiety-producing information or wishes are kept out of conscious awareness. These processes are used by everyone to some degree, but overreliance on them ties up libido, tends to distort reality, and reduces the opportunity to see a full range of personal option. These processes keep the individual from knowing himself, from being congruent, and from changing. The most common defense mechanisms are:

Denial:

This is the process by which an individual protects himself against painful information by refusing to accept its validity. An example of this is when a person who on first hearing that a loved one has died, refuses to believe it.

Displacement:

This is a process by which the individual puts his feelings about one person onto another person or object. An example of this is when a student has had disagreements with a teacher, and then comes home and shouts at his roommate.

Projection:

This is a process by which a person attributes to another person the feelings he is really having himself. An example of this is: I am unconsciously angry with you, but I believe that you are angry with me.

Regression:

This is a process by which an individual reverts back to a more infantile way of meeting his needs. An example of this is when an individual, feeling overwhelmed by a job and personal setbacks, refuses to go to work, stays in bed, snuggles up under the covers, and seeks to be taken care of.

Rationalization:

This is a process by which the individual makes excuses for himself, or justifies his own or someone else's behavior — behavior that would otherwise be considered unacceptable or hurt his self-esteem. An example of this may result when a person is late for a job interview, thereby losing his bid for a job. He may rationalize by telling himself that he did not really want the job. Another example is when a person on a diet may overeat, and then rationalize by telling himself that it was a bad day.

Sublimation:

This is a rechanneling of unacceptable impulses into personally and socially acceptable channels. It is considered to be a healthy process. For example, aggressive impulses might be channeled into a game of handball. Freud felt that all artistic endeavor, work, and hobbies were a function of sublimation. In poor mental adjustment there is little capacity for sublimation.

Identification:

This is the process by which an individual takes on the qualities or attributes of a person he admires. For example, a little boy wears a Superman cape to emulate his hero, or a young lady smokes cigarettes to model after her favorite teacher.

Repression:

Repression is a process by which the ego pushes painful or anxiety-producing material out of consciousness. Some repression is necessary to deal with unacceptable wishes. Repression is at the core of many of the other defense mechanisms.

Fixation:

This is the process by which the individual gets "stuck" at a stage of psychosocial development because there is anxiety associated with moving to the next stage. An example of this is a young lady who can only carry on a flirtatious, superficial relationship with men because of her fear of mature heterosexuality.

Reaction-Formation:

This is a process by which the conscious thought and feelings that develop in the ego are just the opposite of unfelt, unconscious thoughts and wishes. For example, a person who is highly pious and overly moral might be responding to unconscious wishes to engage in immoral behavior.

Conversion (or conversion reaction):

This is a process by which unconscious wishes or thoughts are repressed, then channeled, and make their appearance via a variety of physical or somatic symptoms. An example of this is when an individual who has an unconscious wish to "walk out on" his spouse develops a hysterical paralysis of the lower limbs.

Appendix F
Person Drawings

The pictures in this appendix are presented to exemplify the patient's expression of his image and his concerns as they are presented in figure drawings. These drawings were used as tools for interaction and were not interpreted by the occupational therapist. They facilitated a shared discussion of self-image, roles, interests, likes and dislikes, and patient concerns.

The Patient and His Environment

Patients may depict their environment or objects within the environment that represent a conflict, concern, or problem that they are experiencing.

Figure F-1. The patient (a 15 year old girl) depicts her dilemma as being between continuing her life style as a runaway and staying at home following the rules of her parents. She drew the "welcome" mat, and stated that she wished there was such a mat at her home.

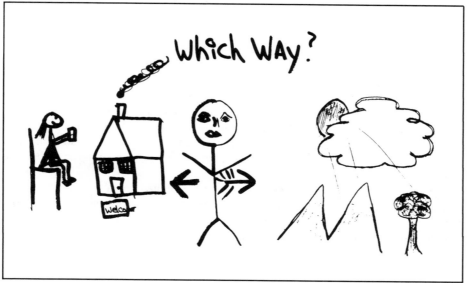

Figure F-1. Dilemma.

Figure F-2. Hold and treat.

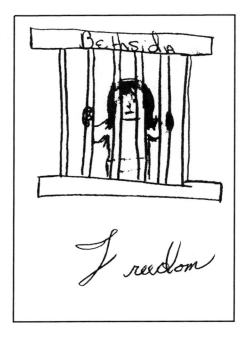

Figure F-2. The patient (a 15 year old girl) reflects her attitude about her "hold and treat" status (hospital commitment). Her primary concern was her loss of "freedom," rather than the reasons for her hospitalization — drug and alcohol abuse, promiscuity, being overweight, and her parents' refusal to have her return home to live.

Figure F-3. The patient (a 20 year old male) identified himself as a "biker." (A biker is a person who owns a motorcycle and may belong to a particular motorcycle gang or identify with a special group of people. He may choose a transient life style, have an antisocial attitude, and seek power.) This patient was in the hospital for an inability to control his aggression.

Figure F-4. The patient (a 30 year old female) is hospitalized for depression. She states that the chair in her drawing is her only support and that she needs something to lean on. She expressed feelings of being overwhelmed by the demands of her husband, the responsibilities of her job, and that she had multiple financial concerns.

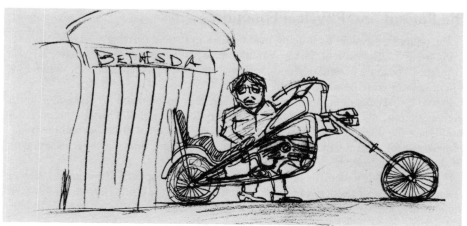

Figure F-3. Biker.

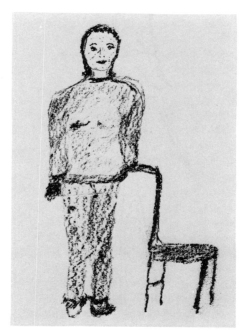

Figure F-4. Chair.

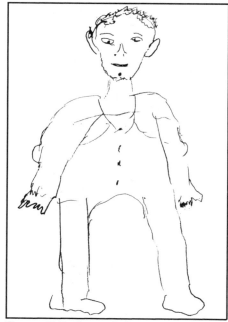

Figure F-5. Organic brain syndrome.

The Patient and Physical Function

The patient's physical well-being may be seen in patient drawings.

Figure F-5. The patient, a 69 year old male with organic brain syndrome, was hospitalized because of agitation and paranoia. His drawing is typical of one drawn by a patient with organic problems.

Figure F-6. The patient (an 18 year old female) was hospitalized for depression and a suicide attempt. She is hemiplegic due to surgery for removal of a benign tumor. After completing the drawing, she shared her feelings regarding her disability and the hopelessness she felt. Physically, she was more capable than her drawing suggests and than her discussion indicated.

Figure F-7. The patient (a 19 year old female) was hospitalized for anorexia. Her weight at the time of his drawing was 85 pounds. During the discussion which followed this drawing, she verbalized many angry feelings.

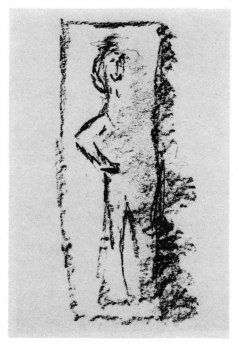

Figure F-6. Hemiplegia.

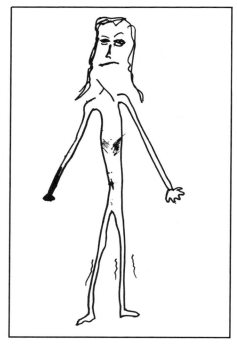

Figure F-7. Anorexia.

The Patient and Symbolic Drawings

The drawings presented in this section are symbolic. Patients who may or may not be reality oriented may choose to express their feelings, concerns, or problems symbolically. Patients who are diagnosed as "psychotic" may have lucid periods. Thus, the patient may be asked to do a self-portrait during the evaluation process, or the drawing may be requested after the patient is stabilized on his medications. The occupational therapist may limit the discussion of symbolism if the discussion increases the patient's confusion, promotes agitation, or is otherwise to the detriment of the patient.

Figure F-8. The patient (a 30 year old male) was diagnosed as "psychotic," or not reality oriented. He drew himself as a tree, and expressed the dichotomy of his conflict in the angel-devil drawings. His discussion focused on issues of right and wrong, good and evil, and God and the devil. The therapist chose to limit the discussion of religious issues and helped him to verbalize his conflicts regarding "right" or "wrong" choices that were affecting his job performance and daily function at home.

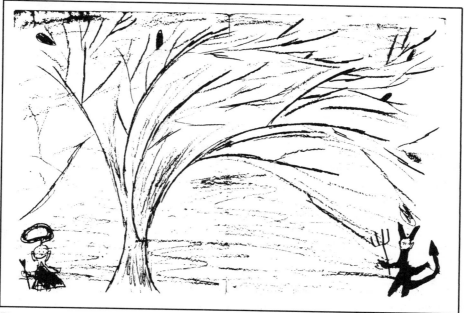

Figure F-8. Tree.

Figure F-9. Symbolic rectangle.

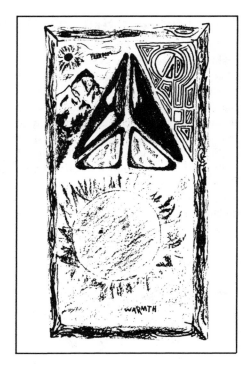

Figure F-9. The patient (a 19 year old male) was hospitalized for depression and psychotic episodes due to drug abuse. Through his symbolic self-portrait, he expressed his feelings and identity through his concerns which related to political and social movements.

Figures F-10A and F-10B. The patients (ages 20 and 30 years old, respectively) were psychotic at the time of the drawings. Each drew herself symbolically and wished to discuss, at length, the symbolism. When this occurs, the therapist must determine the benefits of the discussion to the patient and its usefulness to treatment planning. The therapist may limit the discussion.

Figure F-11. The patient (an 18 year old male) depicted his concerns through symbols that he added to his person drawing. He drew a light bulb and shared his concern with "thoughts that go on in my head"; he described himself as "always getting into trouble," as expressed through "horns" and the "halo" in the drawing.

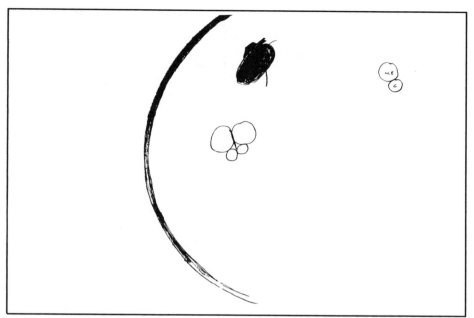

Figure F-10A. Symbolism.

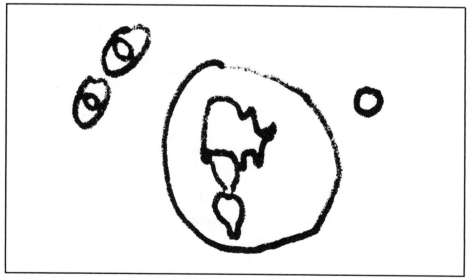

Figure F-10B. Symbolism.

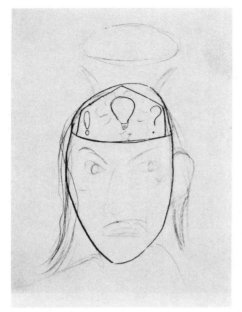

Figure F-11. Light bulb.

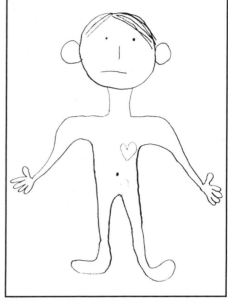

Figure F-12. Heart and male organ.

The Patient and Drawing Emphases

Patients also express concerns and problems through emphases in drawings which may be represented by accentuating body parts, colors used, and pressure of the lines drawn.

Figure F-12. The patient (an 18 year old male) drew body parts to express his concern regarding his male identity and to express "if I'm alive I have a heart."

Figure F-13. The patient (a 28 year old male) drew his heart and expressed his fear that "something was wrong with his heart." Anxiety was his chief complaint.

Figure F-14. The patient (a 16 year old male) was hospitalized for bipolar depression, manic phase, and verbalized his multiple concerns regarding homosexuality. Note the spontaneous elaboration of the drawing to the right of the main figure.

The Patient and Similarity of Drawings

Figures F-15A and F-15B. These two drawings were made by two women of triplets (both 19 years old). The women were not in treatment at the same time, but were both hospitalized within the same one and a half year time period. Both were experiencing the adjustment problems of young adulthood.

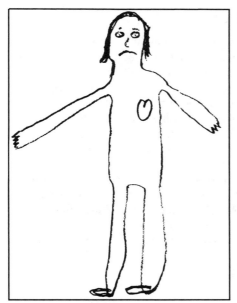

Figure F-13. Heart—anxiety.

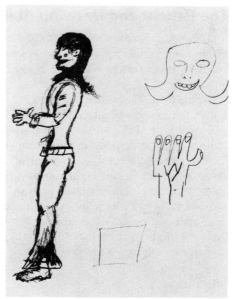

Figure F-14. Homosexuality.

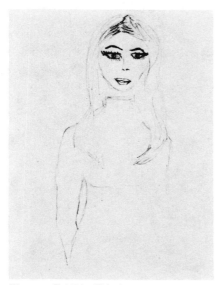

Figure F-15A. Triplets.

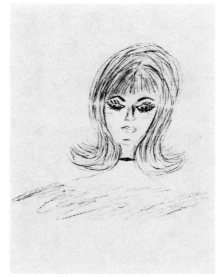

Figure F-15B. Triplets.

The Patient and Drawing Ability

The patient need not have artistic ability in order to represent himself and information that promotes understanding of the patient and his problems. Sometimes the patient has creativity that produces a drawing, but he may be unable or unwilling to share his view of himself.

Figure F-16. The patient (a 21 year old man) was hospitalized for depression. He drew a stick figure and verbalized his concerns about "no job and no plans for the future."

Figure F-17. The patient (a young woman) was hospitalized for depression, and has artistic ability as depicted in her sketch of a girl. She later committed suicide.

Figures F-18A and F-18B. The patient (a 15 year old female) was hospitalized for drug abuse, psychotic episodes, running away from home, and school truancy. She has artistic ability, which is demonstrated in both of her drawings. The symbolic picture was completed shortly after admission to the hospital, and the picture of the young girl was done after six months of treatment. Through symbolism, she discussed wanting to be "like the virgin to crush out all evil... like Robin Hood to be able to give to the poor... give freedom to men and women."

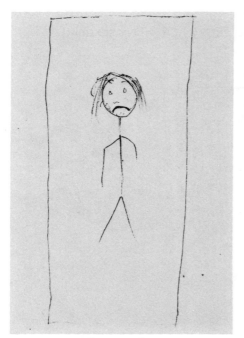

Figure F-16. Depression.

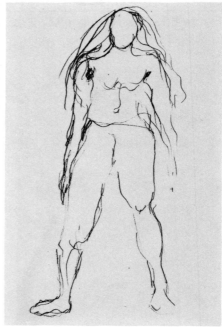

Figure F-17. Suicide.

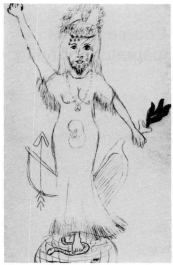

Figure F-18A. Girl at admission.

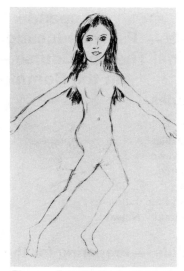

Figure F-18B. Girl after six months.

Appendix G
Sample — Psychoeducational Course Model
Occupational Therapy Course — Independent Living
in the Community

Course Modules

General Budget Principles
Community Residence
Preparing for the Move
Community Resources
Money Management
Meal Planning and Preparation
Friends and Community Network
Recreation

Sample Module — Preparing for the Move

Goals include establishing knowledge, developing and practicing skills, and identifying and clarifying values and attitudes.

Knowledge:

1. The patient will identify the furniture, equipment, and supplies needed for his community residence.

2. The patient will identify the public services needed for his residence, and the advance arrangements needed for telephone, gas, electric services, and newspaper.

3. The patient will identify the community resources near his residence, and the nearest physician, dentist, medical emergency services, supermarket, shopping center, discount stores, library, and recreation facility.

Skill:

4. The patient will make an itemized list of moving costs.

Attitude:

5. The patient will identify the value of planning and budgeting to reduce stress and ease his move into the community.

Learning Activities:

1. Conduct a brainstorming session in which patients in the group make a list of the possible furniture, equipment, and supplies needed for an apartment.

2. Using the general list compiled during brainstorming, each patient will make an individual list for his residence, identifying bathroom, kitchen, bedroom, and living room needs.

3. Using newspapers, the *Sears Catalog*, *Montgomery Ward Catalog*, or other consumer information, each patient will list the cost of each item on the supply-equipment list and determine the total cost of his apartment needs.

386

4. Each patient will then evaluate independently, or with the assistance of the therapist or his peers, the compatibility of the furniture, supply, and equipment costs with his monthly budget. (The budget would have been established during a previous module, "Budgeting Principles.")

5. Conduct a brainstorming session in which patients in the group make a list of the necessary community facilities, advanced arrangements, and costs for these facilities, i.e., telephone, gas, lights, and television.

6. Using the telephone directory, city maps, and newspapers, the patients will learn to use the physician and dentist referral resource, and identify where supermarkets, secondhand furniture stores, shopping centers, discount stores, church, and library are located.

7. Assign as homework that two or more patients visit some of the community resources previously listed in learning activity six.

Learning Resources:

(Examples of materials that may be used by the therapist during class experiences.)

1. Handout — Budget format for itemized lists and costs

2. Newspapers, magazines, catalogues, and telephone directory;

3. Sample utility bills to explain facility costs; and

4. Mover's pamphlet from local moving company.

Knowledge Gained:

Budget principles;

Community resources; and

Basic principles of home management.

Skills Practiced or Learned:

1. Group and individual decision making;

2. Task oriented problem solving;

3. Budget analysis and implementation; and

4. Communication skills.

Note: The patient's needs and abilities, the group composition, and the treatment setting will determine learning goals, course modules, the learning activities, and the learning resources that the occupational therapist may use. These are not all inclusive, but are a representative sample.

This sample educational model is based upon information shared with the authors by Ms. Judith Talbot, OTR, West Haven Veterans Administration Hospital, New Haven, Connecticut.

Appendix H
Seven Adaptive Skills

Perceptual-Motor Skill

The ability to receive, integrate, and organize sensory stimuli in a manner which allows for the planning of purposeful movement.

1. The ability to integrate primitive postural reflexes, to react appropriately to vestibular stimuli, to maintain a balance between the tactile subsystems, to perceive form, and to be aware of auditory stimuli.

2. The ability to control extraocular musculature, to integrate the two sides of the body, and to focus on auditory stimuli.

3. The ability to perceive visual and auditory figure-ground, to be aware of body parts and their relationships, and to plan gross motor movements.

4. The ability to perceive space, to plan fine motor movements, and to discriminate among auditory stimuli.

5. The ability to discriminate between right and left, and to remember auditory stimuli.

6. The ability to use abstract concepts, to scan, integrate, and synthesize auditory stimuli, and to give auditory feedback.

Cognitive Skill

The ability to perceive, represent, and organize objects, events, and their relationships in a manner which is considered appropriate by one's cultural group.

1. The ability to use inherent behavioral patterns for environmental interaction.

2. The ability to interrelate visual, manual, auditory, and oral responses.

3. The ability to attend to the environmental consequence of actions with interest, to represent objects in an exoceptual manner, to experience objects, to act on the bases of egocentric causality, and to seriate events in which the self is involved.

4. The ability to establish a goal and intentionally carry out means, to recognize the independent existence of objects, to interpret signs, to imitate new behavior, to apprehend the influence of space, and to perceive other objects as partially causal.

5. The ability to use trial and error problem solving, to use tools, to perceive variability in spatial positions, to seriate events in which the self is not involved, and to perceive the causality of other objects.

6. The ability to represent objects in an image manner, to make believe, to infer a cause given its effect, to act on the bases of combined spatial relations, to attribute omnipotence to others, and to perceive objects as permanent in time and place.

7. The ability to represent objects in an endoceptual manner, to differentiate between thought and action, and to recognize the need for causal sources.

8. The ability to represent objects in a denotative manner, to perceive the viewpoint of others, and to decenter.

9. The ability to represent objects in a connotative manner, to use formal logic, and to work in the realm of the hypothetical.

Drive-Object Skill

The ability to control drives and select objects in such a manner as to ensure adequate need satisfaction.

1. The ability to form a discontinuous, libidinal object relationship.
2. The ability to form a continuous, part-libidinal object relationship.
3. The ability to invest aggressive drive in an external object.
4. The ability to transfer libidinal drive to objects other than the primary object.
5. The ability to invest libidinal energy in appropriate abstract objects and to control aggressive drive.
6. The ability to engage in total and diffuse libidinal object relationships.

Dyadic Interaction Skill

The ability to participate in a variety of dyadic relationships.

1. The ability to enter into association relationships.
2. The ability to interact in an authority relationship.
3. The ability to interact in a chum relationship.
4. The ability to enter into a peer, authority relationship.
5. The ability to enter into an intimate relationship.
6. The ability to engage in a nurturing relationship.

Group Interaction Skill

The ability to be a productive member of a variety of primary groups.

1. The ability to participate in a parallel group.
2. The ability to participate in a project group.
3. The ability to participate in an egocentric-cooperative group.
4. The ability to participate in a cooperative group.
5. The ability to participate in a mature group.

Self-Identity Skill

The ability to perceive the self as an autonomous, holistic, and acceptable object which has permanence and continuity over time.

1. The ability to perceive the self as a worthy object.
2. The ability to perceive the assets and limitations of the self.
3. The ability to perceive the self as self-directed.
4. The ability to perceive the self as a productive, contributing member of a social system.

5. The ability to perceive the self.

6. The ability to perceive the aging process of the self in a rational manner.

Sexual Identity Skill

The ability to perceive one's sexual nature as good, and to participate in a heterosexual relationship which is oriented to the mutual satisfaction of sexual needs.

1. The ability to accept and act upon the bases of one's pregenital sexual nature.

2. The ability to accept sexual maturation as a positive growth experience.

3. The ability to give and receive sexual gratification.

4. The ability to enter into a sustained heterosexual relationship.

5. The ability to accept physiological and psychological changes that occur at the time of the climacteric.

Reproduced with permission. Mosey A: *Three Frames of Reference for Mental Health*. Thorofare, New Jersey: Charles B. Slack, Incorporated, 1970, pp. 134-136.

Note: In Mosey, A. *Psychosocial Components of Occupational Therapy,* New York, Raven Press, 1986 there are six adaptive skills: sensory integration skill, cognitive skill, dyadic interaction skill, group interaction skill, self-identity skill, and sexuality identity skill.

Appendix I
Commonly Assessed Sensory, Motor, and Cognitive Tasks

Visual Perception:

Focus on a single stimulus
Scan a visual field
Identify shapes and colors
Identify common objects, shown individually
Identify object (from photograph or in actual presentation) from a variety of perspectives
Identify objects or shapes depicted in distracting visual field
Describe the purpose of objects viewed
Remember visual data

Visual-Motor Synthesis:

Write familiar schemes (i.e., name)
Copy simple shapes
Duplicate with blocks a two-dimensional or three-dimensional pattern
Draw a designated object without the aid of a pattern to copy

Auditory Perception:

Comprehend familiar schemes, i.e., "Hello, what is your name?"
Localize where sounds are coming from
Attend to one auditory stimulus and screen out irrelevant ones
Comprehend complex or new auditory scheme
Recall auditory information

Auditory Motor Synthesis:

Follow simple, familiar commands, (i.e., wave goodbye or shake hands
Duplicate a rhythm with finger (or pencil); change rhythm as therapist changes it
Follow commands, less familiar schemes, i.e., touch your right elbow with your left hand

Spatial Relationship Synthesis:

Follow direction to go left, right, up, or down
Mimic hand directions of interviewer
Deal with spatial ideas, (i.e., tell time, draw hands on a clock)

Place objects above, below, or to the right of
Understand arithmetic computations

Body-Awareness Synthesis:

Cross body midline in reaching, and in tasks
Name body parts
Indicate where body parts are in space (eyes closed)
Imitate postures of interviewer sitting across from or next to the individual assessed
Draw an integrated person-symbol

Vestibular-Kinesthetic Synthesis:

Maintain balance (one leg and two legs, eyes open)
Maintain balance (one and two legs, eyes closed)
Maintain trunk balance when interviewer applies pressure (individual seated and standing)
Walk straight line (forward and backward)

Tactile Perception:

Recognize tactile qualities (cold, warm, pressure, or pain
Locate tactile stimuli applied to body
Indicate specified fingers
Recognize textures (rough, smooth, or bumpy)
Discriminate objects by shape and feel

Motor Synthesis:

Initiate and stop movement of large muscle bodies
Use both sides of the body in purposeful movement
Cross body midline
Accomplish gross-motor purposeful movement (i.e., jump, hop, skip, clap, and catch a large ball)
Use smaller muscle groups in purposeful movement (i.e., write name or open lock with key)
Persist in motor task (i.e., keep hand in air until therapist says to put it down)

Cognition/Attention:

Maintain eye contact
Attend to visual stimulus
Attend to interviewer's verbal directions
Attend to conversation in a group structure
Sustain involvement in a task (1 minute, 10 minutes, ½ hour)

Cognition/ Concentration:

Sustain involvement in a task (1 minute, 10 minutes, ½ hour)

Able to subtract fron 100 by 7's or from 30 by 3's

Cognition/Orientation:

(To person)

Answers: What is your name? Your occupation? How old are you?

Do you remember who I am? What I do? who is that person? (Point to significant other)

(To place)

Answers: Where are you now? What is the name of this hospital (if not at home)?

(To time)

Answers: What day (of the week) is it today?

What is the calendar date?

What is the season of the year?

Cognition/Knowledge:

(See also "memory" and "problem solving" tasks

Seriates numbers

Sorts objects according to same and different

Discusses simple current events

Does simple math

Reads (therapist begins with single words, and then reads phrases and sentences).

Writes

Demonstrates knowledge of motor process(es), procedures, and social expectations in daily encounters

Cognition/Insight and Judgment:

States why in treatment

Describes strengths, limitations, and needs

Discusses family's feelings about treatment

Describes the view others have of him

Interprets proverb

Demonstrates judgment in tasks of daily living, i.e., dresses and grooms appropriately; clothing is clean; asks for assistance from the OTR or nurse as needed; eats adequate meals

Uses tools appropriately (observes safety precautions)

Follows norms of social politeness

Cognition/Memory

(Some common examples, illustrative only)

Personal (and long term):

Gives accurate personal history

Able to describe events of last 24 hours prior to treatment (when an appropriate question)

Can answers: what did you do last Christmas, who were you with, and where were you? (Therapist can use any significant day)

What was for breakfast this morning?

What did we do in therapy yesterday?

Impersonal (and short term):

Remembers three unrelated items: five minutes to ½ hour

Remembers content of paragraph he reads: 2 to 15 minutes

Procedural-motoric (long term):

Demonstrates how to dial a phone or find a phone number

Demonstrates how to play checkers, play badminton, or pot a plant (if this was a skill formerly in his learning repertoire)

Sensory-perceptual (short or long term):

Demonstrates way to hospital room (or other familiar site)

Can find bathroom, dining room, or other landmark in the hospital or his home

Accurately recalls what is heard or seen in his environment

Cognition/Problem Solving Tasks:

(Combines knowledge, memory, and insight in higher cognitive function)

Generates one (or more) solutions to:

obtain an unknown phone number, trace a route on a city map, read a bus schedule, and describe how to get from one place to another

Balances a simple checkbook ledger

Makes change

States what he would do in a medical emergency

Constructs a 3-D box, given a piece of paper, tape, and scissors

Analysis of Activity Complexity

Parameters	Less Complex	More Complex
Sensory	Requires attention to primarily one sensory mode	Requires multisensory integration
	Requires little attention to detail	Requires attention to detail or subtle change
	Sensory input given slowly and boldly	Sensory input given quickly and less boldly
	Errors easily perceptible	Errors difficult to discern
Temporal	Can be completed in short time	Task extends over time
	New information given slowly	New information given quickly
	Task can be done slowly	Task to be done quickly
	Allows opportunity for pause or rest	Little opportunity for rest
Motor	Requires gross motor skill	Requires fine motor skill
	High unilateral demand	High bilateral demand
	Makes no use or simple use of tools; use of familiar tools	Complex use of tools; unfamiliar tools
	Highly repetitive	Requires many changes in motor response
	Done slowly	Done quickly
Cognitive	Involves only familiar schemes	Introduces new schemes (novel schemes)
	High degree of predictability	Little predictability
	Can be learned through imitation	Requires creativity and spontaneity
	Uses knowledge already acquired	Requires assimilation of new information
	Depends on ability to perceive concrete relationships	Depends on ability for abstraction
	Cause-effect is obvious	Cause-effect is not obvious

	Requires little memory	Requires sustained memory
	Demands little attention and concentration	Requires attention and concentration
External vs. Internal Control	Obvious benchmarks for passage of time	No obvious benchmarks for time passage
	Has obvious rules	Rules not obvious
	Has written or visual instructions	Instruction retained in one's memory
	Others signal when activity is started and stopped	Person must signal self to stop or start
	Errors pointed out by others	Self perceives errors
Social	Social group limited to two to four members	Social discourse in large group
	Group has familiar others	Group of unfamiliar others
	Task-oriented	Process oriented
	Low expectation for self-disclosure	High expectation for self-disclosure
	Low expectation for cooperation and sharing	High expectation for cooperation and sharing
	Social group has one permanent leader	Changing leadership
	Group homogenous	Group heterogenous
	Minimal change in membership	Social membership changes frequently
	Social "rules" obvious	Social rules subtle

Appendix J
The Apraxias, Agnosias, and Aphasias

Apraxia

Apraxia is the impairment of voluntary or purposeful movement not attributable to muscle deficit, or lack of comprehension.

1. Ideomotor apraxia — The person understands what the therapist asks him to do, but cannot organize the sequence of behavior necessary to accomplish the task, i.e., he may be able to "automatically" put on glasses when he picks up a magazine, but cannot follow the therapist's request that he (intentionally) put on his glasses.

2. Ideational apraxia — The person cannot create the idea of what motor behavior is desired, i.e., when asked to "button your sweater," he cannot create the idea of what is meant by this. However, his well established automatic responses may be retained.

3. Constructional apraxia — The person can demonstrate isolated purposeful movements, but cannot put them together; he cannot apply skills to a new situation, i.e., he is unable to construct a "star" from matches, or draw a clock to show a depicted time, or to assemble Lego© blocks according to a desired pattern.

4. Dressing apraxia — The person has an inability or difficulty with dressing; he does not know which limb goes in which part of his clothing, and he has problem with sequencing the events in dressing.

Agnosia

Agnosia is an impairment in object recognition not due to a deficit in the sensory systems or ignorance.

1. Visual agnosia — The person cannot name objects by sight alone (he may be able to describe their attributes). (Object recognition will typically be better for "real" objects than for "pictures" of objects.)

2. Tactile agnosia — The person cannot recognize an object by touch alone.

3. Prosopagnosia — The person is unable to recognize familiar faces (may be able to identify familiar others when he hears their voice).

4. Finger agnosia — The person is unable to name his own fingers or those of the therapist.

5. Spatial agnosia — The person experiences spatial disorientation, he is unable to find his way around familiar surroundings, and the person loses his understanding of directionality. This may include inability to locate one's own body parts.

6. Unilateral neglect — Related to body agnosia, the person ignores one side of his body, or fails to use it upon command, i.e., when asked to comb his hair, he combs only one side, or to put on his shoes, he puts on only one shoe. The neglected body side may be used appropriately in spontaneous, coordinated acts.

Aphasia

Aphasia is a speech or language disorder, evidenced in problems with word choice, grammar, or comprehension, and is not due to motor disturbance or ignorance.

1. Wernicke's aphasia (also known as receptive aphasia). In this case, the person does not understand what is being said to him. His speech may be fluid and well articulated, but is out of context and is senseless, and he has associated difficulty with naming objects, reading, and writing. This condition leads to unusual and even bizarre behavior.

2. Broca's aphasia — In this case, the person has iimited ability for verbal expression. This can range from a complete "loss of words" to mild problems with word finding. The written and spoken word are well comprehended. Residual speech is more likely to contain nouns and verbs. Automatic phrases like "good-morning" may be retained. Reading, writing, and calculation are impaired.

3. Global aphasia — The most severe aphasia. There is a major deficit in word comprehension and a lack of meaningful speech.

4. Conduction aphasia — The person can produce meaningful spontaneous speech, but cannot repeat back what is told him.

5. Transcortical aphasia — The person can repeat back what he hears, but has difficulty with spontaneous speech production.

The information in this table is compiled from the following:

Strub R, Black FW: *Organic Brain Syndromes: An Introduction to Neurobehavioral Disorders*. Philadelphia: F. A. Davis Company, 1981, pp. 217-236.

Holden U, Woods R: *Reality Orientation: Psychological Approaches to the Confused Elderly*. Edinburgh: Churchill Livingstone, Incorporated, 1982, pp. 114-121.

Luria A: *Higher Cortical Functions in Man*. New York: Basic Books, Incorporated, 1966.

Williams M: *Brain Damage, Behavior, and the Mind*. New York: John Wiley & Sons, Incorporated, 1979, pp. 64-109.

Appendix K
Task Checklist

Directions: Circle number in appropriate column and add for total.	Rarely	Sometimes	Often	Circle rater/student familiarity – 1 2 3 4 5 +	Rarely	Sometimes	Often	Name _____ Rater _____ Date _____	Rarely	Sometimes	Often
I. ENTRY LEVEL				**IV. RELATIONSHIP LEVEL**				**VII. ACHIEVEMENT LEVEL**			
States desire to attend	0	1	2	Seeks approval	0	1	2	Assumes self-responsibility	0	1	2
Stays through classes	0	1	2	Accepts feedback	0	1	2	Completes tasks	0	1	2
Hallucinates/delusional	2	1	0	Is outgoing and friendly	0	1	2	Manages stress	0	1	2
Is easily distracted	2	1	0	Interacts with peers	0	1	2	Is able to abstract	0	1	2
Stays on topic/coherent	0	1	2	Seeks reinforcement	0	1	2	Is self-motivated	0	1	2
Is disruptive/combative	2	1	0	Works productively 1-1	0	1	2	Generalizes	0	1	2
Speaks & acts at normal pace	0	1	2	Gives compliments	0	1	2	Competent in ADL skills	0	1	2
Observes limits	0	1	2	Receives compliments	0	1	2	Makes discharge plans	0	1	2
Affect is appropriate	0	1	2	Uses staff appropriately	0	1	2	Seeks independence	0	1	2
Threatens suicide	2	1	0	Shares feelings with others	0	1	2	Generates + self-statements	0	1	2
TOTAL		2	0	TOTAL		1	9	TOTAL		1	0
II. ACCEPTANCE LEVEL				**V. EXPLORATORY LEVEL**				**SUMMARY GRAPH**			
Attentive	0	1	2	Asks questions	0	1	2				
Suspicious, guarded	2	1	0	Seeks new situations	0	1	2				
Answers questions	0	1	2	Makes suggestions	0	1	2				
Engages others	0	1	2	Tries new behaviors	0	1	2				
Is rude or indifferent	2	1	0	Requests feedback	0	1	2				
Keeps appointments	0	1	2	Initiates activities	0	1	2				
Withdraws/lacks trust	2	1	0	Reveals feelings	0	1	2				
Refuses feedback	2	1	0	Considers goals	0	1	2				
Denies problems	2	1	0	Role plays	0	1	2				
Accepts contacts with staff	2	1	0	Expresses concern for others	0	1	2				
TOTAL		2	0	TOTAL		1	8				
III. ORDER LEVEL				**VI. MASTERY LEVEL**							
Appears neat and orderly	0	1	2	Makes decisions	0	1	2				
Follows rules	0	1	2	Problem solves	0	1	2				
Adheres to schedule	0	1	2	Exercises good judgment	0	1	2				
Acts impulsively	2	1	0	Sets treatment goals	0	1	2				
Organizes tasks	0	1	2	Self-reinforces	0	1	2				
Is rigid or compulsive	2	1	0	Generates alternatives	0	1	2				
Follows directions	0	1	2	Verbalizes spontaneously	0	1	2				
Complies with treatment	0	1	2	Is able to relax	0	1	2				
Is punctual	0	1	2	Exerts self-control	0	1	2				
Attends regularly	0	1	2	Takes notes/completes	0	1	2				
TOTAL		2	0	assignments TOTAL		1	4				

Summary Graph columns: I II III IV V VI VII (scale 0–20)

Reprinted with permission from the *American Journal of Occupational Therapy* Lillie, M.D., Armstrong H.E. Contributions to the development of psychoeducational approaches to mental health service, 36(7):438-443, 1982 p. 441.

Index

Abstraction, as cognitive function, 305-306
Activities therapy, evolution of, 4
Activity (See also Purposeful activity)
  as a means to competency, 264-265
  as a means to control negative feelings, 265
  as a means of expression, 58
  as educational modules, 171-172
  as homework (See also Homework, in
    cognitive behavioral treatment), 172
  as occupation, 264
  as reinforcement, 103
  as therapy, 351
  establishing behavioral components of,
    102-103
  function in cognitive behavioral treatment,
    171-172
  function in developmental framework, 219-221
  function in object relations framework, 57-59
  in sensory-integrative treatment, 236-237
  processing of, 59-60
  product orientation within, 264
  role development within, 59
  to achieve an end product, 103
  to assess knowledge and skills, 171
  to increase ego function, 58-59
  to increase knowledge and competence, 171
  to regain mastery and control, 58
  to teach needed skills, 102
Activity groups (See also Groups and Treatment
  groups), 73-74
  assertiveness training, 117-119
  prevocational, 115-116
  processing of, 74
  resocialization, 116-117
Adaptive function, DSM III definition of, 268

Adaptive skills
  establishing the existence of, 225-226
  failure to learn, 206
  Mosey's identification of (See also Appendix
    H), 208-209
Affective changes
  associated with brain impairment, 307
  responding to those of brain impairment,
    320-322
Aggression, 42
Agnosia, definition of (See also Appendix J),
  294-295
Allen, C (See Voluntary motor behavior; Cognitive
  dsyfunction; Treatment process; Assessment
  procedures and instruments), 210-212
Amplification, as a treatment strategy, 316
Anticipated consequences, 159
Anxiety
  desensitization for, 96
  existential, 51
  Freudian view of, 46
Aphasia, definition of (See also Appendix J), 297
Apraxia, definition of (See also Appendix J), 296
Assessment (See also Evaluation)
  behavioral guidelines for, 103-104
  diagnosis, 173-174
  in cognitive-behavioral framework, 173-175
  object relations guidelines for, 60-61
  of environment with the brain impaired
    patient, 312-313
  of social function with brain impairment,
    307-308
  screening for occupational disorder, 265
  with the brain impaired individual (See also
    Appendix I), 307-308

Assessment in developmental treatment, 223-224
Assessment of cognition
    medical aspect of, 147-148
    occupational therapist's role in, 149-150
    problem solving as a means for, 151
Assessment
    of cognitive structures, 175
    of person-environment match, 175-176
    to determine a life theme, 175
Assessment procedures and instruments, 61-62,
    105-110, 176-177, 226-227, 265-268, 308-312
    Adolescent Role Assessment, 227
    Adult Psychiatric Sensory Integration
        Evaluation (See Schroeder Block Campbell
        Adult Psychiatric Evaluation)
    Allen's Cognitive Level Test, 176-177, 227
    Allen's Lower Cognitive Level Test, 177
    Azima battery, 62-63
    Bay Area Functional Performance Evaluation,
        266, 309-310
    Bender Gestalt test, 310
    Benton Neuropsychological Assessment,
        311-312
    Comprehensive Evaluation of Basic Living
        Skills, 267
    Comprehensive Occupational Therapy
        Evaluation, 110
    Developmental Task Level of Adolescent
        Girls, 266
    Ehrenberg Comprehensive Assessment
        Process, 63
    Environmental Questionnaire, 267
    Fidler Activity Laboratory, 63
    Fidler and Fidler projective, 62
    Figure drawing (See also Figure drawing), 64
    Goodman battery, 63
    Hemphill battery, 63
    Interest Check List, 267-268
    Inventory of Depersonalization and
        Oocupational Skill Loss During
        Hospitalization, 267
    Inventory of Occupational Choice Skills,
        266-267
    King Person Symbol, 63
    Kohlman Evaluation of Living Skills, 110
    Lerner Magazine Picture Collage, 63
    Lifestyle Performance Profile, 227
    Magazine method of testing, 310
    Mosey's projective, 62
    Occupational Case Analysis and Interview and
        Rating Scale, 266
    Occupational Role History, 266
    Person drawing, 310
    Schroeder Block Campbell Sensory
        Integration Evaluation, 227, 310-311
    Scorable Self Care Evaluation, 110-111
    self inventory, 106
    Sensory Motor Cognitive Assessment, 227
    Shoemyen battery, 63
    simulated experiences, 109-110
    Task Check List (See also Appendix K), 176
Attachment, 133-134
Attention
    as a function of cognition, 300
    selective, 144
Attention span, 144
Attentional dysfunction, compensation for, 300
Automaticity, in everyday behavior, 174-175

Backward chaining, 92-93
Bandura, A (See also Social learning theory),
    157-160
Bara, B (See also Problem solving), 146
Beck, A (See also Cognitive therapy, Beck's),
    165-166
Behavior (See also Learning)
    adaptive and maladaptive, 98
    how learned, 86-87
    shaping of, 92-93
Behavior therapy
    citations regarding in the occupational therapy
        literature, 85-86
    contrast with feeling-orientation, 97-98
Behavioral data base, example of, 105-107
Behavioral frame of reference
    contributions of, 119-120
    definition of, 85
    limitations of, 120-123
Behavioral rehearsal (See also Modeling), 101
Bibliotherapy, 179
Biofeedback, 96-97
Body awareness
    compensation for dysfunction in, 296
    synthesis of, 295
Boulding's hierarchal levels, 253
Brain (See also Treatment process, strategies for
    working with the brain impaired; Central nervous
    system; Brain impairment), 284-287

functional adaptation in, 286-287
lateralization, 79-80, 284
system complex in, 286
Brain impairment
affective changes associated with, 287-292
role of environment with, 291-292
Brainstorming, 317

Causality, in thinking, 135
Central nervous system (CNS) (See also Brain;
Brain impairment; Treatment process, strategies
for working with the brain impaired)
plasticity of, 285-287
Chaining (See also Learning, building chains of),
92-93
Clark, P (See Human development through
occupation), 254
CNS
bilaterality in, 285-286
compensation within, 286-287
Cognition (See also Cognitive development,
Knowledge, Memory, Metacognition), 127-128,
299-302
assimilation and accommodation in, 129
concrete operations in, 138
current view of, 128
development of in infancy, 132
development of in early childhood, 134-138
development of in later childhood, 138
development of in adolescence and adulthood,
140-143
effect on goal setting, 161-162
equilibration in, 129
information-processing view of, 128-129
general occupational therapy definition of, 150
motivation for, 130
structural organismic perspective of, 129-131
summary of basic infantile, 134
summary of early childhood, 138
summary of later childhood, 140-141
summary of young adult, 143
Cognitive-behavioral frame of reference
contributions of, 185
definition of, 156, 174
limitations of, 184-185
Cognitive development, social, 133
Cognitive dissonance, role in building moral and
social reasoning levels, 234
Cognitive dysfunction

Allen's view of, 210
biologic component of, 210-212
cognitive behavioral view of, 168
controversial issues in, 232, 24
personality variables in, 149
Cognitive map, Tolman's, 122
Cognitive schemes, 129
Cognitive skills, biologic changes in, 211
Cognitive therapy
Beck's, 165-166
contrast with Rational Emotive Therapy (See
also Table 6-1), 166-168
Collective unconscious, 49
Community mental health movement, 3-4
Compensation, as cognitive function, 138-139
Competence
cognitive behavioral view of, 169
levels of, 187
occupational behavior view of, 268
Concentration, as a function of cognition, 300-301
Confabulation, 283-284
Consciousness, Freudian levels of, 42
Consensual validation, 73-74
Continuing Relationship Maintainance, 342-343
Contract
behavioral, 112
social, 160
Coping skills therapies, 157
Corrective emotional experience, 73
Cybernetics, in occupational behavior, 257

Disorder
occupational behavior classifications, 258
occupational behavior definition of, 257-258
Decatastrophizing, 183
Defense mechanisms (See also Appendix E), 46
Development
barriers to, 219
mediating factors in understanding, 207-208
Developmental frame of reference
contributions of, 241-242
definition of, 194-195
limitations of, 242-243
Developmental tasks
definition of, 195, 199, 200, 202
psychological issues in, 203
recurrent, 205
Tables 7-1 and 7-2, 201, 204
Developmental theory, occupational therapy

contributors to, 194-195
Developmental profile, 224-226
Differentiation, 137

Eclecticism, in object relations framework, 39-40,
    76-77
Educational essentials, 10
Ego psychology, 275
Ellis, A (See also Rational emotive therapy),
    163-165
Empathy, as decentration, 140
Enabling skills, in the process of development,
    195-196, 208
Enactive learning, 187
Environment, role in the developmental process,
    218
Erikson, E (See also Developmental tasks,
    psyohological issues in), 202-203
Ethics
        medical (See also Patient rights), 6-7
        relating to suicide, 343-344
        statement for the profession (See also
            Appendix A), 9
Evaluation
        creating climate for the, 64
        goals for object relations practice, 68
Existential humanism (See also Humanism), 49-52
        historical roots of, 49
        parallels with occupational therapy, 52

Feedback, role of in relearning, 315-316
Figure drawing (See also Assessment procedures
    and instruments, Person drawing)
        developmental aspect of, 80-81
        example of (See also Appendix F), 67
        guidelines for discussion, 66-67
        patient therapist dialogue in, 67-68
        presentation of task, 65
        used in screening for suicide, 344
Frames of reference, discussion of term, 5
Freud, S (See also Stage theory, Anxiety, Defence
    mechanisms, Psychoanalytical method,
    Symbols), 40-41
        disenchantment with, 75-76
        influence in society, 40-41
Functions, in cognition, 135

Gender identification, 80
        criticism of Freud's view of, 53-54

current view of, 54
Freudian view, 44
General systems theory, 253, 257
Generalization, role of in relearning, 317-318
Generativity vs. stagnation, 203
Generic model, of a profession, 275
Geriatric psychiatry, 55
Groups (See also Treatment groups and Activity
    groups), 22-31
        activity, 24-25
        as a laboratory for living, 23
        as a social microcosm, 73
        characteristics of, 25
        communication in, 28
        content and process within, 28-29
        degrees of interaction in, 71-72
        development of process, 29
        developmental, 24
        documentation of, 30-31
        feedback within, 73-74
        gatekeeping in, 27
        life development intervention, 239-140
        psychoeducational (See also Treatment
            process, psychoeducation for suicide),
            182-183
        role of the therapist in, 26
        safety within, 27-28
        styles of leadership in, 26-27
        task, 23-24
        taxonomy of, 23-25
        universality of experience in, 28
Growth facilitating environment, 222
Guided search, 317

Habits, occupational behavior view of (See also
    Learning, habits), 260
Habituation, within the CNS, 315
Havighurst, R (See also Life stages, Havighurst's),
    205
Hemispherectomy, 286
Hewett, F (See also Competence, levels of), 187
Highlighting, See also Amplification, 316
Homework
        cognitive-behavioral, 164
        in cognitive-behavioral treatment, 172, 179
Human development through occupation (HDTO)
        (See also Table 8-1), 254
Humanism (See also Existential humanism),
        influence in occupational therapy, 1-2

Identification, 137
Identity vs. role confusion, 203
Identities, in cognition, 135
Imitation
    complex, 137
    simple, 132
Individuation, 48, 198
Insight
    behavioral view of, 123
    clinical view of, 304-305
    cognitive-behavioral view of, 161-162
Instrumental conditioning (See also Learning, operant conditioning in), 88
Integration (Jungian view of), 198
Integrity vs. despair, 203
Intelligence, four classes of functional, 149
Interpropositional thinking, 139
Intimacy vs. isolation, 203
Inversion, as cognitive function, 138

Journals and newsletters, professional evolution of, 10-11
Judgment, clinical view of, 304-305
Jung, C (See also Life stages and symbols), 196-198
    influence on Herman Hesse, 244
    influence on society, 47-48

Kiev, A (See also Treatment process, psychoeducation model for suicide), 335-336
King, LJ (See also Sensory-integration treatment), 216-217
Knowledge (See also Cognition, Metacognition, Memory), 130-131
    categories of, 302
    explicit, 151-152, 301
    fund of, 302
    physical, 130, 132, 134
    quantity and quality of, 130-131
    tacit, 151-152, 301
Knowledge deficits, compensation for, 302
Kohlberg, L (See also Moral reasoning; Moral development; Treatment process, for building moral and social reasoning), 212-216

Language (See also Speech synthesis), 133
    as functional communication, 298
    development of in infancy, 133
    development of metaphorical, 142

distinguishing among listeners in, 136
    social and private use of, 133
Learning (See also Behavior), 86-87
    building chains of, 92-93
    classical conditioning in, 87
    cues, 88
    discrimination in, 88
    from vicarious experience, 161
    generalization in, 87
    habits, 87
    operant conditioning in, 88
    response, 86
    spontaneous recovery in, 87
    stimulus, 86
    vicarious (See also Modeling), 93
Learning lab, 23
Learning modules, 182
Legislation, pertaining to occupational therapy, 7
Levinson, D (See also Life stages), 199
Libidinal energy (See also Psychic energy), 40-42
Life development intervention
    creating dollars for, 240-241
    individual empowerment within, 239
    purpose of, 238-240
    stages of, 238-239
Life stage, definition of, 195
Life stage theory, contributors to, 196
Life stages
    Havighurst's, 205
    Jungian, 196-198
    Levinson's, 199-201
    midlife, 199-201
    polarities in, 199
    transitional stress in, 199, 201-202
    transitional vs. stable, 199
Limbic system, 287
Logic, idiosyncratic nature of in suicide, 333
Luria, A (See also CNS, plasticity of), 285

Magical thinking, 135
Man, as machine (See also Cognition, information-processing view of), 128-129
Marker events, 205-207
    definition of, 195
    within the profession, 7-10
Memory
    classifications according to length of storage, 152
    components of, 302-304

construction and reconstruction in, 145
hardware of, 145
episodic, 145
personal association in, 303-304
semantic, 145
temporal aspects of, 303
Memory loss, compensation for, 304
Memory strategies, 146, 319
Mental status exam, 148
Mentor relationship, 201
Metacognition, 144-145
Metamemory, 146
Modeling, 93094
in cognitive-behavioral treatment, 180
intervening role of cognition in, 159
of gradual mastery, 159
social influences in, 94
the scientist's attitude, 169-170
Modeling and physical guidance (See also Physical guidance), 180
Moore, J (See also CNS, plasticity of), 285
Moral development
impact on occupational therapy treatment process, 215-216
Kohlbergian stages in, 212-214
recent changes in theory, 244-245
summary of principles guiding, 214-215
Moral reasoning (See also Moral development), 212
Mosey, A (See also Adaptive skills, and Appendices C, D, and H), 225-226
Motor impersistance, 296
Motor synthesis (See also Apraxia), 296-297
Motor synthesis dysfunction, compensation for, 295-296

Neugarten, B (See also Marker events), 205-207

Object, in occupational behavior frame of reference, 276
Object choice
biological determination in, 54
fixation in, 44-46
flexibility of, 42
Object relations frame of reference, definition of, 39
Occupation, definitions of), 259
Occupational behavior
contributions of, 273
definitions of, 259

limiting professional practice to, 254
limitations of, 273-274
summary of current emphases, 271-273
Occupational behavior frame of reference, definition of, 251-252
Occupational choice, stages in the development of, 262-264
Occupational choice counseling, 263-264
Occupational performance (See also Occupational behavior and Occupation), 258-259
Occupational roles
beliefs regarding, 261
taxonomy of, 261
Order, occupational behavior definition of, 257
Organic brain syndromes (See also Brain; Treatment process, strategies for working with the brain inpaired; Central nervous system; Brain impairment), 281-283
DSM III catagories of, 282
Orientation, 301

Paradigm
discussion of term, 5
Kuhn's, 275
of occupational behavior, 252-253
Patient-activity match, 3
Patient rights, 178-179
historical changes in, 7
in token economies, 95-96
Patient vs. client, contrast of terms, 5-7
Perception, 143
Perseveration
definition of, 296-297
Figure 9-1, 297
Personology, 276
Pharmacology
in health treatment, 211, 245
long term effects of, 217
Physical guidance, in relearning (See also Modeling), 316-317
Play-work skill continuum, 9
Press, 276
Principles of hierarchy, 269
Principles of restoring order, Table 8-2, 270
Problem oriented record, 112
Problem solving
Bara's categories of, 146
clinical view of, 306-307
process of, 146-147

Problem solving therapies, 157
Procedural-motoric knowledge, 302
Process schizophrenia, physical characteristics of, 216-217
Process schizophrenia vs. reactive schizophrenia, contrast of terms, 245
Professional issues
    current, 10
    regarding multiple frames of reference, 347-350
Projection, 47
Propositional beliefs, 302
Psychic energy, 40-42
    ego, 41-42
    id, 41-42
    superego, 42
Psychoanalysis
    differences from occupational therapy, 76
    transference within, 47
Psychoanalytic method, 46-47
Psychological testing, 148
Psychosocial occupational therapy
    parameteters of, 351
    promise/reality, 354-355
    summary of guiding theoretical principles, 353-354
Pyschotherapy (See also Therapy)
    current trends in, 52
    shortened length of, 55-56
Punishment, learning view of, 91-92
Purposeful activity (See also Activity), 31-35
    as an agent of change, 32-35
    boundaries created by, 34
    definition of, 31-32
    process within, 32-35
    safe environment for, 33-34
    valuing of, 34

Rational emotive therapy
    ABC theory in, 163
    disputing irrational beliefs in, 164
    masturbatory thinking in, 163
    unconditional acceptance in, 164
Rational psychotherapies, 157
Rational restructuring, 183
Readiness, in skill development, 219
Re-attribution, 183
Reality testing, 41
Reality orientation, as a relearning strategy, 318-319
Referent non-referent array, 136

Regression, 209
Reilly, M, influence in occupational behavior frame of reference, 252
Reinforcement
    external, 159
    guidelines for using, 90-91
    intervening role of cognition in, 159
    kinds of, 89-90
    negative (adverse stimulus), 122
    schedules of, 90-91
    social learning hierarchy of, 160-161
    vicarious, 159
Representative assembly, of the profession, 9
Repression, 146
Reticular activating system, 287
Retraining, repetition within as a treatment principle, 315
Role, occupational behavior definition of (See also Occupational roles), 260-261
Role of the occupational therapist
    as participant observer, 57
    in behavioral therapy, 89-91, 101
    in cognitive behavioral treatment, 169-171
    in dealing with sex stereotypes, 54
    in object relations frame of reference, 57
    in occupational behavior frame of reference, 262-264
    in referring the suicidal patient, 339-340
    in suicide prevention, 334-335
    in the developmental frame of reference, 222-223
    setting limits with the suicidal patient, 338-339
    summary of, 352

Satiation, 91
Scientific movement, influence in occupational therapy, 2-3
Screening tool, definition of, 225
Self
    adaptation in the, 218
    as an open system, 257
    behavioral view of the, 97-98
    changes in the second half of life, 48-49
    cybernetic cycle within the (Figure 8-1), 257
    deep change within the, 183-184
    development of ideal, 140
    extroversion vs. introversion in the, 48, 197
    habituation subsystem within the, 260-262

holism of, 50-51, 244
holism of in CNS disorder, 283-284
holism of in organic brain impairment, 287
interests of the, 260
intrinsic motivation within the, 218, 257, 275
man as machine, 275
peripheral change within, 183-184
performance subsystems within the, 262
personal causation in, 260
polarities of the, 47
rational and a-rational, 197
search for automomous identity in the, 142
subsystems of the, 259-262
uniqueness of the, 56
values in, 260
volition subsystem in, 259-260
Self actualization, 51, 56
Self concept, dimensions of mature, 142
Self control
    as cognitive-behavioral issue, 155
    as reinforcement, 160
Self produced consequences, 159
Sensory dysfunction, compensation for, 294
Sensory-integration treatment
    as a strategy with the brain impaired patient,
        320
    theoretical basis for, 216-217
Sensory perception, 293-295
Sensory-perceptual knowledge, 302
Sensory synthesis, 293-295
Separation-individuation, 44-55
Shaping (See also Behavior, shaping of), 92
Sign learning, 276
Simplification, as a treatment principle, 314
Skills, occupational behavior catagories of, 262
Social learning paradigm
    correlation of events within, 159
    diagnosis of, 158
Social learning theory
    Bandura's, 157-160
    relevance to occupational therapy, 162-163
Social perspective, 212
Speech synthesis dysfunction, compensation for
    (See also Language and Aphasia), 299
Spatial relationship synthesis, 295
Splinter skills, 102
Stage theory, Freudian, 43-46
Standards of Practice (See also Appendix B), 9
Subjectivity

in development of cognition, 129
in existential humanism, 50
in object relations frame of reference, 74-75
Substitution, as a relearning strategy, 316
Suicidal crisis, effects on therapeutic milieu,
    341-342
Suicidal depression, as a chronic problem, 342
Suicidal patient
    ambivalence in, 335
    characteristic emotions and cognition of,
        331-333
    dependency needs of, 337
    temporal distortions in, 332
Suicide
    as rebirth, 343
    beliefs regarding psychology of (See also
        Suicide crisis and Suicidal patient), 328-329
    danger signals of impending, 340-341
    demography of, 329-330
    on a continuum of self-destructive behaviors,
        328
    talking with patient about, 337-338
Suicide crisis
    as a loss of equilibrium (See also Figure 10-1),
        333-334
    nature of, 329
Suicide education, therapist need for, 327-328
Suicide wish, clarifying the existence of, 339-341
Symbolic-representation intelligence, 133
Symbolism, in occupational behavior, 275-276
Symbols
    Freudian dream, 46
    guidelines for exploration of, 71
    interpretation of, 70-71
    Jungian, 49

Temporal orientation, 260
Theoretical imperialism, 274
Therapeutic relationship
    authenticity in the, 50
    behaviorally oriented interaction in, 114-115
    boundaries related to suicide, 342
    caring in, 18-19
    definition of, 16
    elements of, 15-16
    in existential humanism, 50-51
    limitations of, 21-22
    moral-development influence in, 215-216
    mutual reciprocity in, 57

open communication in, 19-20
role of therapist in, 15-16
safety in, 17-19
tentativeness within, 20-21
trust in, 18
unconditional positive regard in, 50-51
understanding within, 20
valuing, 18-20
with the suicidal patient, 337-339
Therapy (See also Psychotherapy)
here and now in, 51, 53, 80
Time management counseling, 263
Token economies, 94-96
Tolman, E (See also Cognitive map), 122
Transcendence, 48, 198
Transference (See also Psychoanalysis, transference
within), 47
Transformations, in cognition, 138
Treatment goals, 68-69
contrast of developmental vs. behavioral,
227-228
establishing priorities with the brain impaired
patient, 313-314
in behavioral practice, 111-112
in cognitive-behavioral treatment, 177-178
in developmental frame of reference, 227-229
in occupational behavior, 268
to change behavior and thoughts, 177-178
to reestablish cognitive self regulation, 177
Treatment Groups (See also Groups and Activity
groups), 72
around meal preparation, 73
gardening, 73
Treatment process
Allen's cognitive, 230
behavioral guidelines for, 113-114
class format within (See also Learning
modules), 181
climate in, 69-70
developmental aspects in occupational
behavior, 269
films and visual media in, 180
for building moral and social reasoning, 234
for increasing self-knowledge, 70

for superficial or deep change, 183-184
guiding assuptions in behavioral framework,
103-104
guiding assuptions in cognitive behavioral
frame of reference, 172-173
guiding assuptions in developmental
framework, 221-222
guiding assuptions in object relations frame
of reference, 60-61
guidelines for dealing with the suicidal
patient, 339-342
in cognitive behavioral frame of reference,
179-183
in developmental frame of reference, 229-230
in occupational behavior frame of reference
(See also Principles of hierarchy and
Principles of restoring order), 268-271
Leva's cognitive, 232-234
listening for "musts" in, 178-179
principles related to sensory-integration, 236
psychoeducational model for suicide), 335-336
socialization within, 271
stategies for working with brain impairment,
314
therapist participation in (See also Modeling),
69-70
to build adaptive skills, 237-238
to develop assertive beliefs, 179-180
to identify cognitive distortions, 180-182

Veatch, R (See Ethics, medical), 6
Vestibular kinesthetic synthesis, 295-296
Vestibular regulating system, in sensory-
integration, 217
Vocational rehabilitation, evolution of in
occupational therapy, 3-4
Voluntary motor behavior, assessment of,
210-212

Wilcox, W (See also Social perspective; Moral
development; Treatment process, for
building moral and social reasoning),
212-216
Wyatt vs. Stickney, 95